BEFORE WE ARE BORN

Essentials of Embryology
and Birth Defects

Keith L. Moore

Recipient of the inaugural Henry Gray/Elsevier Distinguished Educator Award in 2007 — the American Association of Anatomists' highest award for excellence in human anatomy education at the medical/dental, graduate, and undergraduate levels of teaching.

American Association of Anatomists

BEFORE WE ARE BORN

Essentials of Embryology and Birth Defects

7th Edition

Keith L. Moore, PhD, FIAC, FRSM

Professor Emeritus, Division of Anatomy, Department of
Surgery
Faculty of Medicine, University of Toronto,
Toronto, Ontario, Canada
Former Professor and Head, Department of Anatomy,
University of Manitoba, Winnipeg, Manitoba, Canada
Former Professor and Chairman, Department of
Anatomy and Cell Biology, University of Toronto,
Toronto, Ontario, Canada

T.V.N. Persaud, MD, PhD, DSc, FRCPath (Lond.)

Professor Emeritus and Former Head, Department of
Human Anatomy and Cell Science
Professor of Pediatrics and Child Health
Associate Professor of Obstetrics, Gynecology,
and Reproductive Sciences, Faculty of Medicine,
University of Manitoba
Winnipeg, Manitoba, Canada
Professor of Anatomy and Embryology, St. George's
University, Grenada, West Indies

With the Collaboration of
Mark G. Torchia, MSc, PhD

Associate Professor and Director of Development
Department of Surgery, University of Manitoba
Director of Advanced Technologies, Winnipeg Regional
Health Authority
Winnipeg, Manitoba, Canada

SAUNDERS

ELSEVIER

1600 John F. Kennedy Boulevard
Suite 1800
Philadelphia, PA 19103-2899

BEFORE WE ARE BORN: ESSENTIALS OF EMBRYOLOGY AND BIRTH DEFECTS, SEVENTH EDITION

ISBN: 978-1-4160-3705-7
International Edition: 978-0-8089-2398-5

Notice

Neither the Publisher nor the Authors assume any responsibility for any loss or injury and/or damage to persons or property arising out of or related to any use of the material contained in this book. It is the responsibility of the treating practitioner, relying on independent expertise and knowledge of the patient, to determine the best treatment and method of application for the patient.

The Publisher

Previous editions copyrighted 2003, 1998, 1993, 1989, 1983, 1974

Library of Congress Cataloging-in-Publication Data
Moore, Keith L.
  Before we are born : essentials of embryology and birth defects / Keith L. Moore, T.V.N. Persaud; with the collaboration of Mark G. Torchia. – 7th ed.
       p. ; cm.
  Includes bibliographical references and index.
  ISBN-13: 978-1-4160-3705-7
  ISBN-10: 1-4160-3705-5
  1. Embryology, Human. 2. Abnormalities, Human. I. Persaud, T. V. N.
II. Torchia, Mark G. III. Title.
  [DNLM: 1. Embryonic Development. 2. Abnormalities. 3. Embryology–methods.
4. Fetal Development. QS 604 M822b 2008]

QM601.M757 2008
612.6'4–dc22

2006039362

Acquisitions Editor: Inta Ozols/Madelene Hyde
Developmental Editor: Kathryn DeFrancesco
Project Manager: Bryan Hayward
Interior and Cover Designer: Steven Stave

Printed in Canada

Last digit is the print number: 9   8   7   6   5   4   3   2   1

In Memory of Marion Moore

Marion was my best friend, confidante, colleague, and wife for 57 years. She was the mother of our five children and grandmother of our nine grandchildren. Her assistance with the editing and preparation of earlier editions of this and other books was invaluable. Marion, you will always be in our thoughts and in our hearts. You will be surely missed but never forgotten.

Keith L. Moore

Preface

Before We Are Born has been completely updated and redesigned in an easy-to-read format. It provides medical and other students in the health professions with the essentials of normal and abnormal development. This concise work is a digest of our larger book, The Developing Human: Clinically Oriented Embryology, eighth edition, and is suited for a one-semester course and for reviewing.

An important feature of this book is the section entitled Clinically Oriented Questions, which appears at the end of each chapter. In addition, available through Elsevier's studentconsult.com website are many new clinical cases and questions with answers and explanations. These will benefit students preparing for USMLE Step 1 and similar examinations. Accompanying this edition of Before We Are Born is an innovative set of full-color animations that will help students understand the complexities of embryological development. Also, many of the illustrations in the book have been improved with three-dimensional renderings and bold, effective color.

The teratology content has been updated because the study of abnormal development is required for understanding the causes of birth defects and how these may be prevented. Molecular aspects of developmental biology have been highlighted throughout the book, especially in the areas that appear promising for clinical medicine and future research. Every chapter has been revised thoroughly to reflect new research findings and their clinical significance. The chapters are organized to present clearly a systematic and logical approach to human prenatal development.

Keith L. Moore
Vid Persaud

Acknowledgments

Many colleagues and students have made invaluable contributions to this newest edition of *Before We Are Born*. We are indebted to the following colleagues (listed alphabetically) for critical reviewing of chapters, making suggestions for improvement of this book, or providing some of the new figures: Dr. Steve Ahing, Faculty of Dentistry, University of Manitoba, Winnipeg, Manitoba; Dr. Albert Chudley, Departments of Pediatrics and Child Health, Biochemistry and Medical Genetics, University of Manitoba, Winnipeg, Manitoba; Dr. Blaine M. Cleghorn, Faculty of Dentistry, Dalhousie University, Halifax, Nova Scotia; Dr. Raymond Gasser, Department of Cell Biology and Anatomy, Louisiana State University School of Medicine, New Orleans, Louisiana; Dr. Brian K. Hall, Department of Biology, Dalhousie University, Halifax, Nova Scotia; Dr. Boris Kablar, Department of Anatomy and Neurobiology, Dalhousie University, Halifax, Nova Scotia; Dr. Deborah Levine, Beth Israel Deaconess Medical Center, Boston, Massachusetts; Dr. Edward A. Lyons, University of Manitoba, Winnipeg, Manitoba; Professor Bernard J. Moxham, Cardiff School of Biosciences, Cardiff University, Cardiff, Wales; Dr. Valerie Dean O'Loughlin, Department of Anatomy and Cell Biology, Medical Sciences, Indiana University, Bloomington, Indiana; Dr. Stuart Morrison, Department of Radiology, Cleveland Clinic, Cleveland, Ohio; Dr. Drew Noden, Department of Biomedical Sciences, Cornell University, College of Veterinary Medicine, Ithaca, New York; Dr. Maria Patestas, Des Moines University, Des Moines, Iowa; Professor T.S. Ranganathan, St. George's University, School of Medicine, Grenada; Dr. Gregory Reid, Department of Obstetrics, Gynecology and Reproductive Sciences, University of Manitoba, Winnipeg, Manitoba; Dr. Norman Rosenblum, The Hospital for Sick Children and Department of Pediatrics, University of Toronto, Toronto, Ontario; Dr. J. Elliott Scott, Departments of Oral Biology and Human Anatomy & Cell Science, University of Manitoba, Winnipeg, Manitoba; Dr. Robert Semo, Department of Obstetrics and Gynecology, University of California, San Diego, California; Dr. Richard Shane Tubbs, Children's Hospital, University of Alabama at Birmingham, Birmingham, Alabama; Dr. Christopher von Bartheld, Department of Physiology and Cell Biology, University of Nevada School of Medicine, Reno, Nevada; and Professor Christoph Viebahn, Department of Anatomy and Embryology, Göttingen University, Göttingen, Germany.

The new illustrations were prepared by Hans Neuhart, President of the Electronic Illustrators Group in Fountain Hills, Arizona. The stunning collection of animations was created by *Emantras*, and for skillfully reviewing them we thank Dr. David L. Bolender, Department of Cell Biology, Neurobiology, and Anatomy, Medical College of Wisconsin, Milwaukee, Wisconsin.

We are greatly indebted to Ms. Inta Ozols, Executive Medical Editor, and Ms. Madelene Hyde, Publisher, for their insight, encouragement, and many suggestions. We wish to thank Ms. Kathryn DeFrancesco, our Developmental Editor, for her specialist advice and skillful editing. For coordinating work relating to the animations, we would like to thank Ms. Carol Emery. Finally, our special thanks also go to the production staff, particularly Mr. Bryan Hayward, Project Manager, and Ms. Linnea Hermanson, Production Editor. This new edition of *Before We Are Born* is largely the result of their professional dedication and technical expertise.

Keith L. Moore
Vid Persaud

Contents

INTRODUCTION TO HUMAN EMBRYOLOGY

Human development begins when an **oocyte** (ovum) from a female is fertilized by a **sperm** (spermatozoon) from a male. Development involves many changes that transform a single cell, the **zygote**, into a multicellular human being. Embryology is concerned with the origin and development of a human being from a zygote to birth. The stages of development before birth are shown in Figures 1-1 and 1-2.

■ EMBRYOLOGIC TERMINOLOGY

Most embryologic terms have Latin (L.) or Greek (Gr.) origins.

Oocyte (L. *ovum*, egg). This term refers to the female germ cell produced by the *ovaries*. When mature, the cell is called a *secondary oocyte*.

Sperm (Gr. *sperma*). This term refers to the male germ cell produced by the *testes*. Numerous sperms (L. *spermatozoa*) are expelled from the male urethra during ejaculation.

Embryo. This term refers to the developing human during all of its early stages of development (e.g., zygote, morula, blastocyst).

Zygote. This cell, formed by the union of an oocyte and a sperm, is the beginning of a new human being. The expression *fertilized ovum* refers to a secondary oocyte that has been impregnated by a sperm; when fertilization is complete, the oocyte becomes a zygote.

Fertilization Age. It is difficult to determine exactly when fertilization (conception) occurs because the process cannot be observed in vivo (within the living body). Physicians calculate the age of the embryo or fetus from the first day of the last normal menstrual period. This is the **gestational age**, which is approximately 2 weeks longer than the *fertilization age* because the oocyte is not fertilized until approximately 2 weeks after the preceding menstruation (see Fig. 1-1).

Cleavage. Mitotic cell division, or cleavage of the zygote, forms embryonic cells called *blastomeres*. The size of the early embryo remains the same because the blastomeres become smaller with each succeeding cell division.

Morula. When cleavage produces 12 to 32 blastomeres, the embryo is called a *morula*. It is so called because the cluster of cells resembles the fruit known as a mulberry or blackberry (L. *morus*). The morula begins to form approximately 3 days after fertilization, just as the embryo enters the uterus via the uterine tube.

Blastocyst. After the morula enters the uterus, a fluid-filled cavity—the **blastocystic cavity**—forms inside the morula. The embryo is now called a *blastocyst*, which contains an inner cell mass, or **embryoblast,** that forms the embryo.

Conceptus. This term refers to the entire products of conception from fertilization onward (the embryo) and its membranes (e.g., the placenta).

Primordium. This term refers to the beginning or first discernible indication of an organ or structure.

Fetus. After the embryonic period (8 weeks), the developing human is called a *fetus.* During the fetal period (ninth week to birth), differentiation and growth of the tissues and organs formed during the embryonic period occur. Functional maturation of the organs and the rate of body growth are remarkable, especially during the third and fourth months (see Fig. 1-2), and weight gain is phenomenal during the terminal months.

Trimester. This period consists of 3 calendar months. Obstetricians commonly divide the 9-month gestation period into three trimesters. The most critical stages of development occur during the first trimester, when embryonic and early fetal development is occurring.

Abortion. This term refers to the expulsion from the uterus of an embryo or fetus before it is viable (i.e., mature enough to survive outside the uterus).

■ IMPORTANCE OF AND ADVANCES IN EMBRYOLOGY

The study of prenatal stages of development helps us understand the normal relationships of adult body structures and the causes of congenital anomalies. Much of the modern practice of obstetrics involves applied, or **clinical, embryology.** Because some children may have disorders, such as spina bifida and congenital heart disease, that result from maldevelopment, the significance of embryology is readily apparent to pediatricians. Advances in surgery, especially in procedures involving the prenatal and pediatric age groups, have made knowledge of human development more clinically significant.

Rapid advances in the field of molecular biology have led to the use of sophisticated techniques (e.g., **recombinant DNA technology**, chimeric models, transgenics, and **stem cell manipulation**) in research laboratories to explore such diverse issues as the genetic regulation of morphogenesis, the temporal and regional expression of specific genes, and the mechanisms by which cells are committed to form the various parts of the embryo. For the first time, researchers are beginning to understand how, when, and where selected genes are activated and expressed in the embryo during normal and abnormal development.

The critical role of genes, **signaling molecules**, receptors, and other molecular factors in regulating early embryonic development is rapidly being delineated. In 1995, Edward B. Lewis, Christiane Nüsslein-Volhard, and Eric F. Wieschaus were awarded the Nobel Prize in Physiology or Medicine for their discovery of genes that control embryonic development. Such discoveries are contributing to a better understanding of the causes of spontaneous abortion and congenital anomalies.

In 1997, Ian Wilmut and colleagues were the first to produce a mammal (a sheep dubbed **Dolly**) by cloning using the technique of somatic cell nuclear transfer. Since then, other animals have been cloned successfully from cultured differentiated adult cells. Interest in human cloning has generated considerable debate because of social, ethical, and legal implications. Moreover, there is concern that cloning may result in an increase in the number of infants born with birth defects and serious diseases.

Human embryonic stem cells are pluripotential and capable of developing into diverse cell types. The isolation and culture of human embryonic stem cells may hold great promise for the development of molecular therapies as a result of the sequencing of the human genome.

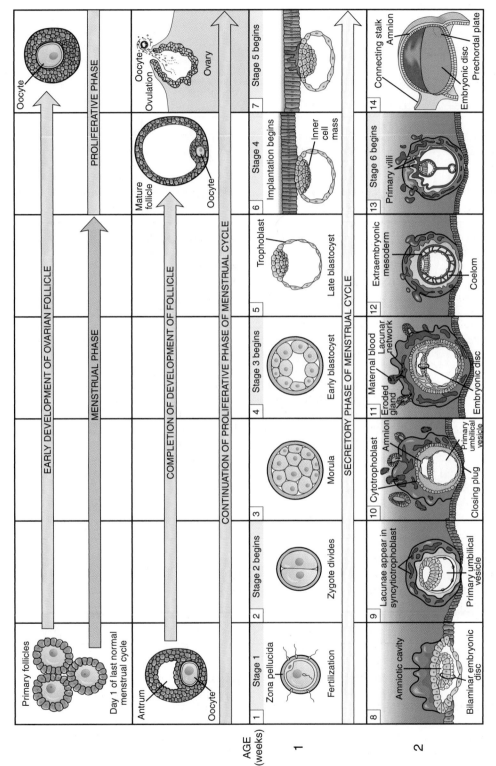

FIGURE 1–1. Early stages of human embryonic development. Development of an ovarian follicle containing an oocyte, ovulation, and the phases of the menstrual cycle are shown. Development begins at fertilization, approximately 14 days after the onset of the last normal menstrual period. Cleavage of the zygote in the uterine tube, implantation of the blastocyst, and early development of the embryo are also shown.

15
First missed
menstrual period

Primitive streak

16 Stage 7 begins

Arrows indicate migration of mesenchymal cells

17 Trilaminar embryo

Amnion

Migration of cells from primitive streak

18 Stage 8 begins

Neural plate

Primitive streak

Length: 1.5 mm

19
Neural plate
Neural groove
Somite
Primitive node
Primitive streak

20 Stage 9 begins

Brain
Neural groove
Somite
Thyroid gland begins to develop

21
Neural groove
First pairs of somites
Primitive streak
Connecting stalk

22 Stage 10 begins

Heart begins to beat

Neural folds fusing

23 Rostral neuropore

Primordia of eye and ear present.

Caudal neuropore

24 Stage 11 begins

Heart bulge
Rostral neuropore closes
2 pairs of pharyngeal arches

25

Otic pit

3 pairs of pharyngeal arches

26 Stage 12 begins

Upper limb bud

Indicates actual size

27
Fore-brain
Pharyngeal arches
Site of otic (ear) pit

CRL = crown-rump length

28 Stage 13 begins

CRL: 4.0 mm

29

CRL: 5.0 mm

30

31
Nasal pit
Developing eye
Primordial mouth

32 Stage 14 begins

Eye
Upper limb bud
Lower limb bud
Heart

33 Stage 15 begins

Hand-plate

CRL: 7.0 mm

34 Cerebral vesicles distinct

Foot-plate present

35

Eye

Cord

CRL: 8.0 mm

36

Oral and nasal cavities confluent

37 Stage 16 begins

Ear
Eye
Foot-plate

CRL: 9.0 mm

38

Large head

Upper lip and nose formed

39

CRL: 10.0 mm

40

Eye
External acoustic meatus
Digital rays
Foot plate

41 Stage 17 begins

Digital rays

Ventral view

42

Ear
Eye

CRL: 13.0 mm

3
4
5
6

FIGURE 1-1.—cont'd

TIMETABLE OF HUMAN PRENATAL DEVELOPMENT
7 – 38 weeks

FIGURE 1-1.—cont'd

Eleventh Week to Full Term

11   12   16   20   24   28   32   36   38   **Full Term**

FIGURE 1–2. The embryonic period terminates at the end of the eighth week; by this time, the beginnings (primordia) of all essential structures are present. The fetal period, extending from the ninth week to birth, is characterized by growth and elaboration of structures. Sex is clearly distinguishable by 12 weeks. Fetuses are viable 22 weeks after fertilization, but the chance of survival is not good until the fetus is several weeks older. The 11- to 38-week fetuses pictured are shown at approximately half their actual sizes.

■ DESCRIPTIVE TERMS

In anatomy and embryology, special terms of position, direction, and various planes of the body are used. Descriptions of the adult are based on the *anatomical position*, the position in which the body is erect, the upper limbs are at the sides, and the palms are directed anteriorly (see Fig. 1-3*A*). The descriptive terms of position, direction, and planes used for embryos are shown in Figure 1-3*B* to *E*.

FIGURE 1–3. Illustrations of descriptive terms of position, direction, and planes of the body. **A,** Lateral view of an adult in the anatomical position. **B,** Lateral view of a 5-week embryo. **C** and **D,** Ventral views of a 6-week embryo. The *median plane* is an imaginary vertical plane of section that passes longitudinally through the body, dividing it into right and left halves. A *transverse plane* refers to any plane that is at right angles to both the median and the frontal planes. **E,** Lateral view of a 7-week embryo. A *frontal (coronal) plane* is any vertical plane that intersects the median plane at a right angle and divides the body into front (anterior, or ventral) and back (posterior, or dorsal) parts. In describing development, it is necessary to use words denoting the position of one part to another, or to the body as a whole. For example, the vertebral column (spine) develops in the dorsal part of the embryo, and the sternum (breast bone) in the ventral part of the embryo.

1. What is the difference between the terms *conceptus* and *embryo*? What are the *products of conception?*
2. Why do we study human embryology? Does it have any practical value in medicine and other health sciences?
3. Physicians date a pregnancy from the first day of the last normal menstrual period, as explained earlier, but the embryo does not start to develop until approximately 2 weeks later. Why do physicians use this terminology?

The answers to these questions are at the back of the book.

HUMAN REPRODUCTION

Human reproduction begins with *fertilization* of an **oocyte** by a **sperm**. Each of these cells brings a half share of genetic information so that the new cell, a **zygote**, receives all the genetic information required for directing the development of a new human being.

Puberty begins when secondary sex characteristics (e.g., pubic hair) appear, typically between the ages of 12 and 15 years in females and 13 and 16 years in males. **Menarche** (first menstruation) may occur as early as 8 years of age, and puberty in females is largely completed by age 16 years. In males, puberty ends when mature sperms are formed.

■ THE REPRODUCTIVE ORGANS

Each sex has reproductive organs (Fig. 2-1) that produce and transport germ cells (gametes) from the gonads (testes or ovaries) to the site of fertilization in the uterine tube.

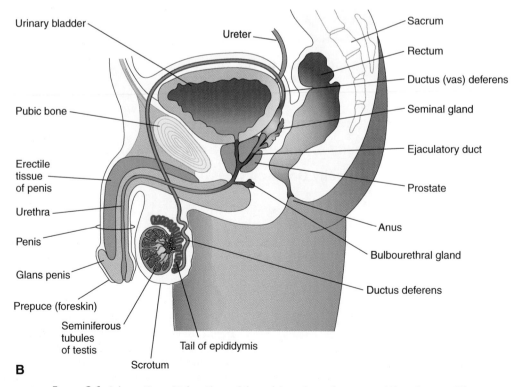

FIGURE 2-1. Schematic sagittal sections of the pelvic regions of a woman (**A**) and a man (**B**).

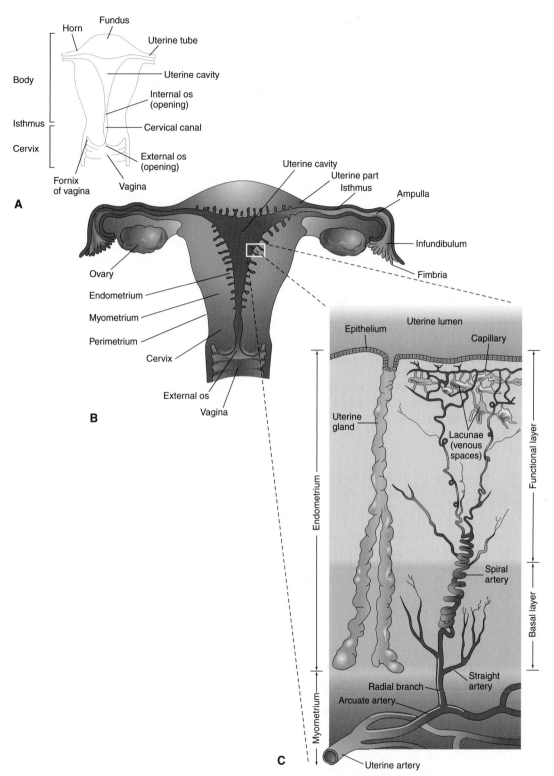

FIGURE 2-2. Female reproductive organs. **A,** Parts of the uterus. **B,** Diagrammatic coronal section of the uterus, uterine tubes, and vagina. The ovaries are also shown. **C,** Enlargement of the area outlined in **B.** The functional layer of the endometrium is sloughed off during menstruation, the monthly endometrial shedding of tissue and discharge of bloody fluid from the uterus and vagina.

Female Reproductive Organs

The Vagina

The vagina (see Fig. 2-1*A*) serves as the excretory passage for menstrual fluid, receives the penis (see Fig. 2-1*B*) during sexual intercourse, and forms the inferior part of the birth canal.

The Uterus

The uterus is a thick-walled, pear-shaped organ (see Fig. 2-2*A* and *B*) and consists of two main parts:
● The **body,** the expanded superior two thirds
● The **cervix,** the cylindrical inferior third
   The **fundus** is the rounded part of the uterine body that lies superior to the orifices of the uterine tubes.

The **body of the uterus** narrows from the fundus to the **isthmus**, the constricted region between the body and the **cervix**. The lumen of the cervix, the cervical canal, has a constricted opening, the *os (ostium)* at each end. The **internal os** communicates with the cavity of the body of the uterus, whereas the **external os** communicates with the vagina. The walls of the body of the uterus consist of three layers:

● **Perimetrium**, a thin external layer of peritoneum
● **Myometrium**, a thick smooth muscle layer
● **Endometrium**, a thin internal mucous membrane

At the peak of its development, the endometrium is 4 to 5 mm thick. During the luteal (secretory) phase of the menstrual cycle (see Fig. 2-8), three layers of the endometrium can be distinguished microscopically (see Fig. 2-2C) into the following:

● A **compact layer**, consisting of densely packed connective tissue around the neck of the uterine glands
● A **spongy layer**, composed of edematous connective tissue containing the dilated, tortuous bodies of the uterine glands
● A **basal layer**, containing the blind ends of the uterine glands

The basal layer of the endometrium has its own blood supply and is not cast off during menstruation. The compact and spongy layers, known collectively as the *functional layer*, disintegrate and are shed at menstruation and after *parturition* (delivery of an infant).

The Uterine Tubes

The uterine tubes, measuring 10 cm long and 1 cm in diameter, extend laterally from the **horns** (Latin, *cornua*) of the uterus (see Fig. 2-2A). Each tube opens into a horn of the uterus at its proximal end and into the peritoneal cavity at its distal end. *The uterine tube is divided into four parts: infundibulum, ampulla, isthmus, and uterine part.* The tubes carry oocytes from the ovaries and sperms entering from the cervix to reach the fertilization site in the ampulla of the uterine tube (see Fig. 2-2B). The uterine tube then conveys the dividing zygote to the uterine cavity.

The Ovaries

The **ovaries** are almond-shaped glands located on each side of the uterus that produce **oocytes** (see Fig. 2-2). When released from the ovary at *ovulation*, the secondary oocyte passes into one of two trumpet-shaped *uterine tubes*. These tubes open into the *uterus*, which protects and nourishes the embryo and fetus until birth. The ovaries also produce estrogen and progesterone, the hormones responsible for the development of secondary sex characteristics and regulation of pregnancy.

Female External Sex Organs

The female external sex organs are known collectively as the **vulva**, or pudendum (Fig. 2-3). The **labia majora**, fatty external folds of skin, conceal the vaginal orifice, the opening of the vagina. Inside these labia are two smaller folds of mucous membrane, the **labia minora**. The

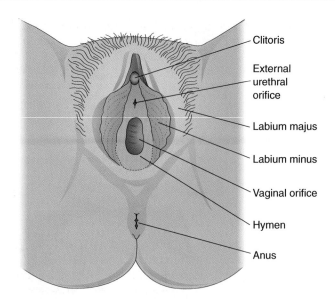

FIGURE **2-3.** External female genitalia. The labia are spread apart to show the external urethral and vaginal orifices.

clitoris, a small erectile organ, is situated at the superior junction of these folds. The vagina and urethra open into a cavity, the **vestibule** (the cleft between the labia minora). The vaginal orifice varies with the condition of the **hymen**, a fold of mucous membrane that surrounds the vaginal orifice.

Male Reproductive Organs

The male reproductive system (see Fig. 2-1B) includes the penis, testes, epididymis, ductus (vas) deferens, prostate, seminal glands, bulbourethral glands, ejaculatory ducts, and urethra. The testes are oval glands that are suspended in the scrotum.

Each **testis** consists of many highly coiled seminiferous tubules that produce sperms. Immature sperms pass from the testis into a single, complexly coiled tube, the **epididymis**, where they are stored. From the epididymis, the **ductus deferens** carries the sperms to the ejaculatory duct. The ductus descends into the pelvis, where it fuses with the duct of the seminal gland to form the **ejaculatory duct**, which enters the urethra.

The **urethra** is a tube that leads from the urinary bladder to the outside of the body; its spongy part runs through the penis. Within the **penis**, three columns of *erectile tissue* surround the urethra. During sexual excitement, this tissue fills with blood, causing the penis to become erect. Semen consists of sperms mixed with fluid produced by the *seminal glands, bulbourethral glands*, and *prostate*.

■ GAMETOGENESIS

The sperm and oocyte are highly specialized gametes, or germ cells (Fig. 2-4). Each of these cells contains half the number of required chromosomes (i.e., 23 instead of 46).

The number of chromosomes is reduced during a special type of cell division called **meiosis**. This type of cell division occurs during **gametogenesis** (formation of germ cells). In males, this process is termed **spermatogenesis**; in females, it is known as **oogenesis** (Fig. 2-5). This process, which involves the chromosomes and cytoplasm of the gametes, prepares these sex cells for their role in fertilization.

Meiosis

Meiosis consists of two meiotic cell divisions (Fig. 2-6), during which the chromosome number of the germ cells is reduced to one half (23, the *haploid* number) the number present in other cells in the body (46, the *diploid* number).

During the **first meiotic division**, the chromosome number is reduced from diploid to haploid. Homologous chromosomes (one from each parent) pair during prophase and then separate during anaphase, with one representative of each pair going to each pole of the meiotic spindle. The spindle connects to the chromosome at the centromere. At this stage, they are double chromatid chromosomes. The X and Y chromosomes are not homologs; however, they have homologous segments at the tips of their short arms. They pair in these regions only. By the end of the first meiotic division, each new cell formed (secondary spermatocyte or secondary oocyte) has the haploid chromosome number (double chromatid chromosomes); therefore, each new cell contains half the number of chromosomes of the preceding cell (primary spermatocyte or primary oocyte). This separation, or disjunction, of paired homologous chromosomes is the physical basis of segregation, or separation, of allelic genes during meiosis.

The **second meiotic division** follows the first division, without a normal interphase (i.e., without an intervening step of DNA replication). Each chromosome divides, and each half, or *chromatid*, is drawn to a different pole of the meiotic spindle; thus, the haploid number of chromosomes (23) is retained, and each daughter cell formed by meiosis has the reduced haploid number of chromosomes, with one representative of each chromosome pair (now a single chromatid chromosome). The second meiotic division is similar to ordinary mitosis, except that the chromosome number of the cell entering the second meiotic division is haploid.

Meiosis is a significant process of cell division because:
- It provides for *constancy of the chromosome number* from generation to generation by reducing the chromosome number from diploid to haploid, thereby producing haploid gametes.
- It allows *random assortment of maternal and paternal chromosomes* between the gametes.
- It relocates segments of maternal and paternal chromosomes by *crossing over of chromosome segments*, which "shuffles" the genes and produces a recombination of genetic material.

Spermatogenesis

Primordial sperms—spermatogonia—are transformed into mature germ cells, or sperms. This maturation process begins at puberty. Before maturation, these spermatogonia remain dormant in the seminiferous tubules of the testes from the late fetal period until puberty, at which time they begin to increase in number. After several mitotic cell divisions,

FIGURE 2-4. Male and female gametes, or germ cells. **A,** The parts of a human sperm (×1250). The head, composed mostly of the nucleus, is partly covered by the acrosome, an organelle containing enzymes. The tail of the sperm consists of three regions: middle piece, principal piece, and end piece. **B,** A sperm drawn to approximately the same scale as the oocyte. **C,** A human secondary oocyte (×200), shown surrounded by the zona pellucida and the corona radiata.

NORMAL GAMETOGENESIS

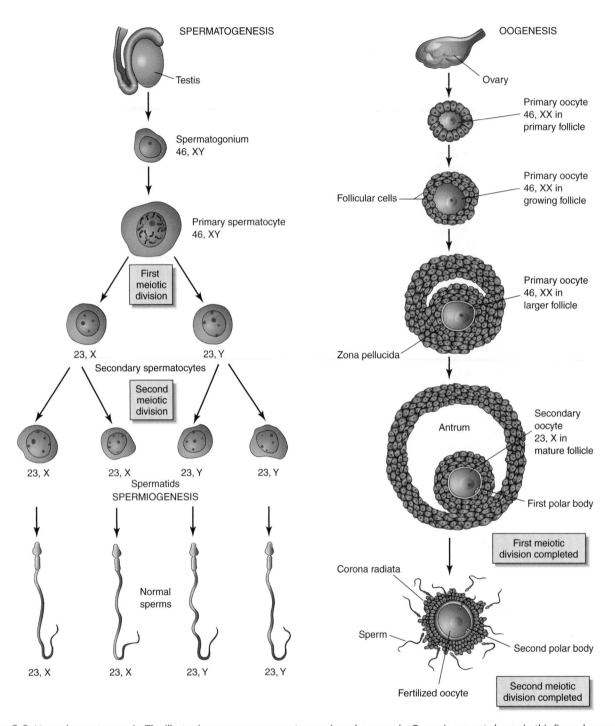

FIGURE 2-5. Normal gametogenesis. The illustrations compare spermatogenesis and oogenesis. Oogonia are not shown in this figure because they differentiate into primary oocytes before birth. The chromosome complement of the germ cells is shown at each stage. The number designates the total number of chromosomes, including sex chromosome(s) (shown after the comma). Note: (1) After the two meiotic divisions, the diploid number of chromosomes, 46, is reduced to the haploid number, 23; (2) four sperms form from one primary spermatocyte, whereas only one secondary oocyte results from maturation of a primary oocyte; (3) the cytoplasm is conserved during oogenesis to form one large cell, the oocyte. The polar bodies are small, nonfunctional cells that eventually degenerate.

the spermatogonia grow and undergo gradual changes that transform them into **primary spermatocytes**—the largest germ cells in the seminiferous tubules. Each primary spermatocyte subsequently undergoes a reduction division—the *first meiotic division*—to form two haploid **secondary spermatocytes**, which are approximately half the size of primary spermatocytes. Subsequently, the secondary spermatocytes undergo a *second meiotic division* to form four haploid **spermatids**, which are approximately half the size of secondary spermatocytes. During this division, no

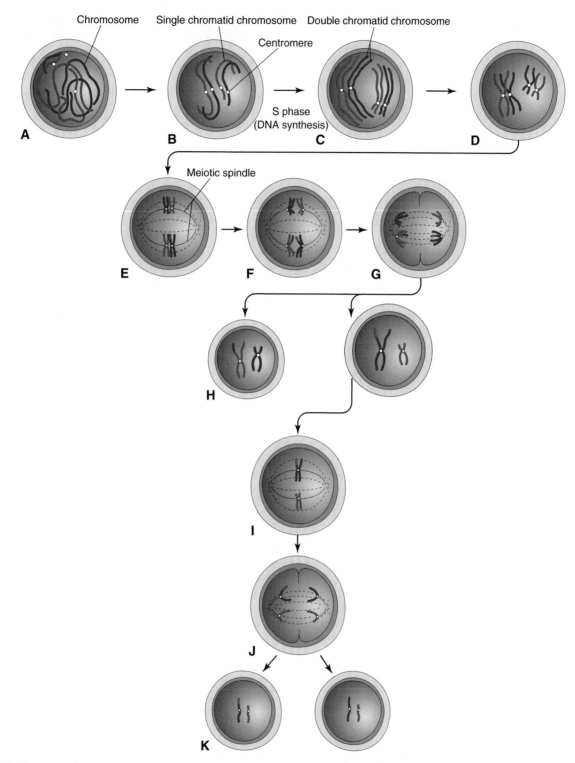

FIGURE 2-6. Diagrammatic representation of meiosis. Two chromosome pairs are shown. **A–D,** Stages of prophase of the first meiotic division. The homologous chromosomes approach each other and pair; each member of the pair consists of two chromatids. Observe the single crossover in one pair of chromosomes, resulting in the interchange of chromatid segments. **E,** Metaphase. The two members of each pair become oriented on the meiotic spindle. **F,** Anaphase. **G,** Telophase. The chromosomes migrate to opposite poles. **H,** Distribution of parental chromosome pairs at the end of the first meiotic division. **I–K,** Second meiotic division, which is similar to mitosis, except that the cells are haploid.

further reduction occurs in the number of chromosomes. The spermatids are gradually transformed into four mature sperms during a process known as **spermiogenesis**. During this metamorphosis (change in form), the nucleus condenses, the acrosome forms, and most of the cytoplasm is shed. Spermatogenesis, including spermiogenesis, requires approximately 2 months for completion and normally continues throughout the reproductive life of a male. When spermiogenesis is complete, sperms enter the lumina of the seminiferous tubules. The sperms then move to the epididymis (see Fig. 2-1*B*), where they are stored and become functionally mature.

When ejaculated, the **mature sperm** is a free-swimming, actively motile cell *consisting of a head and a tail* (see Fig. 2-4*A*). *The neck of the sperm is the junction between the head and the tail.* The head, forming most of the bulk of the sperm, contains the nucleus. The anterior two thirds of the head is covered by the **acrosome**, a caplike organelle containing enzymes that facilitate sperm penetration during fertilization. The tail provides the motility of the sperm, assisting with its transport to the site of fertilization in the ampulla of the uterine tube. *The tail consists of three segments*: the middle piece, principal piece, and end piece. The middle piece contains the energy-producing mitochondria, which fuel the lashing movements of the tail.

Oogenesis

Oogenesis refers to the sequence of events by which oogonia are transformed into **oocytes** (see Fig. 2-5). This maturation process begins during the fetal period, but is not completed until after puberty. During early fetal life, primordial ova—oogonia—proliferate by mitosis and enlarge to form **primary oocytes**. By birth, all primary oocytes have completed the prophase of the *first meiotic division*. These oocytes remain in prophase until puberty. Shortly before ovulation, a primary oocyte completes the first meiotic division (see Fig. 2-5). Unlike the corresponding stage of spermatogenesis, the division of cytoplasm is unequal. The **secondary oocyte** receives almost all the cytoplasm, whereas the **first polar body** receives very little, causing it to degenerate after a short time. At ovulation, the nucleus of the secondary oocyte begins the *second meiotic division*, but progresses only to metaphase.

If the secondary oocyte is fertilized by a sperm, the second meiotic division is completed and a **second polar body** is also formed (see Fig. 2-5). The secondary oocyte released at ovulation is surrounded by a covering of amorphous material known as the **zona pellucida** and a layer of follicular cells called the **corona radiata** (see Fig. 2-4*C*). The secondary oocyte is large, being just visible to the unaided eye. Up to 2 million primary oocytes are usually present in the ovaries of a newborn infant. Most of these oocytes regress during childhood so that, by puberty, no more than 40,000 remain. Of these, only approximately 400 mature and are expelled at ovulation.

Comparison of Male and Female Gametes

Compared with the sperm, the oocyte is massive and immotile (see Fig. 2-4*B* and *C*), whereas the microscopic sperm is highly motile. The mature oocyte also has an abundance of cytoplasm, whereas the sperm has very little. In terms of sex chromosome constitution, **there are two kinds of normal sperm** (see Fig. 2-5): 22 autosomes plus an X sex chromosome (i.e., 23, X), and 22 autosomes plus a Y sex chromosome (23, Y). **There is only one kind of normal secondary oocyte**: 22

ABNORMAL GAMETOGENESIS

During gametogenesis, homologous chromosomes sometimes fail to separate—known as **nondisjunction**—and as a result, some gametes have 24 chromosomes and others only 22 (Fig. 2-7). If a gamete with 24 chromosomes unites with a normal one with 23 chromosomes, a zygote with 47 chromosomes results, as occurs in infants with **Down syndrome** (see Fig. 19-2). This condition is called **trisomy** because of the presence of three representatives of a particular chromosome instead of the usual two. If a gamete with only 22 chromosomes unites with a normal gamete, a zygote with 45 chromosomes results. This condition is known as **monosomy** because only one representative of the particular chromosomal pair is present. Up to 10% of sperms in an ejaculate may be grossly abnormal (e.g., having two heads), but it is generally believed that these abnormal sperms do not fertilize oocytes owing to their lack of normal motility.

---

autosomes plus an X sex chromosome (i.e., 23, X). *The difference in sex chromosome complement forms the basis of primary sex determination.*

■ FEMALE REPRODUCTIVE CYCLES

Commencing at puberty, females undergo monthly reproductive cycles regulated by the **hypothalamus**, **pituitary gland**, and **ovaries** (Fig. 2-8). These cycles prepare the reproductive system for pregnancy. *Gonadotropin-releasing hormone* is synthesized by neurosecretory cells in the hypothalamus. It stimulates the release of two hormones (gonadotropins) that are produced by the anterior pituitary and act on the ovaries:

● *Follicle-stimulating hormone* stimulates the development of the ovarian follicles and the production of **estrogen** by the follicular cells.
● *Luteinizing hormone* serves as the "trigger" for ovulation and stimulates the follicular cells and corpus luteum to produce **progesterone**.

These ovarian hormones also produce growth of the follicles and the endometrium.

The Ovarian Cycle

Follicle-stimulating hormone and luteinizing hormone produce cyclic changes in the ovaries (development of the ovarian follicles, ovulation, and formation of the corpus luteum), collectively known as the **ovarian cycle**. During each cycle, follicle-stimulating hormone promotes growth of several primary follicles (see Fig. 2-8); however, only one of them usually develops into a mature follicle and ruptures.

ABNORMAL GAMETOGENESIS

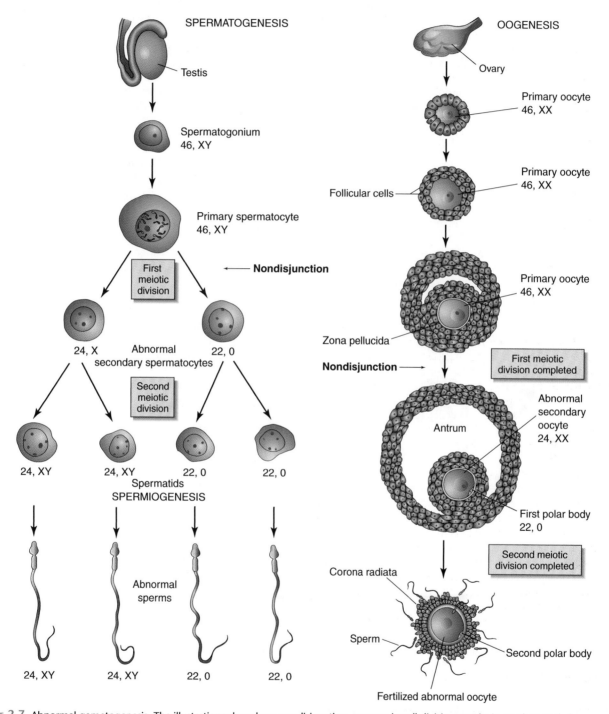

FIGURE 2-7. Abnormal gametogenesis. The illustrations show how nondisjunction, an error in cell division, results in an abnormal chromosome distribution in germ cells. Although nondisjunction of sex chromosomes is illustrated, a similar defect may occur during the division of autosomes. When nondisjunction occurs during the first meiotic division of spermatogenesis, one secondary spermatocyte contains 22 autosomes plus an X and a Y chromosome, whereas the other one contains 22 autosomes and no sex chromosome. Similarly, nondisjunction during oogenesis may give rise to an oocyte with 22 autosomes and two X chromosomes (as shown) or one with 22 autosomes and no sex chromosome.

Follicular Development

Development of an ovarian follicle (Figs. 2-8 and 2-9) is characterized by:

- Growth and differentiation of a primary oocyte
- Proliferation of follicular cells
- Formation of the zona pellucida
- Development of a connective tissue capsule surrounding the follicle—the *theca folliculi*

The **theca folliculi** differentiates into two layers: an internal vascular and glandular layer—called the *theca interna*—and a capsule-like layer known as the *theca externa*. Thecal cells are believed to produce an angiogenic factor that promotes growth of blood vessels in the theca interna; these vessels provide nutritive support for follicular development.

Ovulation

The follicular cells divide actively, producing a stratified layer around the oocyte (see Fig. 2-9*A*). Subsequently, fluid-filled spaces appear around the follicular cells, which coalesce to form a single cavity, the **antrum**, containing **follicular fluid**. After the antrum forms, the ovarian follicle is called a **secondary follicle** (see Fig. 2-9*B*). The primary oocyte is surrounded by a mound of follicular cells, known as the **cumulus oophorus**, which projects into the enlarged

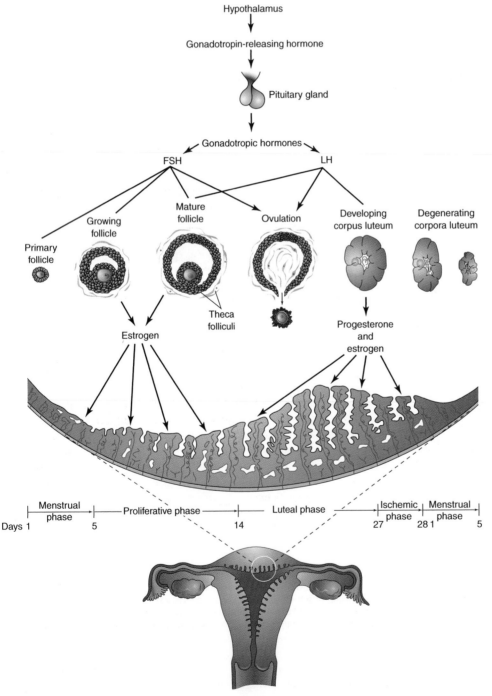

FIGURE 2-8. Illustrations of the interrelationships between the hypothalamus, pituitary gland, ovaries, and endometrium. One complete menstrual cycle and the beginning of another are shown.

FIGURE 2-9. Photomicrographs of sections from adult human ovaries. **A,** Light micrograph of the ovarian cortex demonstrating mostly primordial follicles (P), which are primary oocytes surrounded by follicular cells (×270). **B,** Light micrograph of a secondary follicle. Observe the primary oocyte and the follicular fluid surrounded by membrana granulosa (×132). (From Gartner LP, Hiatt JL: Color Textbook of Histology, 2nd ed. Philadelphia, WB Saunders, 2001.)

MITTELSCHMERZ AND OVULATION

A variable amount of abdominal pain, called *mittelschmerz*, accompanies ovulation in some women. Mittelschmerz may be used as a sign of ovulation; however, there are better indicators, such as the slight drop in basal body temperature, followed by a sustained rise after ovulation.

ANOVULATION AND HORMONES

Some women do not ovulate because of an inadequate release of gonadotropins. In some of these women, ovulation can be induced by the administration of gonadotropins or an ovulatory agent, resulting in maturation of several ovarian follicles and multiple ovulations. The incidence of multiple pregnancy increases when ovulation is induced.

ANOVULATORY MENSTRUAL CYCLES

In anovulatory cycles, the endometrial changes are minimal; the proliferative endometrium develops as usual, but no ovulation occurs and no corpus luteum forms. Consequently, the endometrium does not progress to the luteal phase; it remains in the proliferative phase until menstruation begins. The estrogen in oral contraceptives, with or without progesterone, suppresses ovulation by acting on the hypothalamus and pituitary gland, inhibiting secretion of gonadotropin-releasing hormone, follicle-stimulating hormone, and luteinizing hormone.

---

antrum. The follicle continues to enlarge and soon forms a bulge on the surface of the ovary (Fig. 2-10*A*). A small, oval, avascular spot, the stigma, soon appears on this bulge. Before ovulation, the secondary oocyte and some cells of the cumulus oophorus detach from the interior of the distended follicle (see Fig. 2-10*B*).

Ovulation follows within 24 hours of a surge of luteinizing hormone production. This surge, elicited by the high estrogen level in the blood (Fig. 2-11), appears to cause the stigma to rupture, expelling the secondary oocyte with the follicular fluid (see Fig. 2-10*D*).

The expelled secondary oocyte is surrounded by the zona pellucida and one or more layers of follicular cells, which are radially arranged to form the corona radiata (see Fig. 2-4*C*) and the cumulus oophorus.

The Corpus Luteum

Shortly after ovulation, the ovarian follicle collapses (see Fig. 2-10*D*). Under the influence of luteinizing hormone, the walls of the follicle develop into a glandular structure, the corpus luteum, which secretes primarily progesterone, but also some estrogen.

If the oocyte is fertilized, the corpus luteum enlarges to form a *corpus luteum of pregnancy* and increases its hormone production. Degeneration of the corpus luteum is prevented by *human chorionic gonadotropin* (hCG) (see Chapter 4).

If the oocyte is not fertilized, the corpus luteum begins to involute and degenerate approximately 10 to 12 days after ovulation. It is then called a *corpus luteum of menstruation.* The corpus luteum is subsequently transformed into white scar tissue in the ovary, forming the *corpus albicans* (degenerating corpus luteum).

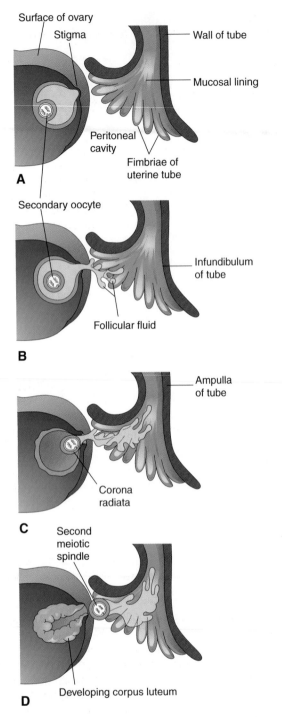

FIGURE 2-10. Diagrams (**A–D**) illustrating ovulation. When the stigma ruptures, the secondary oocyte is expelled from the ovarian follicle with the follicular fluid. After ovulation, the wall of the follicle collapses. The follicular wall is then transformed into a glandular structure called the *corpus luteum.*

The Menstrual Cycle

The menstrual (endometrial) cycle is the period during which the oocyte matures, is ovulated, and enters the uterine tube (Fig. 2-11). The hormones produced by the ovarian follicles and the corpus luteum (estrogen and progesterone) produce cyclic changes in the endometrium

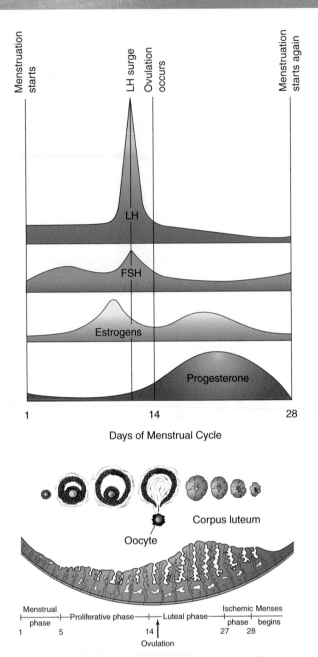

FIGURE 2-11. The blood levels of various hormones during the menstrual cycle. Follicle-stimulating hormone (FSH) stimulates the ovarian follicles to develop and produce estrogens. The level of estrogens rises to a peak just before the luteinizing hormone (LH) surge induces ovulation. Ovulation normally occurs within 24 hours after the LH surge. If fertilization does not occur, the blood levels of circulating estrogens and progesterone fall. This hormone withdrawal causes the endometrium to regress and menstruation to start again.

of the uterus. These monthly changes in the uterine lining constitute the **endometrial,** or **menstrual, cycle** (period). The average menstrual cycle is 28 days (range, 23–35 days), with day 1 of the cycle corresponding to the day on which menstruation begins. Menstrual cycles may normally vary in length by several days in normal women.

Phases of the Menstrual Cycle

The menstrual cycle is divided into three main phases for descriptive purposes only (see Fig. 2-11). In actuality, *the menstrual cycle is a continuous process*; each phase gradually passes into the next one.

MENSTRUAL PHASE

The first day of menstruation (period) is the beginning of the menstrual cycle. The functional layer of the uterine wall is sloughed off and discarded with the menstrual flow, which usually lasts 4 to 5 days. The menstrual flow, or **menses**, discharged through the vagina consists of varying amounts of blood combined with small pieces of endometrial tissue. After menstruation, the eroded endometrium is thin.

PROLIFERATIVE PHASE

The proliferative phase, lasting approximately 9 days, coincides with growth of the ovarian follicles and is controlled by estrogen secreted by these follicles. There is a two- to threefold increase in the thickness of the endometrium during this time. Early during this phase, the surface epithelium of the endometrium regenerates. The glands increase in number and length, and the spiral arteries elongate (see Fig. 2-2C).

LUTEAL PHASE

The luteal (secretory) phase, lasting approximately 13 days, coincides with the formation, function, and growth of the corpus luteum. The progesterone produced by the corpus luteum stimulates the glandular epithelium to secrete a glycogen-rich, mucoid material. The glands become wide, tortuous, and saccular, and the endometrium thickens because of the influence of progesterone and estrogen from the corpus luteum and the increase in fluid in the connective tissue.

If fertilization does not occur:
● The corpus luteum degenerates.
● Estrogen and progesterone levels decrease, and the endometrium enters an *ischemic phase* during the last day of the luteal phase.
● Menstruation occurs.

Ischemia (reduced blood supply) of the spiral arteries occurs by constriction resulting from the decrease in the secretion of progesterone. Hormone withdrawal also results in the stoppage of glandular secretion, a loss of interstitial fluid, and a marked shrinking of the endometrium. Toward the end of the ischemic phase, the spiral arteries become constricted for longer periods. This results in venous stasis and patchy ischemic necrosis (death) in the superficial tissues. Eventually, rupture of vessel walls follows, and blood seeps into the surrounding connective tissue. Small pools of blood form and break through the endometrial surface, resulting in bleeding into the uterine lumen and subsequent drainage from the vagina.

As small pieces of the endometrium detach and pass into the uterine cavity, the torn ends of the arteries bleed into the uterine cavity, resulting in a loss of 20 to 80 mL of blood. Eventually, over 3 to 5 days, the entire compact layer and most of the spongy layer of the endometrium are discarded. Remnants of the spongy and basal layers soon undergo regeneration during the subsequent proliferative phase of the endometrium.

If fertilization occurs:
● Cleavage of the zygote and formation of the blastocyst occur.
● The blastocyst begins to implant on approximately the sixth day of the luteal phase.
● Human chorionic gonadotropin (hCG) keeps the corpus luteum secreting estrogens and progesterone.
● The luteal phase continues, and menstruation does not occur.

During pregnancy, the menstrual cycles cease and the endometrium passes into a pregnancy phase. With the termination of pregnancy, the ovarian and menstrual cycles resume after a variable time. If pregnancy does not occur, the reproductive cycles normally continue until the permanent cessation of the menses—**menopause**—usually between the ages of 48 and 55 years.

■ TRANSPORTATION OF THE GAMETES

Oocyte Transport

During ovulation, the fimbriated (fringed) end of the uterine tube comes in close proximity to the ovary (see Fig. 2-10). The fingerlike processes of the tube, the *fimbriae*, move back and forth over the ovary. The sweeping action of the fimbriae and the fluid currents produced by them "sweep" the secondary oocyte into the funnel-shaped infundibulum of the uterine tube. The oocyte then passes into the ampulla of the tube, primarily as a result of waves of peristalsis—movements of the wall of the tube characterized by alternate contraction and relaxation.

Sperm Transport

From their storage site in the epididymis (see Fig. 2-1B), sperms are rapidly transported to the urethra by peristaltic contractions of the ductus deferens. Secretions from the *seminal glands*, *prostate*, and *bulbourethral glands* are added to sperm-containing fluid (semen) in the ductus deferens and urethra. The number of sperms ejaculated ranges from 200 to 600 million. The sperms pass slowly through the cervical canal by movements of their tails. *Vesiculase*, an enzyme produced by the seminal glands, coagulates some of the *semen* and forms a vaginal plug that may prevent backflow of semen into the vagina. At the time of ovulation, the amount of cervical mucus increases and becomes less viscid, making it more favorable for sperm transport. *Prostaglandins* in the semen stimulate uterine motility and help to move the sperms through the uterus to the site of fertilization in the uterine tube.

The volume of the **ejaculate** ranges from 2 to 6 mL. Sperms move 2 to 3 mm per minute. They move slowly in the acid environment of the vagina, but more rapidly in the alkaline environment of the uterus. Only approximately 200 sperms reach the fertilization site. Most of them degenerate during their passage through the female genital tract.

Semen analysis is an important part of evaluating patients for infertility. Sperms account for less than 5% of the volume of semen. The remainder of the ejaculate consists of the secretions of the seminal glands (60%), prostate (30%), and bulbourethral glands (5%). The ejaculate of normal males usually contains more than 100 million sperms per milliliter of semen. Although there is much variation in individual cases, men whose semen contains a minimum of 20 million sperms per milliliter, or 50 million in the total specimen, are probably fertile. A man with less than 10 million sperms per milliliter of semen is likely to be sterile, especially when the specimen contains immotile and abnormal sperms. For potential fertility, at least 40% of sperms should be motile after 2 hours, and some should be motile after 24 hours. Male infertility may result from endocrine disorders, abnormal spermatogenesis, or obstruction of a genital duct (e.g., the ductus deferens), and it represents the cause of infertility in approximately 30% to 50% of affected couples.

■ MATURATION OF SPERMS

Freshly ejaculated sperms are unable to fertilize oocytes. They must undergo a period of conditioning—**capacitation**—lasting approximately 7 hours. During this period, a glycoprotein coat and seminal proteins are removed from the surface of the sperm's *acrosome*. Capacitated sperms show no morphologic changes, but they exhibit increased activity. Sperms are usually capacitated in the uterus or the uterine tubes by substances secreted by these organs.

■ VIABILITY OF OOCYTES AND SPERMS

Oocytes are usually fertilized within 12 hours of ovulation. In vitro observations have shown that oocytes cannot

The most effective method of contraception in males is **vasectomy** (excision of a segment of the ductus deferens). After vasectomy, there are no sperms in the ejaculate, but the amount of seminal fluid is the same as before the procedure.

be fertilized after 24 hours, and they degenerate shortly thereafter. Some sperms are stored in folds of the mucosa of the cervix, are gradually released into the cervical canal, and then pass from the uterus into the uterine tubes. Semen and oocytes that have been frozen to low temperatures may be kept for many years, and children have been born to women who have been artificially inseminated with semen stored for several years.

CLINICALLY ORIENTED QUESTIONS

1. There have been reports of a woman who claimed that she menstruated throughout her pregnancy. How could this happen?
2. If a woman forgets to take an oral contraceptive and then takes two, is she likely to become pregnant?
3. What is *coitus interruptus*? Some people believe that it is an effective method of birth control. Is this true?
4. What is the difference between spermatogenesis and spermiogenesis?
5. Some say that an intrauterine device (IUD) is a contraceptive. Is this correct?

The answers to these questions are at the back of the book.

3

THE FIRST WEEK OF HUMAN DEVELOPMENT

A zygote, formed by the union of a sperm and an oocyte, is a highly specialized, totipotent cell. It contains chromosomes and genes derived from the mother and the father. The zygote divides many times and is progressively transformed into a multicellular human being through cell division, migration, growth, and differentiation.

■ FERTILIZATION

The usual site of fertilization is in the ampulla, the longest and widest part of the uterine tube (see Fig. 2-2B). If the oocyte is not fertilized here, it slowly passes along the tube into the cavity of the uterus, where it degenerates. Fertilization is a complex sequence of coordinated molecular events that begins with contact between a sperm and an oocyte (Fig. 3-1A) and ends with the intermingling of maternal and paternal chromosomes at metaphase of the first mitotic division of the **zygote**. Carbohydrate- and protein-binding molecules on the surface of the gametes are involved in sperm chemotaxis and gamete recognition, as well as in the process of fertilization.

Phases of Fertilization

The phases of fertilization (Figs. 3-1 and 3-2):
● **Passage of a sperm through the corona radiata of the oocyte.** Dispersal of the follicular cells of the corona radiata results mainly from the action of the enzyme *hyaluronidase,* which is released from the acrosome of the sperm. *Tubal mucosal enzymes* also appear to assist hyaluronidase. Additionally, movements of the tail of the sperm are important during penetration of the corona radiata.
● **Penetration of the zona pellucida.** The formation of a pathway through the zona pellucida for the sperm results from the action of enzymes released from the acrosome. The proteolytic enzyme *acrosin* (as well as *esterases* and *neuraminidase*) appears to cause

FIGURE 3-1. Acrosome reaction and sperm penetration of an oocyte. The area outlined in **A** is detailed in **B**. 1, Sperm during capacitation, a period of conditioning that occurs in the female reproductive tract. 2, Sperm undergoing the acrosome reaction during which perforations form in the acrosome. 3, Sperm digesting a path through the zona pellucida by the action of enzymes released from the acrosome. 4, Sperm after entering the cytoplasm of the oocyte. Note that the plasma membranes of the sperm and the oocyte have fused and that the head and tail of the sperm enter the oocyte.

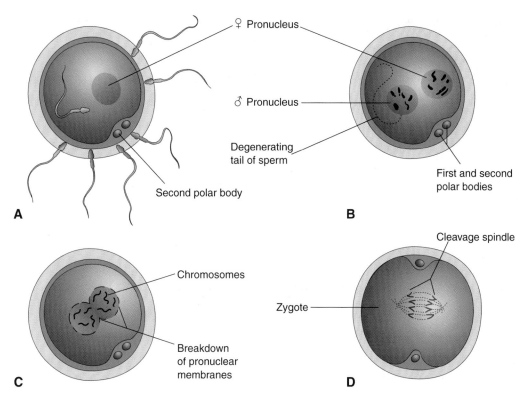

♀ Pronucleus

♂ Pronucleus

Degenerating
tail of sperm

Second polar body

First and second
polar bodies

A

B

Cleavage spindle

Chromosomes

Zygote

Breakdown
of pronuclear
membranes

C

D

FIGURE 3-2. Illustrations of fertilization. **A,** The corona radiata has disappeared, a sperm has entered the oocyte, and the second meiotic division has occurred, resulting in the formation of a mature oocyte. The nucleus of the oocyte is now the female pronucleus. **B,** The sperm head has enlarged to form the male pronucleus. **C,** The pronuclei are fusing. **D,** The zygote has formed; it contains 46 chromosomes, the diploid number.

lysis of the zona pellucida, thereby forming a path for the sperm to follow to the oocyte. Once the sperm penetrates the zona pellucida, a **zona reaction** occurs, changing the physical properties of the zona pellucida and making it impermeable to other sperms.

● **Fusion of the plasma cell membranes of the oocyte and sperm.** The cell membranes break down at the area of fusion. The head and tail of the sperm then enter the cytoplasm of the oocyte, but the plasma membrane of the sperm remains behind (see Figs. 3-1A and B and 3-2A).

● **Completion of the second meiotic division of the oocyte.** The oocyte completes the second meiotic division and forms a mature oocyte and a second polar body (see Fig. 3-2A). The nucleus of the mature oocyte becomes the female pronucleus.

● **Formation of the male pronucleus.** Within the cytoplasm of the oocyte, the nucleus of the sperm enlarges to form the male pronucleus. The tail of the sperm degenerates (see Fig. 3-2B). During growth, the male and female pronuclei replicate their DNA (Fig. 3-2C).

● **Breakdown of the pronuclear membranes.** Condensation of the chromosomes, arrangement of the chromosomes for mitotic cell division, and the first cleavage division of the zygote occur (see Figs. 3-2D and 3-4A). The combination of 23 chromosomes in each pronucleus results in a zygote with 46 chromosomes.

DISPERMY AND TRIPLOIDY

Although several sperms begin to penetrate the zona pellucida, usually only one enters the oocyte and fertilizes it. In *dispermy*, two sperms participate in fertilization, resulting in three sets of chromosomes (triploidy). **Triploid conceptions** account for approximately 20% of spontaneous abortions occurring as a result of chromosomal abnormalities. **Triploid embryos** appear quite normal, but nearly always abort spontaneously. Aborted fetuses with triploidy have severe *intrauterine growth retardation,* with disproportionately small trunks and many other anomalies. A few triploid infants have been born, but all died shortly after birth.

Results of Fertilization

Fertilization:

● Stimulates the secondary oocyte to complete the second meiotic division, producing the second polar body
● Restores the normal diploid number of chromosomes (46) in the zygote
● Results in variation of the human species through mingling of maternal and paternal chromosomes
● Determines the chromosomal sex of the embryo; an X-bearing sperm produces a female embryo and a Y-bearing sperm produces a male embryo

FIGURE 3-3. In vitro fertilization and embryo transfer procedures.

Uterus   Uterine tube

Ovary

Hormonal stimulation of mature oocyte formation, resulting in several mature follicles

Collection of oocytes from follicles with aspirator during laparoscopy

Placement of oocytes in Petri dish with capacitated sperms; in vitro fertilization of oocytes

Cleavage of zygotes in culture medium until four- to eight-cell stages are reached

Speculum in vagina

Uterus   Bladder

Transfer of one to two cleaving embryos into uterine cavity by way of a catheter inserted through the vagina and cervical canal

Catheter

Rectum

FIGURE 3-3. In vitro fertilization and embryo transfer procedures.

● Causes metabolic activation of the oocyte, which initiates cleavage (of the zygote)

The zygote is genetically unique because half of its chromosomes come from the mother and half are derived from the father. This mechanism forms the basis for biparental inheritance and variation of the human species. Meiosis allows independent assortment of maternal and paternal chromosomes among the germ cells. Crossing over of chromosomes, by relocating segments of the maternal and paternal chromosomes, "shuffles" the genes, thereby producing a recombination of genetic material (see Fig. 2-6).

IN VITRO FERTILIZATION AND EMBRYO TRANSFER

The process of in vitro fertilization (IVF) of oocytes and transfer of either the dividing (cleaving) zygotes or a blastocyst into the uterus has provided an opportunity for many couples who are infertile. The first of these IVF babies was born in 1978. The steps involved in IVF and embryo transfer are summarized in Figure 3-3. The incidence of multiple pregnancies is higher with IVF than when pregnancy results from normal ovulation. The incidence of spontaneous abortion of transferred embryos is also higher in IVF.

The technique of **intracytoplasmic sperm injection** involves injecting a sperm directly into the cytoplasm of the mature oocyte. This procedure is invaluable in cases of infertility resulting from blocked uterine tubes or oligospermia (reduced number of sperms).

■ CLEAVAGE OF THE ZYGOTE

Cleavage consists of repeated mitotic divisions of the zygote, resulting in a rapid increase in the number of cells. Division of the zygote begins approximately 30 hours after fertilization.

These cells—called **blastomeres**—become smaller with each cleavage division (Fig. 3-4A to D). Cleavage normally occurs as the zygote passes through the uterine tube. During cleavage, the zygote is still contained within the zona pellucida.

After the eight-cell stage, the blastomeres change their shape and tightly align themselves against each other—**compaction**—to form a compact ball of cells. This phenomenon may be mediated by cell surface adhesion glycoproteins. Compaction permits greater cell-to-cell interaction and is a prerequisite for segregation of the internal cells that form the inner cell mass (see Fig. 3-4E). When there are 12 to 32 blastomeres, the conceptus is called a **morula**. The inner cells of the morula—the inner cell mass, or **embryoblast**—are surrounded by a layer of flattened blastomeres that form the trophoblast.

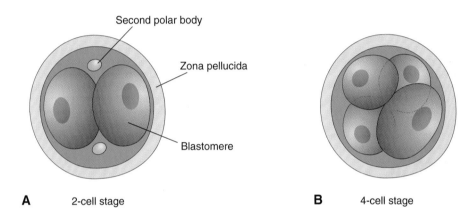

A — 2-cell stage
B — 4-cell stage

FIGURE 3-4. Illustrations of cleavage of the zygote and formation of the blastocyst. **A–D** show various stages of cleavage. The period of the morula begins at the 12- to 32-cell stage and ends when the blastocyst forms. **E** and **F** show sections of blastocysts. The zona pellucida disappears by the late blastocyst stage (5 days). The polar bodies shown in **A** are small, nonfunctional cells that soon degenerate. Blastocyst formation normally occurs in the uterus. Although cleavage increases the number of blastomeres, note that each of the daughter cells is smaller than the parent cells. As a result, there is no increase in the size of the developing embryo until the zona pellucida degenerates.

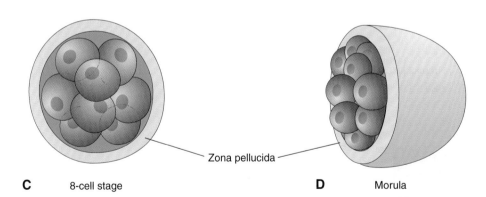

C — 8-cell stage
D — Morula

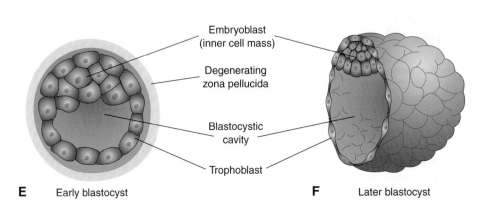

E — Early blastocyst
F — Later blastocyst

An immunosuppressant protein—the **early pregnancy factor**—is secreted by the trophoblastic cells and appears in the maternal serum within 24 to 48 hours after fertilization. The early pregnancy factor forms the basis for a pregnancy test applicable during the first 10 days of development.

■ FORMATION OF THE BLASTOCYST

Shortly after the morula enters the uterus (approximately 4 days after fertilization), uterine fluid passes through the zona pellucida to form a fluid-filled space—the **blastocystic cavity**—inside the morula (see Fig. 3-4E). As fluid increases in the cavity, the blastomeres are separated into two parts:

● The **trophoblast**, the thin outer cells that give rise to the embryonic part of the placenta

● The **embryoblast**, a group of centrally located blastomeres that is the primordium of the embryo

At this stage, the conceptus, or embryo, is called a **blastocyst**. The embryoblast now projects into the blastocystic cavity, and the trophoblast forms the wall of the blastocyst (see Fig. 3-4E and F). After the blastocyst has floated in the uterine fluid for approximately 2 days, the zona pellucida degenerates and disappears. Shedding of the zona pellucida, or "hatching of the blastocyst," has been observed in vitro. Shedding of the zona pellucida permits the blastocyst to increase rapidly in size. While floating freely in the uterine cavity, the embryo derives nourishment from secretions of the uterine glands.

Approximately 6 days after fertilization, the blastocyst (usually adjacent to the embryoblast) attaches to the endometrial epithelium (Fig. 3-5A). As soon as it attaches to the

A

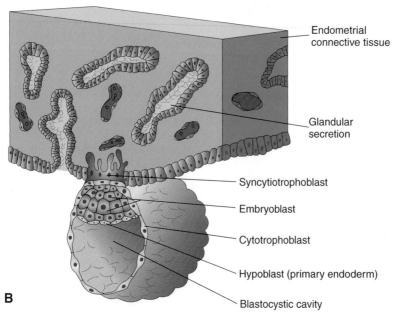

B

FIGURE 3-5. Attachment of the blastocyst to the endometrial epithelium during the early stages of its implantation. **A,** At 6 days, the trophoblast is attached to the endometrial epithelium at the embryonic pole of the blastocyst. **B,** At 7 days, the syncytiotrophoblast has penetrated the epithelium and has started to invade the endometrial connective tissue.

PREIMPLANTATION DIAGNOSIS OF GENETIC DISORDERS

Using currently available techniques of micromanipulation and DNA application, a cleaving zygote known to be at risk for a specific genetic disorder may be diagnosed before implantation during IVF. The sex of the embryo can be determined from a blastomere taken from a six- to eight-cell zygote and analyzed by DNA amplification of sequences from the Y chromosome. This procedure has been used to determine chromosomal sex in cases in which a male embryo would be at risk for a serious X-linked disorder.

ABNORMAL EMBRYOS AND SPONTANEOUS ABORTIONS

Many early embryos abort spontaneously. The early implantation stages of the blastocyst are critical periods of development that may fail to occur because of inadequate production of progesterone and estrogen by the corpus luteum (see Fig. 2-8). Clinicians occasionally see a patient whose last menstrual period was delayed by several days and whose last menstrual flow was unusually profuse. Very likely, such patients have had an early spontaneous abortion. The overall early spontaneous abortion rate is believed to be approximately 45%. Early spontaneous abortions occur for a variety of reasons, an important one being the presence of **chromosomal abnormalities**.

---

epithelium, the trophoblast starts to proliferate rapidly and differentiate into two layers (see Fig. 3-5B):
- The **cytotrophoblast**, the inner layer of cells
- The **syncytiotrophoblast**, the outer layer consisting of a multinucleate protoplasmic mass formed by the fusion of cells

The fingerlike processes of the syncytiotrophoblast extend through the endometrial epithelium and invade the endometrial connective tissue. By the end of the first week, the blastocyst is superficially implanted in the compact layer of the endometrium and is deriving its nourishment from the eroded maternal tissues. The highly invasive syncytiotrophoblast rapidly expands adjacent to the embryoblast—the **embryonic pole**. The syncytiotrophoblast produces proteolytic enzymes that erode the maternal tissues, enabling the blastocyst to "burrow" into the endometrium. At the end of the first week, a cuboidal layer of cells, called the **hypoblast**, appears on the surface of the embryoblast, facing the blastocystic cavity (see Fig. 3-5B). Comparative embryologic data suggest that the hypoblast arises by delamination (separation of blastomeres) from the embryoblast.

CLINICALLY ORIENTED QUESTIONS

1. Although women do not commonly become pregnant after they are 48 years old, very elderly men can still impregnate women. Why is this? Is there an increased risk of Down syndrome or other congenital anomalies in the child when the father is older than 50 years of age?
2. Are there oral contraceptives for men? If not, what is the reason?
3. Is a polar body ever fertilized? If so, does the fertilized polar body give rise to a viable embryo?
4. What is the most common cause of spontaneous abortion during the first week of development?
5. Some clinicians have speculated that a woman could have dissimilar twins as a result of one oocyte being fertilized by a sperm from one man and another one being fertilized by a sperm from another man. Is this possible?
6. When referring to a zygote, do the terms *cleavage* and *mitosis* mean the same thing?
7. How is the cleaving zygote nourished during the first week?
8. Is it possible to determine the sex of a cleaving zygote developing in vitro? If so, what medical reasons would there be for doing so?

The answers to these questions are at the back of the book.

THE SECOND WEEK OF HUMAN DEVELOPMENT

Implantation of the blastocyst is completed during the second week of embryonic development. As this crucial process occurs, changes occur in the embryoblast, producing a bilaminar embryonic disc composed of two layers, the epiblast and the hypoblast (Fig. 4-1). The **embryonic disc** gives rise to the germ layers that form all the tissues and orans of the embryo. Extraembryonic structures forming during the second week include the amniotic cavity, amnion, umbilical vesicle (yolk sac), connecting stalk, and chorionic sac.

Implantation of the blastocyst begins at the end of the first week. The actively erosive **syncytiotrophoblast** invades the endometrial connective tissue that supports the uterine capillaries and glands. As this occurs, the blastocyst slowly embeds itself in the endometrium. Syncytiotrophoblastic cells from this region displace endometrial cells in the central part of the implantation site. The endometrial cells undergo *apoptosis* (programmed cell death), which facilitates implantation. Proteolytic enzymes produced by the syncytiotrophoblast are involved in this process. The uterine connective tissue cells around the implantation site become loaded with glycogen and lipids and assume a polyhedral appearance. Some of these cells—**decidual cells**—degenerate adjacent to the penetrating syncytiotrophoblast. The syncytiotrophoblast engulfs these degenerating cells, providing a rich source of *embryonic nutrition*. As the blastocyst implants, more trophoblast contacts the endometrium and continues to differentiate into two layers (see Fig. 4-1A and B):

- The **cytotrophoblast**, a layer of mononucleated cells that is mitotically active and forms new trophoblastic cells that migrate into the increasing mass of syncytiotrophoblast, where they fuse and lose their cell membranes
- The **syncytiotrophoblast**, a rapidly expanding, multinucleated mass in which no cell boundaries are discernible

The syncytiotrophoblast produces a hormone, **human chorionic gonadotropin** (hCG), which enters the maternal blood in the lacunae in the syncytiotrophoblast (see Fig. 4-1C); hCG maintains the endocrine activity of the corpus luteum in the ovary during pregnancy and forms the basis for pregnancy tests. Highly sensitive radioimmunoassays are available for detecting hCG. Enough hCG is produced by the syncytiotrophoblast at the end of the second week to yield a positive pregnancy test, even though the woman is probably unaware that she is pregnant.

■ FORMATION OF THE AMNIOTIC CAVITY AND EMBRYONIC DISC

As implantation of the blastocyst progresses, changes occurring in the embryoblast result in the formation of a flattened, almost circular, bilaminar plate of cells—the **embryonic disc**—consisting of two layers (Figs. 4-1A and 4-2B):

- The **epiblast**, the thicker layer, consists of high, columnar cells related to the amniotic cavity.
- The **hypoblast**, the thinner layer, consists of small, cuboidal cells adjacent to the exocoelomic cavity.

Concurrently, a small cavity appears in the embryoblast, which is the primordium of the **amniotic cavity** (see Fig. 4-1A). Soon, amniogenic (amnion-forming) cells called

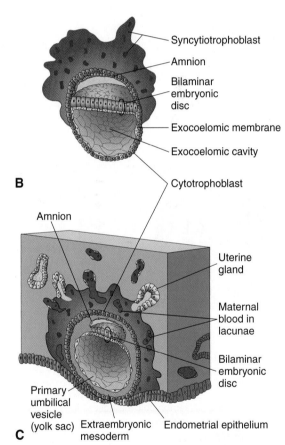

FIGURE 4-1. Implantation of a blastocyst. The actual size of the conceptus is approximately 0.1 mm. **A,** Illustration of a section of a partially implanted blastocyst (approximately 8 days after fertilization). Note the slitlike amniotic cavity. **B,** Illustration of a slightly older blastocyst (endometrium not shown). **C,** Illustration of a section through a blastocyst at approximately 9 days. Note the lacunae appearing in the syncytiotrophoblast. The term *yolk sac* is a misnomer because it contains no yolk.

amnioblasts separate from the epiblast and organize to form a thin membrane, the **amnion**, which encloses the amniotic cavity (see Fig. 4-1A).

The epiblast forms the floor of the amniotic cavity and is continuous peripherally with the amnion. The hypoblast

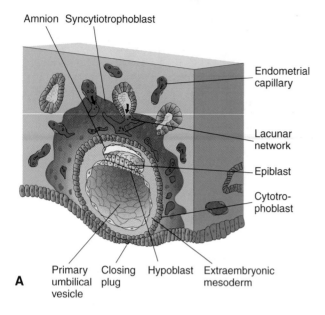

A

Amnion Syncytiotrophoblast

Endometrial capillary

Lacunar network

Epiblast

Cytotrophoblast

Primary umbilical vesicle Closing plug Hypoblast Extraembryonic mesoderm

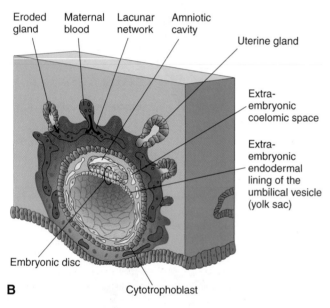

B

Eroded gland Maternal blood Lacunar network Amniotic cavity

Uterine gland

Extra-embryonic coelomic space

Extra-embryonic endodermal lining of the umbilical vesicle (yolk sac)

Embryonic disc

Cytotrophoblast

FIGURE 4-2. Illustration of sections of two implanted blastocysts at 10 days (**A**) and 12 days (**B**). These stages of development are characterized by the formation of lacunar networks—the communication of the blood-filled lacunae. In **B**, note that spaces have appeared in the extraembryonic mesoderm, indicating the beginning of the formation of the extraembryonic coelom.

forms the roof of the **exocoelomic cavity** and is continuous with the cells that migrated from the hypoblast to form the **exocoelomic membrane**. This membrane surrounds the blastocystic cavity and lines the internal surface of the cytotrophoblast. The exocoelomic membrane and cavity soon become modified to form the **primary umbilical vesicle**. The embryonic disc then lies between the amniotic cavity and the primary umbilical vesicle. The outer layer of cells from the umbilical vesicle endoderm forms a layer of loosely arranged connective tissue, the **extraembryonic mesoderm**, which surrounds the amnion and the umbilical vesicle, formerly called the **yolk sac** (see Fig. 4-1C).

As the amnion, embryonic disc, and primary umbilical vesicle form, isolated cavities called **lacunae** appear in the syncytiotrophoblast (see Figs. 4-1C and 4-2). The lacunae soon become filled with a mixture of maternal blood from ruptured endometrial capillaries and cellular debris from eroded uterine glands. The fluid in the lacunae, sometimes called *embryotroph*, passes to the embryonic disc by diffusion. The communication of the eroded uterine vessels with the lacunae represents the *beginning of uteroplacental circulation*. When maternal blood flows into the lacunae, oxygen and nutritive substances become available to the extraembryonic tissues over the large surface of the syncytiotrophoblast. Oxygenated blood passes into the lacunae from the spiral endometrial arteries in the endometrium; deoxygenated blood is removed from the lacunae through endometrial veins.

The 10-day human embryo is completely embedded in the endometrium (see Fig. 4-2A). For approximately 2 days, there is a defect in the endometrial epithelium that is filled by a **closing plug**, a fibrinous coagulum of blood. By day 12, an almost completely regenerated uterine epithelium covers the closing plug (see Fig. 4-2B). As the conceptus implants, the endometrial connective tissue cells undergo a transformation known as the **decidual reaction**. The cells swell because of the accumulation of glycogen and lipid in their cytoplasm, and they are then known as *decidual cells*. The primary function of the decidual reaction is to provide an immunologically privileged site for the conceptus.

In a **12-day embryo**, adjacent syncytiotrophoblastic lacunae have fused to form **lacunar networks** (see Fig. 4-2B), giving the syncytiotrophoblast a spongelike appearance. The lacunar networks, which are particularly prominent around the embryonic pole, are the *primordia of the intervillous space of the placenta* (see Chapter 8). The endometrial capillaries around the implanted embryo first become congested and dilated to form sinusoids, which are thin-walled terminal vessels that are larger than ordinary capillaries. The syncytiotrophoblast then erodes the sinusoids, and maternal blood flows into the lacunar networks. The degenerated endometrial stromal cells and glands, together with the maternal blood, provide a rich source of material for *embryonic nutrition*. Growth of the bilaminar embryonic disc is slow compared with the growth of the trophoblast.

As changes occur in the trophoblast and endometrium, the extraembryonic mesoderm increases and isolated extraembryonic coelomic spaces appear within it (see Fig. 4-2B). These spaces rapidly fuse to form a large, isolated cavity, the **extraembryonic coelom** (Fig. 4-3A). This fluid-filled cavity surrounds the amnion and the umbilical vesicle, except where they are attached to the chorion by the **connecting stalk**. As the extraembryonic coelom forms, the primary umbilical vesicle decreases in size and a smaller, **secondary umbilical vesicle** forms (see Fig. 4-3B). During formation of the secondary umbilical vesicle, a large part of the primary umbilical vesicle is pinched off. The human umbilical vesicle (yolk sac) contains no yolk. It may have a role in the selective transfer of nutritive materials to the embryonic disc. The trophoblast absorbs nutritive fluid from the lacunar networks in the syncytiotrophoblast; the fluid is then transferred to the embryo.

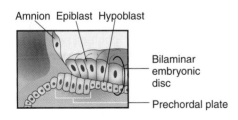

FIGURE 4-3. Sections of implanted human embryos. **A,** At 13 days, note the decrease in the relative size of the primary umbilical vesicle and the early appearance of the primary chorionic villi. **B,** At 14 days, note the newly formed secondary umbilical vesicle and the location of the prechordal plate. **C,** Detailed view of the prechordal plate area outlined in **B.**

■ DEVELOPMENT OF THE CHORIONIC SAC

The end of the second week is characterized by the appearance of **primary chorionic villi** (Figs. 4-3*A* and 4-4*A* and *C*). Proliferation of the cytotrophoblastic cells produces cellular extensions that grow into the overlying syncytiotrophoblast. The growth of these cytotrophoblastic extensions is believed to be induced by the underlying **extraembryonic somatic mesoderm**. The cellular projections form primary chorionic villi, the first stage in the development of the chorionic villi of the placenta. The extraembryonic coelom splits the extraembryonic mesoderm into two layers (see Fig. 4-3*A* and *B*):

● The *extraembryonic somatic mesoderm*, which lines the trophoblast and covers the amnion
● The *extraembryonic splanchnic mesoderm*, which surrounds the umbilical vesicle

The extraembryonic somatic mesoderm and the two layers of trophoblast form the **chorion**. The chorion forms the wall of the chorionic sac (see Fig. 4-3*A*). The embryo and its amniotic sac and umbilical vesicle are suspended in the **chorionic cavity** by the connecting stalk (see Figs. 4-3*B* and 4-4*B*). The amniotic sac and the umbilical vesicle are analogous to two balloons pressed together (at the site of the embryonic disc) and suspended by a cord (the connecting stalk) from the inside of a larger balloon (the chorionic sac). Transvaginal ultrasonography (endovaginal sonography) is used to measure the diameter of the chorionic (gestational) sac. This measurement is valuable for evaluating early embryonic development and pregnancy outcome.

The **14-day embryo** still has the form of a flat, bilaminar, embryonic disc, but endodermal cells in a localized area are now columnar and form a thickened circular area called the **prechordal plate** (see Fig. 4-3*B* and *C*). This plate indicates the future site of the mouth and is an *important organizer of the head region.*

■ IMPLANTATION SITES OF THE BLASTOCYST

Implantation of the blastocyst begins at the end of the first embryonic week and normally occurs in the endometrium of the uterus, usually superiorly in the body of the uterus and slightly more often on the posterior than on the anterior wall.

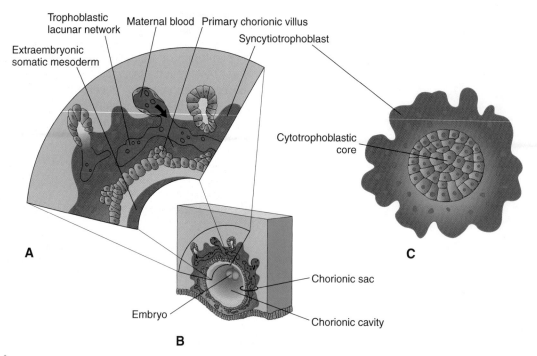

Figure 4-4. **A,** Illustration of a section (outlined in **B**) of the wall of the chorionic sac. **B,** Illustration of a 14-day conceptus showing the chorionic sac and the chorionic cavity. **C,** Transverse section through a primary chorionic villus.

EXTRAUTERINE IMPLANTATION SITES

Blastocysts may implant outside the uterus. Extrauterine implantations result in **ectopic pregnancies**; most ectopic implantations occur in the uterine tube (Figs. 2-2B and 4-5A and B). Ectopic tubal pregnancy occurs in approximately 1 in 200 pregnancies in North America. A woman with a tubal pregnancy has the usual signs and symptoms of pregnancy, but she may also experience abdominal pain and tenderness because of distention of the uterine tube, abnormal bleeding, and irritation of the pelvic peritoneum.

There are *several causes of tubal pregnancy*; however, they are often related to factors that delay or prevent transport of the cleaving zygote to the uterus (e.g., blockage of the uterine tube caused by scarring secondary to infection in the abdominopelvic cavity). Ectopic tubal pregnancies usually result in rupture of the uterine tube and hemorrhage into the peritoneal cavity during the first 8 weeks, followed by death of the embryo. Tubal rupture and hemorrhage constitute a threat to the mother's life.

INHIBITION OF IMPLANTATION

The administration of relatively *large doses of estrogen* ("morning-after pills") for several days, beginning shortly after unprotected sexual intercourse, usually does not prevent fertilization, but often prevents implantation. Normally, the endometrium progresses to the luteal (secretory) phase of the menstrual cycle as the zygote forms, undergoes cleavage, and enters the uterus. A large amount of estrogen, however, disturbs the normal balance between estrogen and progesterone that is necessary to prepare the endometrium for implantation. An **intrauterine device** inserted into the uterus through the vagina and cervix usually interferes with implantation by causing a local inflammatory reaction. Some intrauterine devices contain slow-release progesterone, which interferes with the development of the endometrium so that implantation does not usually occur.

FIGURE 4-5. **A,** Coronal section of the uterus and the uterine tube illustrating an ectopic pregnancy in the ampulla of the tube. **B,** Ectopic tubal pregnancy (6 weeks). The sonogram of the uterine tube *(left)* shows a small gestational sac *(arrow).* (**B,** Courtesy of E.A. Lyons, MD, Department of Radiology, Health Sciences Centre, University of Manitoba, Winnipeg, Manitoba, Canada.)

CLINICALLY ORIENTED QUESTIONS

1. What is meant by the term *implantation bleeding*? Is this the same as *menses* (menstrual fluid)?
2. Can a drug taken during the first 2 weeks of pregnancy cause abortion of the embryo?
3. Can an ectopic pregnancy occur in a woman who has an intrauterine device?
4. Can a blastocyst that implants in the abdomen develop into a full-term fetus?
5. Can combined intrauterine and ectopic pregnancy occur?

The answers to these questions are at the back of the book.

5

THE THIRD WEEK OF HUMAN DEVELOPMENT

Rapid development of the embryo from the embryonic disc is characterized by the following:
● Appearance of the primitive streak
● Development of the notochord
● Differentiation of the three germ layers

The third week of embryonic development occurs during the week after the first missed menstrual period, that is, 5 weeks after the onset of the last normal menstrual period. Cessation of menstruation is usually the first indication that a woman may be pregnant.

Approximately 3 weeks after conception, a normal pregnancy can be detected with ultrasonography (Fig. 5-1).

■ GASTRULATION: FORMATION OF THE GERM LAYERS

Gastrulation is the process by which the bilaminar embryonic disc (Fig. 5-2A to H) is converted into a trilaminar embryonic disc. This process is the beginning of **morphogenesis** (development of the form and structure of various organs and parts of the body). Gastrulation begins with the formation of the **primitive streak** (see Fig. 5-2B and C). Each of the three germ layers (ectoderm, endoderm, and mesoderm) of the embryonic disc gives rise to specific tissues and organs.
● The **ectoderm** gives rise to the epidermis, the nervous systems, the retina, and various other structures (see Chapter 6).
● The **endoderm** is the source of the epithelial linings of the respiratory and alimentary (digestive) tract, including the glands opening into the gastrointestinal tract and the glandular cells of associated organs, such as the liver and pancreas.
● The **mesoderm** gives rise to smooth muscular coats, connective tissues, and vessels associated with the tissues and organs. The mesoderm also forms most of the cardiovascular system and is the source of blood cells and bone marrow, the skeleton, striated muscles, and the reproductive and excretory organs.

Primitive Streak

At the beginning of the third week, a thickened, linear band of epiblast, the **primitive streak**, appears caudally in the median plane of the dorsal aspect of the embryonic disc (Figs. 5-2 and 5-3A). The primitive streak results from the proliferation and migration of cells of the epiblast to the median plane of the embryonic disc (see Fig. 5-2D). As the primitive streak elongates by the addition of cells to its caudal end, its cranial end proliferates to form a **primitive node** (see Fig. 5-2E and F). Concurrently, a narrow **primitive groove** develops in the primitive streak that ends in a small depression in the primitive node, the **primitive pit** (see Fig. 5-2F). As soon as the primitive streak appears, it is possible to identify the embryo's craniocaudal axis, its cranial and caudal ends, its dorsal and ventral surfaces, and its right and left sides. Shortly after the primitive streak appears, cells leave its deep surface and form **mesoblast**, a loose

FIGURE 5-1. Endovaginal sonogram of a conceptus approximately 3 weeks after conception, showing the amnion (A) and the umbilical vesicle (UV). In addition, the endometrium (E) surrounding the conceptus is visible. (From Filly RA: Ultrasound evaluation during the first trimester of pregnancy. In Callen PW [ed]: Ultrasonography in Obstetrics and Gynecology, 4th ed. Philadelphia, WB Saunders, 2000.)

network of embryonic connective tissue (see Figs. 5-2H and 5-3B) that forms the supporting tissues of the embryo. Under the influence of various embryonic growth factors, **mesenchymal cells** migrate from the primitive streak. These cells have the potential to proliferate and differentiate into diverse types of cells, such as fibroblasts, chondroblasts, and osteoblasts.

The *primitive streak* actively forms **mesoderm** until the early part of the fourth week; thereafter, its production slows down. The streak diminishes in relative size and becomes an insignificant structure in the sacrococcygeal region of the embryo (Fig. 5-4A to D).

SACROCOCCYGEAL TERATOMA

Remnants of the primitive streak may persist and give rise to a large tumor known as a *sacrococcygeal teratoma* (Fig. 5-5). Because it is derived from pluripotent primitive streak cells, the tumor contains tissues derived from all three germ layers in incomplete stages of differentiation. Sacrococcygeal teratomas are the most common tumors in newborn infants and have an incidence of approximately 1 in 35,000 neonates. These tumors are usually surgically excised promptly, and the prognosis is good.

Notochordal Process and Notochord

Some mesenchymal cells migrate cranially from the primitive node and pit, forming a median cellular cord, the **notochordal process** (Figs. 5-2 G, 5-4B to D, and 5-6A to C). This process soon acquires a lumen, the **notochordal canal** (see Fig. 5-6C to F). The notochordal process grows cranially between the ectoderm and the endoderm until it reaches the **prechordal plate**, a small, circular area

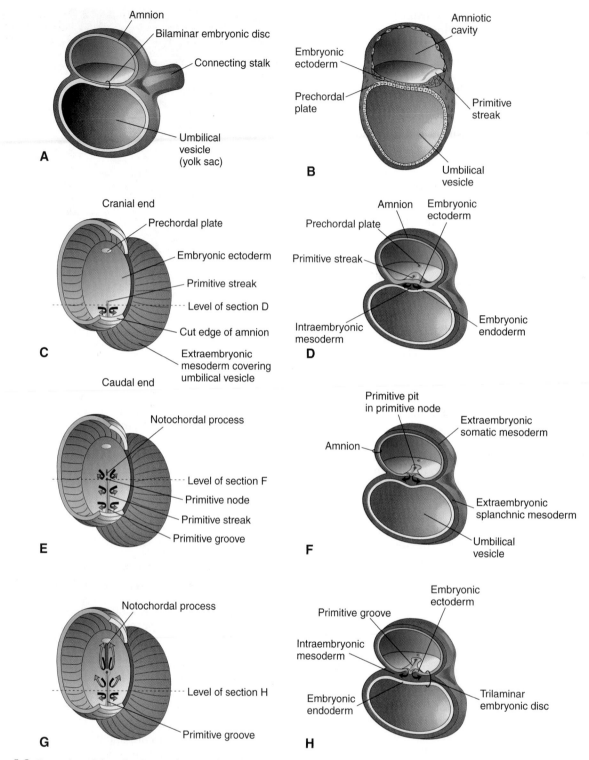

FIGURE 5-2. Formation of the trilaminar embryonic disc (days 15–16). The *arrows* indicate invagination and migration of the mesenchymal cells between the ectoderm and the endoderm. **A, C, E,** and **G,** Dorsal views of the embryonic disc early in the third week, exposed by removal of the amnion. **B, D, F,** and **H,** Transverse sections through the embryonic disc at the levels indicated. The prechordal plate, indicating the head region in **C,** is shown as a light blue oval because it is a thickening of the endoderm that cannot be seen from the dorsal surface.

of cells. The rodlike notochordal process can extend no farther because the prechordal plate is firmly attached to the overlying ectoderm. These fused layers form the **oropharyngeal membrane** (Fig. 5-7*C*) located at the future site of the oral cavity (mouth).

Some mesenchymal cells from the primitive streak and the notochordal process migrate laterally and cranially between the ectoderm and the endoderm until they reach the margins of the embryonic disc, where they are continuous with the extraembryonic mesoderm that covers the amnion and

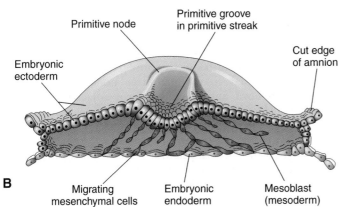

Embryonic ectoderm

Prechordal plate

Cut edge of amnion

Umbilical vesicle covered with extraembryonic mesoderm

Primitive node

Primitive pit

Level of section B

Primitive groove in primitive streak

A

Connecting stalk

Primitive node

Primitive groove in primitive streak

Cut edge of amnion

Embryonic ectoderm

B

Migrating mesenchymal cells

Embryonic endoderm

Mesoblast (mesoderm)

FIGURE 5-3. **A,** Dorsal view of a 16-day embryo. The amnion has been removed to expose the embryonic disc. **B,** Illustration of the cranial half of the embryonic disc during the third week. The disc has been cut transversely to show the migration of mesenchymal cells from the primitive streak to form the mesoblast that soon organizes to form the intraembryonic mesoderm.

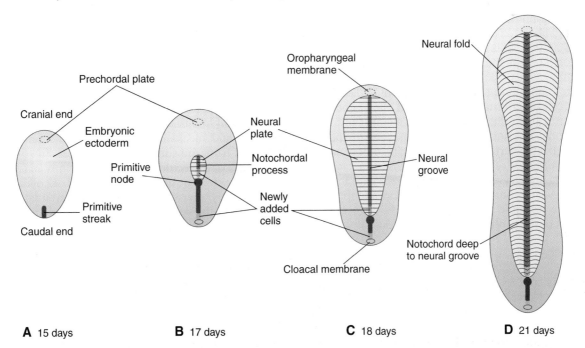

Prechordal plate

Cranial end

Embryonic ectoderm

Primitive node

Primitive streak

Caudal end

Neural plate

Notochordal process

Newly added cells

Oropharyngeal membrane

Cloacal membrane

Neural fold

Neural groove

Notochord deep to neural groove

A 15 days

B 17 days

C 18 days

D 21 days

FIGURE 5-4. Dorsal views of the embryonic disc, showing how it lengthens and changes shape during the third week. The primitive streak lengthens by the addition of cells at its caudal end; the notochordal process lengthens by the migration of cells from the primitive node. The notochordal process and the adjacent mesoderm induce the overlying embryonic ectoderm to form the neural plate, the primordium of the central nervous system. Observe that, as the notochordal process elongates, the primitive streak shortens. At the end of the third week, the notochordal process is transformed into the notochord.

Figure 5-5. A female infant with a large sacrococcygeal teratoma that developed from remnants of the primitive streak. The tumor was surgically removed. (Courtesy of A.E. Chudley, MD, Section of Genetics and Metabolism, Department of Pediatrics and Child Health, Children's Hospital, University of Manitoba, Winnipeg, Manitoba, Canada.)

the umbilical vesicle (see Fig. 5-2D and F). Some cells from the primitive streak migrate cranially on each side of the notochordal process and around the prechordal plate. They meet cranially to form the cardiogenic mesoderm in the **cardiogenic area**, where the primordium of the heart begins to develop at the end of the third week. Caudal to the primitive streak there is a circular area—the **cloacal membrane**—that indicates the future site of the anus (see Figs. 5-6E and 5-7C).

The **notochord** is a cellular rod that:

● Defines the primordial axis of the embryo and gives it some rigidity
● Serves as the basis for the development of the axial skeleton (such as the bones of the head and vertebral column)
● Indicates the future site of the vertebral bodies

The **vertebral column** forms around the notochord, which extends from the oropharyngeal membrane to the primitive node. The notochord degenerates and disappears as the bodies of the vertebrae form, but parts of it persist as the *nucleus pulposus* of each intervertebral disc. *The notochord functions as the primary inductor in the early embryo.* It induces the overlying embryonic ectoderm to thicken and form the **neural plate** (see Figs. 5-4B and C and 5-7A to D), the primordium of the central nervous system.

Allantois

The **allantois** appears on approximately day 16 as a small, sausage-shaped diverticulum (outpouching) that extends from the caudal wall of the umbilical vesicle into the connecting stalk (see Fig. 5-6B, C, and E). The allantois is a large, saclike structure in the embryos of reptiles, birds, and some mammals that has a respiratory function or acts as a reservoir for urine during embryonic life. The allantois remains very small in human embryos because the placenta and amniotic sac take over its functions. The allantois is

involved with early blood formation in the human embryo and is associated with the development of the urinary bladder. The blood vessels of the allantois become the umbilical arteries and veins.

■ NEURULATION: FORMATION OF THE NEURAL TUBE

The processes involved in the formation of the neural plate and neural folds and closure of these folds to form the neural tube constitute neurulation. These processes are completed by the end of the fourth week.

Neural Plate and Neural Tube

As the notochord develops, it induces the embryonic ectoderm over it to thicken and form an elongated plate of thickened neuroepithelial cells called the **neural plate**. The ectoderm of the neural plate (neuroectoderm) gives rise to the central nervous system. The neuroectoderm also gives rise to various other structures, such as the retina. At first, the elongated neural plate corresponds precisely in length to the underlying notochord. It appears cranial to the primitive node and dorsal to the notochord and the mesoderm adjacent to it (see Fig. 5-4B). As the notochord elongates, the neural plate broadens and eventually extends cranially as far as the **oropharyngeal membrane** (see Figs. 5-4C and 5-7C). Eventually, the neural plate extends beyond the notochord (see Figs. 5-7C and E). On approximately day 18, the neural plate invaginates along its central axis to form a median longitudinal **neural groove**, which has **neural folds** on each side (see Fig. 5-7F and G). The neural folds are particularly prominent at the cranial end of the embryo and are the first signs of brain development (Fig. 5-8C). By the end of the third week, the neural folds have begun to move together and fuse, converting the neural plate into a **neural tube** (Figs. 5-8F and 5-9).

Neural tube formation (neural induction) is a complex cellular and multifactorial process involving genes and extrinsic and mechanical factors. The neural tube soon separates from the surface ectoderm (see Fig. 5-9E). The free edges of the ectoderm fuse so that this layer becomes continuous over the neural tube and the back of the embryo. Subsequently, the surface ectoderm differentiates into the epidermis of the skin. Neurulation is completed during the fourth week (see Chapter 6).

Neural Crest Formation

As the neural folds fuse to form the neural tube, some neuroectodermal cells lying along the crest of each neural fold lose their epithelial affinities and attachments to neighboring cells (see Fig. 5-9A to C). As the neural tube separates from the surface ectoderm, **neural crest cells** migrate dorsolaterally on each side of the neural tube. They form a flattened, irregular mass, the **neural crest**, between the neural tube and the overlying surface

FIGURE 5-6. Illustrations of the development of the notochordal process. The small sketch at the upper left is for orientation. **A,** Dorsal view of the embryonic disc (at approximately 16 days), exposed by removal of the amnion. The notochordal process is shown as if it were visible through the embryonic ectoderm. **B, C,** and **E,** Median sections, at the same plane as shown in **A,** illustrating successive stages in the development of the notochordal process and canal. The stages shown in **C** and **E** occur at approximately 18 days. **D** and **F,** Transverse sections through the embryonic disc at the levels shown in **C** and **E.**

ectoderm (see Fig. 5-9*D* and *E*). The neural crest soon separates into right and left parts that migrate in a wave to the dorsolateral aspects of the neural tube (see Fig. 5-9*F*). Many neural crest cells migrate widely within the mesenchyme. Neural crest cells differentiate into various cell types (see Fig. 6-4), including the spinal ganglia (dorsal root ganglia) and the ganglia of the autonomic nervous system. The ganglia of cranial nerves V, VII, IX, and X are also partly derived from neural crest cells. Neural crest cells also form the sheaths of the peripheral nerves and the coverings of the brain and spinal cord (at least the pia mater and arachnoid mater). Neural crest cells contribute to the formation of pigment cells, the suprarenal (adrenal) medulla, and several skeletal and muscular components in the head (see Chapter 10).

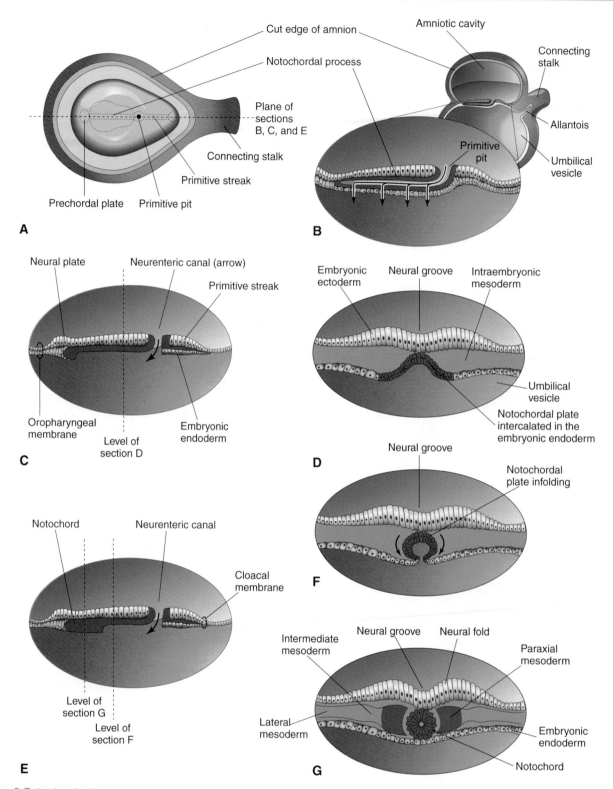

FIGURE 5-7. Further development of the notochord by transformation of the notochordal process. **A,** Dorsal view of the embryonic disc (at approximately 18 days), exposed by removing the amnion. **B,** Three-dimensional median section of the embryo. **C** and **E,** Similar sections of slightly older embryos. **D, F,** and **G,** Transverse sections of the trilaminar embryonic disc shown in **C** and **E.**

■ DEVELOPMENT OF THE SOMITES

As the notochord and the neural tube form, the intra-embryonic mesoderm on each side of them proliferates to form a thick, longitudinal column of **paraxial mesoderm** (see Figs. 5-7G and 5-8B). Each column is continuous laterally with the **intermediate mesoderm**, which gradually thins into a layer of **lateral mesoderm**. The lateral mesoderm is continuous with the extraembryonic mesoderm that covers the umbilical vesicle and amnion.

A

- Cardiogenic area
- Neural plate
- Neural groove
- Neural fold
- Level of section B
- Coelomic spaces
- Cut edge of amnion

B

- Intermediate mesoderm
- Paraxial mesoderm
- Neural groove
- Embryonic ectoderm
- Amnion
- Lateral mesoderm
- Coelomic spaces

C

- Umbilical vesicle covered with extraembryonic mesoderm
- Coelomic spaces
- Level of section D
- First somite
- Connecting stalk

D

- Neural folds
- Intraembryonic somatic mesoderm
- Somite
- Intraembryonic splanchnic mesoderm
- Intraembryonic coelom

E

- Pericardial coelom
- Pericardio-peritoneal canal
- Peritoneal coelom (cavity)
- Level of section F

F

- Somite
- Neural folds about to fuse to form neural tube
- Somatopleure
- Intraembryonic coelom
- Splanchnopleure

FIGURE 5-8. Illustrations of embryos 19 to 21 days old, illustrating the development of the somites and the intraembryonic coelom. **A, C,** and **E,** Dorsal view of the embryo, exposed by removal of the amnion. **B, D,** and **F,** Transverse sections through the embryonic disc at the levels shown. **A,** A presomite embryo of approximately 18 days. **C,** An embryo of approximately 20 days, showing the first pair of somites. A portion of the somatopleure on the right has been removed to show the isolated coelomic spaces in the lateral mesoderm. **E,** A three-somite embryo (approximately 21 days old), showing the horseshoe-shaped intraembryonic coelom, exposed on the right by removal of part of the somatopleure.

Toward the end of the third week, the paraxial mesoderm differentiates and begins to divide into paired cuboidal bodies—called **somites**—on each side of the developing neural tube (see Fig. 5-8C and E). The somites form distinct surface elevations on the embryo and appear somewhat triangular on transverse section (see Fig. 5-8D and F). Because the somites are so prominent during the fourth and fifth weeks, they are used as one of the criteria for determining an embryo's age (see Chapter 6 and Table 6-1). The somites first appear in the future occipital

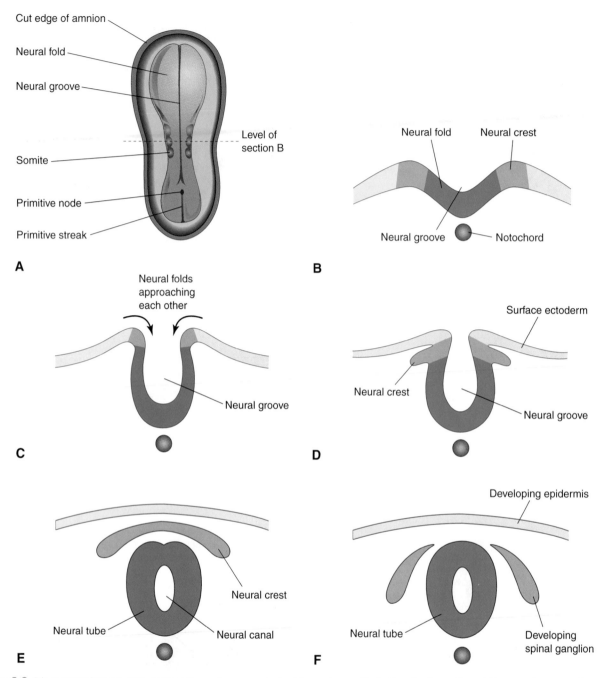

FIGURE 5-9. Diagrammatic transverse sections through progressively older embryos, illustrating the formation of the neural groove, the neural tube, and the neural crest up to the end of the fourth week.

ABNORMAL NEURULATION

Because the neural plate, the primordium of the central nervous system, appears during the third week and gives rise to the neural folds, disturbance of neurulation may result in severe abnormalities of the brain and spinal cord (see Chapter 16). Neural tube defects are among the most common congenital anomalies. Meroencephaly (anencephaly)—partial absence of the brain—is the most severe defect. Available evidence suggests that the primary disturbance affects the neuroectoderm. Failure of the neural folds to fuse and form the neural tube in the brain region results in meroencephaly and spina bifida cystica (see Chapter 16).

region of the embryo, but soon extend craniocaudally and give rise to most of the *axial skeleton* and the associated musculature, as well as to the adjacent dermis of the skin. The first pair of somites appears at the end of the third week (see Fig. 5-8C) near the cranial end of the notochord. Subsequent pairs form in a craniocaudal sequence. *Recent studies indicate that somite formation from the paraxial mesoderm is preceded by expression of the forkhead transcription factors Fox C1 and C2. The craniocaudal segmental pattern of the somites is regulated by the Delta-Notch (Delta 1 and Notch 1) signaling system. A hypothetical molecular oscillator, or clock, has been proposed as the mechanism responsible for the orderly sequencing of the somites.*

■ DEVELOPMENT OF THE INTRAEMBRYONIC COELOM

The intraembryonic coelom (body cavity) first appears as small, isolated, coelomic spaces in the lateral mesoderm and cardiogenic (heart-forming) mesoderm (see Fig. 5-8A to D). These spaces coalesce to form a single, horseshoe-shaped cavity—the **intraembryonic coelom** (see Fig. 5-8E and F)—that divides the lateral mesoderm into two layers:

● A somatic, or *parietal,* layer that is continuous with the extraembryonic mesoderm that covers the amnion
● A splanchnic, or *visceral,* layer that is continuous with the extraembryonic mesoderm that covers the umbilical vesicle

FIGURE 5-10. Successive stages in the development of blood and blood vessels. **A,** The umbilical vesicle (yolk sac) and a portion of the chorionic sac (at approximately 18 days). **B,** Dorsal view of the embryo exposed by removing the amnion. **C** to **F,** Sections of blood islands, showing progressive stages in the development of blood and blood vessels.

The *somatic mesoderm* and the overlying embryonic ectoderm form the body wall, or **somatopleure** (see Fig. 5-8*F*), whereas the *splanchnic mesoderm* and the underlying embryonic endoderm form the wall of the gut, or **splanchnopleure**. During the second month, the intraembryonic coelom is divided into three body cavities: the *pericardial cavity*, the *pleural cavities*, and the *peritoneal cavity*.

■ EARLY DEVELOPMENT OF THE CARDIOVASCULAR SYSTEM

At the end of the second week, embryonic nutrition is obtained from the maternal blood by diffusion through the chorion, extraembryonic coelom, and umbilical vesicle. The early formation of the cardiovascular system correlates with the absence of yolk in the oocyte and umbilical vesicle and the urgent need for transportation of oxygen and nourishment to the embryo from the maternal circulation through the chorion. At the beginning of the third week, blood vessel formation—vasculogenesis—begins in the extraembryonic mesoderm of the umbilical vesicle, connecting stalk, and chorion (Fig. 5-10*A* and *B*). Embryonic blood vessels begin to develop approximately 2 days later. At the end of the third week, a primordial *uteroplacental circulation* had developed (Fig. 5-11).

Vasculogenesis and Angiogenesis

Blood vessel formation in the embryo and the extra-embryonic membranes during the third week may be summarized as follows (see Fig. 5-10*C* to *F*):

Vasculogenesis:
● Mesenchymal cells differentiate into endothelial cell precursors—**angioblasts** (vessel-forming cells)—that aggregate to form isolated angiogenic cell clusters—**blood islands** (see Fig. 5-10*C*).
● Small cavities appear within the blood islands by the confluence of intercellular clefts (see Fig. 5-10*D*).
● Angioblasts flatten to form endothelial cells that arrange themselves around the cavities in the blood islands to form the primordial endothelium (see Fig. 5-10*E*).
● These endothelium-lined cavities soon fuse to form networks of endothelial channels (see Fig. 5-10*F*).

Angiogenesis:
● Vessels sprout into adjacent nonvascularized areas by endothelial budding and fuse with other vessels.

FIGURE 5-11. **A,** Sonogram of a 5-week embryo (7.2 mm) and its attached umbilical vesicle within its chorionic (gestational) sac. The pulsating heart of the embryo was visualized using Doppler ultrasonography. **B,** A sketch of the sonogram, provided for orientation and identification of the structures. CRL, crown-rump length. (From Moore KL, Persaud TVN, Shiota K: Color Atlas of Clinical Embryology, 2nd ed. Philadelphia, WB Saunders, 2000. Courtesy of E.A. Lyons, MD, Professor of Radiology and Obstetrics and Gynecology, Health Sciences Centre, University of Manitoba, Winnipeg, Manitoba, Canada.)

Decidua basalis
Long axis of embryo
7.3 mm crown-rump length
Heart seen with Doppler ultrasound
Umbilical vesicle
Chorionic (gestational) sac
Chorionic cavity

B

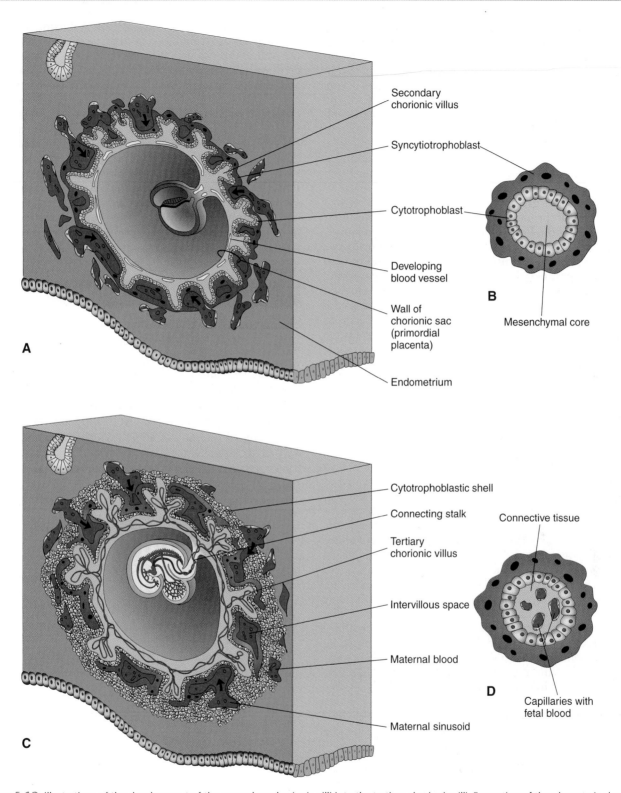

FIGURE 5-12. Illustrations of the development of the secondary chorionic villi into the tertiary chorionic villi. Formation of the placenta is also shown. **A,** Sagittal section of an embryo (at approximately 16 days). **B,** Section of a secondary chorionic villus. **C,** Section of an implanted embryo (at approximately 21 days). **D,** Section of a tertiary chorionic villus. By the end of the third week, a primordial uteroplacental circulation has developed.

Blood cells develop from specialized endothelial cells of vessels (*hemangioblasts*) on the umbilical vesicle and allantois at the end of the third week (see Fig. 5-10*E* and *F*). Blood formation (**hematogenesis**) does not begin within the embryo until the fifth week. This process occurs first in various parts of the embryonic mesenchyme, chiefly the liver, and later, in the spleen, bone marrow, and lymph nodes. Fetal and adult erythrocytes are derived from different hematopoietic progenitor cells (**hemangioblasts**). The mesenchymal cells that surround the primordial endothelial blood vessels also differentiate into the muscular and connective tissue elements of the vessels.

The **heart** and **great vessels** form from mesenchymal cells in the heart primordium—**cardiogenic area** (see Figs. 5-8*A* and 5-10*B*). Paired, endothelium-lined channels—endocardial **heart tubes**—develop during the third week and fuse to form a **primordial heart tube**. The tubular heart joins with blood vessels in the embryo, connecting stalk, chorion, and umbilical vesicle to form a **primordial cardiovascular system** (Fig. 15-12*C*). By the end of the third week, the blood is circulating, and the heart begins to beat on day 21 or 22. Thus, the cardiovascular system is the first organ system to reach a functional state. The embryonic heartbeat can be detected by Doppler ultrasonography during the fifth week, approximately 7 weeks after the last normal menstrual period (see Fig. 5-11).

■ DEVELOPMENT OF THE CHORIONIC VILLI

Shortly after the **primary chorionic villi** are formed at the end of the second week, they begin to branch. Early in the third week, mesenchyme grows into the primary villi, forming a core of loose mesenchymal (connective) tissue (see Fig. 5-12*A* and *B*). The villi at this stage—**secondary chorionic villi**—cover the entire surface of the chorionic sac (see Fig. 5-12*A*). Some mesenchymal cells in the villi soon differentiate into capillaries and blood cells (see Fig. 5-12*D*). When capillaries are visible in the villi, they are called **tertiary chorionic villi** (see Fig. 5-12*C*). The capillaries in the chorionic villi fuse to form **arteriocapillary networks** that soon become connected with the embryonic heart through vessels that differentiate in the mesenchyme of the chorion and connecting stalk (see Fig. 5-12*C*). By the end of the third week, embryonic blood begins to flow slowly through the capillaries in the chorionic villi. Oxygen and nutrients in the maternal blood in the intervillous space diffuse through the walls of the villi and enter the embryo's blood (see Fig. 5-12*C*). Carbon dioxide and waste products diffuse from blood in the fetal capillaries through the wall of the villi into the maternal blood. Concurrently, cytotrophoblastic cells of the chorionic villi proliferate and extend through the syncytiotrophoblast to form a **cytotrophoblastic shell**, which gradually surrounds the chorionic sac and attaches it to the endometrium (see Fig. 5-12*C*). Villi that attach to the maternal tissues through the cytotrophoblastic shell are called **stem chorionic villi** (anchoring villi). The villi that grow from the sides of the stem villi are called **branch chorionic villi** (terminal villi). It is through the walls of the branch villi that the main exchange of material between the blood of the mother and the embryo takes place. The branch villi are bathed in continually changing maternal blood in the **intervillous space**.

ABNORMAL GROWTH OF THE TROPHOBLAST

Sometimes the embryo dies and the chorionic villi do not complete their development; that is, they do not become vascularized to form tertiary villi. These degenerating villi may form cystic swellings, called **hydatidiform moles,** which resemble a bunch of grapes. These moles exhibit variable degrees of trophoblastic proliferation and produce excessive amounts of human chorionic gonadotropin. In 3% to 5% of such cases, these moles develop into malignant trophoblastic lesions called **choriocarcinomas.** These tumors invariably metastasize (spread) by way of the blood to various sites, such as the lungs, vagina, liver, bone, intestine, and brain.

CLINICALLY ORIENTED QUESTIONS

1. Can drugs and other agents cause congenital anomalies of the embryo if they are present in the mother's blood during the third week? If so, what organs would be most susceptible?
2. Are there increased risks for the embryo associated with pregnancies in women older than 40 years of age? If so, what are they?

The answers to these questions are at the back of the book.

HUMAN DEVELOPMENT DURING WEEKS FOUR TO EIGHT

All major external and internal structures are established during the fourth to eighth weeks. By the end of this **organogenetic period**, all of the main organ systems have begun to develop. Exposure of embryos to teratogens during this period may cause major congenital anomalies. **Teratogens** are agents, such as drugs and viruses, that produce or increase the incidence of congenital anomalies (see Chapter 19). As the tissues and organs form, the shape of the embryo changes so that, by the eighth week, the embryo has a distinctly human appearance.

■ FOLDING OF THE EMBRYO

A significant event in the establishment of body form is folding of the flat trilaminar embryonic disc into a somewhat cylindric embryo (Fig. 6-1). Folding results from rapid growth of the embryo, particularly the brain and the spinal cord. Folding at the cranial and caudal ends and at the sides of the embryo occurs simultaneously. Concurrently, a relative constriction occurs at the junction of the embryo and the umbilical vesicle. Folding of the ends of the embryo ventrally produces head and tail folds that cause the cranial and caudal regions to move ventrally as the embryo elongates cranially and caudally (see Fig. 6-1A_2 to D_2).

Head and Tail Folds

By the beginning of the fourth week, the neural folds in the cranial region form the **primordium of the brain.** Later, the developing forebrain grows cranially beyond the oropharyngeal membrane and overhangs the developing heart. Concomitantly, the primordial heart and the oropharyngeal membrane move onto the ventral surface of the embryo (Fig. 6-2). During lateral (longitudinal) folding, part of the endoderm of the umbilical vesicle is incorporated into the embryo as the **foregut** (see Fig. 6-2C). The foregut lies between the brain and the heart, and the oropharyngeal membrane separates the foregut from the primordial mouth, or stomodeum.

Folding of the caudal end of the embryo results primarily from growth of the distal part of the neural tube, the primordium of the spinal cord. As the embryo grows, the tail region projects over the **cloacal membrane** (future site of the anus) (Fig. 6-3B). During folding, part of the endodermal germ layer is incorporated into the embryo as the **hindgut** (see Fig. 6-3C). The terminal part of the hindgut soon dilates to form the **cloaca** (see Fig. 6-3B and C). The connecting stalk (primordium of the umbilical cord) is now attached to the ventral surface of the embryo, and the allantois—an endodermal diverticulum of the umbilical vesicle—is partially incorporated into the embryo (see Figs. 6-1D_2 and 6-3C).

Lateral Folds

Folding of the sides of the embryo results from rapid growth of the spinal cord bond somites, which produces right and left **lateral folds** (see Fig. 6-1A_3 to D_3). The lateral body wall folds toward the median plane, rolling the edges of the embryonic disc ventrally and forming a roughly cylindric embryo. As the abdominal walls form, part of the endoderm germ layer is incorporated into the embryo as the midgut. Initially, there is a wide connection between the **midgut** and the umbilical vesicle (see Fig. 6-1A_2). After lateral folding, the connection is reduced to an omphaloenteric duct, or yolk stalk (see Fig. 6-1C_2). The region of attachment of the amnion to the ventral surface of the embryo is also reduced to a relatively narrow umbilical region (see Fig. 6-1D_2 and D_3). As the **umbilical cord** forms from the connecting stalk, ventral fusion of the lateral folds reduces the region of communication between the intraembryonic and extraembryonic coelomic cavities (see Fig. 6-1C_2). As the amniotic cavity expands and obliterates most of the extraembryonic coelom, the amnion forms the epithelial covering of the umbilical cord (see Fig. 6-1D_2).

■ GERM LAYER DERIVATIVES

The three germ layers (ectoderm, mesoderm, and endoderm) formed during gastrulation give rise to the primordia of all tissues and organs. The specificity of the germ layers, however, is not rigidly fixed. The cells of each germ layer divide, migrate, aggregate, and differentiate in rather precise patterns as they form the various organ systems (organogenesis). The main germ layer derivatives are shown in Figure 6-4.

■ CONTROL OF EMBRYONIC DEVELOPMENT*

Development results from genetic plans in the chromosomes. Knowledge of the genes or hereditary units that control human development is increasing. Most information about developmental processes has come from studies of other organisms, especially fruit flies (*Drosophila*) and mice, because of ethical issues associated with the use of human embryos for laboratory studies. Most developmental processes depend on a precisely coordinated interaction of genetic and environmental factors. Several control mechanisms guide differentiation and ensure synchronized development, such as tissue interactions, regulated migration of cells and cell colonies, controlled proliferation, and programmed cell death. Each system of the body has its own developmental pattern, but most processes of morphogenesis are similar and are relatively simple. Underlying all of these changes are basic regulating mechanisms.

Embryonic development is essentially a process of growth and increasing complexity of structure and function. Growth is achieved by mitosis (the somatic reproduction of cells), together with the production of extracellular matrices, whereas complexity is achieved through morphogenesis and differentiation. The cells that make up the tissues of very early embryos are pluripotential;

*The authors are grateful to Dr. Michael Wiley, Professor of Anatomy and Director of the Division of Anatomy, Department of Surgery, Faculty of Medicine, University of Toronto, for his assistance in preparing this section.

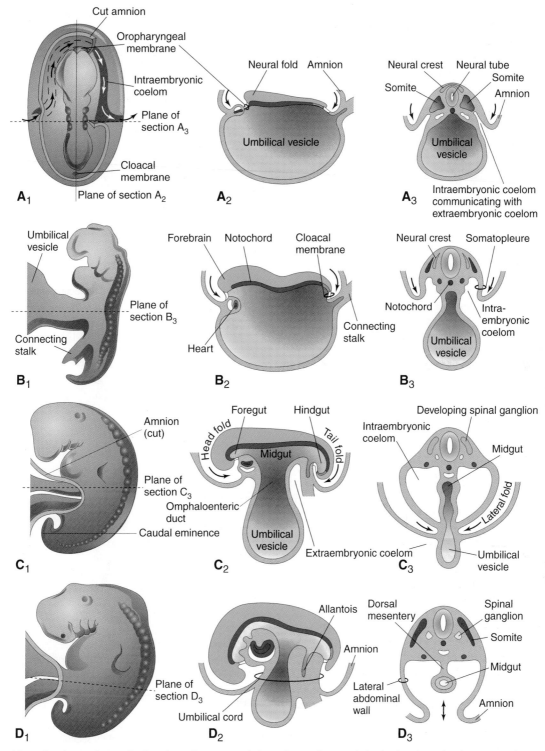

FIGURE 6-1. Folding of embryos during the fourth week. **A₁,** Dorsal view of an embryo early in the fourth week. Three pairs of somites are visible. The continuity of the intraembryonic coelom and the extraembryonic coelom is shown on the right side by removal of a part of the embryonic ectoderm and mesoderm. **B₁, C₁,** and **D₁,** Lateral views of embryos at 22, 26, and 28 days, respectively. **A₂, B₂, C₂,** and **D₂,** Sagittal sections at the plane shown in **A₁. A₃, B₃, C₃,** and **D₃,** Transverse sections at the levels indicated in **A₁** to **D₁.**

that is, depending on the circumstances, they are able to follow more than one pathway of development. This broad developmental potential becomes progressively restricted as tissues acquire the specialized features necessary for increased sophistication of structure and function. Such restriction presumes that choices must be made to achieve

tissue diversification. Most evidence indicates that these choices are determined not as a consequence of cell lineage, but rather in response to cues from the immediate surroundings, including the adjacent tissues. As a result, the architectural precision and coordination that are often required for the normal function of an organ appear to be

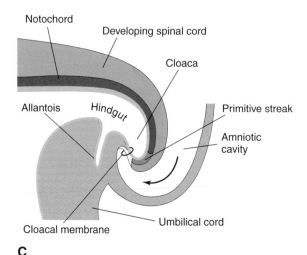

FIGURE 6-2. Folding of the cranial end of the embryo. **A,** Dorsal view of an embryo at 21 days. **B,** Sagittal section of the cranial part of the embryo at the plane shown in **A,** showing the ventral movement of the heart. **C,** Sagittal section of an embryo at 26 days. Note that the septum transversum, heart, pericardial coelom, and oropharyngeal membrane have moved onto the ventral surface of the embryo. Observe also that part of the umbilical vesicle is incorporated into the embryo as the foregut.

FIGURE 6-3. Folding of the caudal end of the embryo. **A,** Lateral view of a 4-week embryo. **B,** Sagittal section of the caudal part of the embryo at the beginning of the fourth week. **C,** Similar section at the end of the fourth week. Note that part of the umbilical vesicle is incorporated into the embryo as the hindgut and that the terminal part of the hindgut has dilated to form the cloaca. Observe also the change in position of the primitive streak, allantois, cloacal membrane, and connecting stalk.

achieved by the interaction of its constituent parts during development.

The interaction of tissues during development is a recurring theme in embryology. The interactions that lead to a change in the course of development of at least one of the interactants are called **inductions**. Numerous examples of such inductive interactions can be found in the literature; for example, during the development of the eye, the optic vesicle induces the development of the lens from the surface ectoderm of the head. When the optic

Muscles of head, striated skeletal muscle (trunk, limbs), skeleton except cranium, dermis of skin, and connective tissue

Urogenital system, including gonads, ducts, and accessory glands

Connective tissue and muscle of viscera

Serous membranes of pleura, pericardium, and peritoneum

Primordial heart

Blood and lymphatic cells

Spleen

Suprarenal (adrenal) cortex

Cranium

Connective tissue of head

Dentin

PARAXIAL MESODERM

INTERMEDIATE MESODERM

LATERAL MESODERM

HEAD

Epithelial parts of
Trachea
Bronchi
Lungs

SURFACE ECTODERM

Epidermis, hair, nails, and cutaneous and mammary glands

Anterior part of pituitary gland

Enamel of teeth

Internal ear

Lens of eye

Epithelium of gastrointestinal tract, liver, pancreas, urinary bladder, and urachus

ENDODERM

ECTODERM

NEUROECTODERM

MESODERM

Neural crest

Neural tube

Trilaminar embryonic disc

Epiblast

Embryoblast

Cranial and sensory ganglia and nerves

Central nervous system

Medulla of suprarenal gland

Retina

Pineal body

Epithelial parts of
Pharynx
Thyroid gland
Tympanic cavity
Pharyngotympanic tube
Tonsils
Parathyroid glands

Pigment cells

Posterior part of pituitary gland

Pharyngeal arch cartilages

Head mesenchyme and connective tissue

Bulbar and conal ridges in heart

FIGURE 6-4. Illustration of the derivatives of the three germ layers: ectoderm, endoderm, and mesoderm. Cells from these layers contribute to the formation of different tissues and organs; for example, the endoderm forms the epithelial lining of the gastrointestinal tract and the mesoderm gives rise to connective tissues and muscles.

vesicle is absent, the eye does not develop. Moreover, if the optic vesicle is removed and placed in association with surface ectoderm that is not usually involved in eye development, lens formation can be induced. Clearly then, the development of a lens depends on the ectoderm acquiring an association with a second tissue. In the presence of the neuroectoderm of the optic vesicle, the surface ectoderm of the head follows a pathway of development that it would not otherwise have taken. Similarly, many of the morphogenetic

tissue movements that play such important roles in shaping the embryo also provide for the changing tissue associations that are fundamental to inductive tissue interactions.

The fact that one tissue can influence the developmental pathway adopted by another tissue presumes that a signal passes between the two interactants. Analysis of the molecular defects in mutant strains that show abnormal tissue interactions during embryonic development and studies of the development of embryos with targeted gene mutations have begun to reveal the molecular mechanisms of induction. The mechanism of signal transfer appears to vary with the specific tissues involved. In some cases, the signal appears to take the form of a diffusible molecule (e.g., sonic hedgehog) that passes from the inductor to the reacting tissue. In other instances, the message appears to be mediated through a nondiffusible extracellular matrix that is secreted by the inductor and that comes into contact with the reacting tissue. In still other cases, the signal appears to require physical contact between the inducing tissue and the responding tissue. Regardless of the mechanism of intercellular transfer involved, the signal is translated into an intracellular message that influences the genetic activity of the responding cells.

To be competent to respond to an inducing stimulus, the cells of the reacting system must express the appropriate receptor for the specific inducing signal molecule, the components of the particular intracellular signal transduction pathway, and the transcription factors that mediate the particular response. Experimental evidence suggests that the acquisition of competence by the responding tissue is often dependent on its previous interactions with other tissues. For example, the lens-forming response of the head ectoderm to the stimulus provided by the optic vesicle appears to be dependent on a previous association of the head ectoderm with the anterior neural plate.

■ HIGHLIGHTS OF DEVELOPMENT DURING WEEKS FOUR TO EIGHT

The criteria for estimating developmental stages in human embryos are listed in Table 6-1.

Fourth Week

At the beginning of the fourth week, the embryo is almost straight and has 4 to 12 pairs of somites that produce conspicuous surface elevations (Fig. 6-5A). The neural tube is formed opposite the somites, but it is widely open at the rostral and caudal neuropores (Figs. 6-5B and 6-6A to D). By 24 days, the first pair of *pharyngeal arches* have appeared

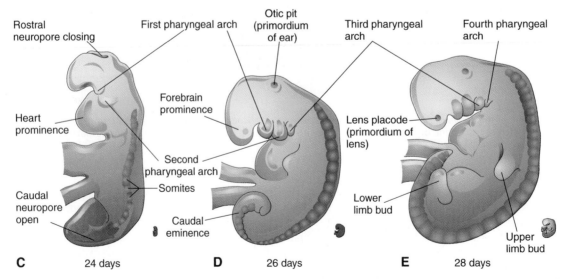

FIGURE 6-5. **A** and **B,** Dorsal views of embryos early in the fourth week, showing 8 and 12 somites, respectively. **C, D,** and **E,** Lateral views of older embryos, showing 16, 27, and 33 somites, respectively. The rostral neuropore is normally closed by 25 to 26 days, and the caudal neuropore is usually closed by the end of the fourth week.

TABLE 6-1. Criteria for Estimating Developmental Stages in Human Embryos

AGE (DAYS)	FIGURE REFERENCE	CARNEGIE STAGE	NO. OF SOMITES	LENGTH (MM)*	MAIN EXTERNAL CHARACTERISTICS[†]
20–21	6–1A₁ 6–2A	9	1–3	1.5–3.0	Flat embryonic disc. Deep neural groove and prominent neural folds. One to three pairs of somites are present. Head fold is evident.
22–23	6–5A 6–6A, C	10	4–12	2.0–3.5	Embryo is straight or slightly curved. Neural tube is forming or has formed opposite somites, but is widely open at the rostral and caudal neuropores. First and second pairs of pharyngeal arches are visible.
24–25	6–5C 6–7A	11	13–20	2.5–4.5	Embryo is curved owing to head and tail folds. Rostral neuropore is closing. Otic placodes are present. Optic vesicles have formed.
26–27	6–5D 6–8A	12	21–29	3.0–5.0	Upper limb buds appear. Rostral neuropore is closed. Caudal neuropore is closing. Three pairs of pharyngeal arches are visible. Heart prominence is distinct. Otic pits are present.
28–30	6–5E 6–9A	13	30–35	4.0–6.0	Embryo has C-shaped curve. Caudal neuropore is closed. Upper limb buds are flipper-like. Four pairs of pharyngeal arches are visible. Lower limb buds appear. Otic vesicles are present. Lens placodes are distinct. Tail-like caudal eminence is present.
31–32	6–10A	14	‡	5.0–7.0	Upper limbs are paddle-shaped. Lens pits and nasal pits are visible. Optic cups are present.
33–36		15		7.0–9.0	Handplates have formed; digital rays are present. Lens vesicles are present. Nasal pits are prominent. Lower limbs are paddle-shaped. Cervical sinuses are visible.
37–40		16		8.0–11.0	Footplates have formed. Pigment is visible in the retina. Auricular hillocks are developing.
41–43	6–11A	17		11.0–14.0	Digital rays are clearly visible in handplates. Auricular hillocks outline the future auricle of the external ear. Trunk is beginning to straighten. Cerebral vesicles are prominent.
44–46		18		13.0–17.0	Digital rays are clearly evident in footplates. Elbow region is visible. Eyelids are forming. Notches are between the digital rays in the hands. Nipples are visible.
47–48		19		16.0–18.0	Limbs extend ventrally. Trunk is elongating and straightening. Midgut herniation is prominent.
49–51		20		18.0–22.0	Upper limbs are longer and are bent at the elbows. Fingers are distinct but webbed. Notches are between the digital rays in the feet. Scalp vascular plexus appears.
52–53		21		22.0–24.0	Hands and feet approach each other. Fingers are free and longer. Toes are distinct but webbed. Stubby caudal eminence (tail) is present.
54–55		22		23.0–28.0	Toes are free and longer. Eyelids and auricles of the external ears are more developed.
56	6–12A	23		27.0–31.0	Head is more rounded and shows human characteristics. External genitalia still have sexless appearance. Distinct bulge is still present in the umbilical cord, caused by herniation of the intestines. Caudal eminence ("tail") has disappeared.

*The embryonic lengths indicate the usual range. In stages 9 and 10, the measurement is greatest length; in subsequent stages, crown–rump measurements are given.
[†]Based on O'Rahilly R, Müller F: Developmental Stages in Human Embryos. Washington, Carnegie Institute of Washington, 1987; and Gasser RF: Digitally Reproduced Embryonic Morphology DVDs. Computer Imaging Laboratory, Cell Biology and Anatomy, New Orleans, LA, LSU Health Sciences Center.
‡At this stage and subsequent stages, the number of somites is difficult to determine and so is not a useful criterion.

FIGURE 6-6. A, Dorsal view of a five-somite embryo at Carnegie stage 10, approximately 22 days, showing the neural folds and the neural groove. The neural folds in the cranial region have thickened to form the primordium of the brain. **B,** Illustration of the structures shown in **A.** Most of the amniotic and chorionic sacs have been cut away to expose the embryo. **C,** Dorsal view of a 10-somite embryo at Carnegie stage 10, approximately 23 days. The neural folds have fused opposite the somites to form the neural tube (primordium of the spinal cord in this region). The neural tube is in open communication with the amniotic cavity at the cranial and caudal ends through the rostral and caudal neuropores, respectively. **D,** Diagram of the structures shown in **C.**

(Fig. 6-7*A* and *B*). The embryo is now slightly curved because of the head and tail folds. The developing heart produces a large ventral prominence and pumps blood (see Fig. 6-5*C*). Three pairs of **pharyngeal arches** are visible by 26 days' gestation (Fig. 6-8*A* and *B*; see also Fig. 6-5*D*), and the rostral neuropore is closed. The **forebrain** produces a prominent elevation of the head, and folding of the embryo imparts a characteristic C-shaped curvature to the embryo. A long, curved **caudal eminence** (tail-like structure) is present. **Upper limb buds** are recognizable by day 26 or 27 as

Rostral
neuropore
closing

Forebrain

1st pharyngeal
arch

Amnion

Heart
prominence

Somites

Neural tube in
region of developing
spinal cord

Caudal neuropore

Connecting
stalk

A

B

Actual size 3.0 mm

FIGURE 6-7. **A,** Dorsal view of a 13-somite embryo at Carnegie stage 11, approximately 24 days. The rostral neuropore is closing, but the caudal neuropore is wide open. **B,** Illustration of the structures shown in **A**. The embryo is curved because of folding at the cranial and caudal ends.

small swellings on the ventrolateral body walls (Fig. *6-5D* and *E*; Fig. *6-9A* and *B*). The **otic pits**, the primordia of the internal ears, are also visible. Ectodermal thickenings, called **lens placodes**, indicating the future lenses of the eyes, are visible on the sides of the head. The fourth pair of pharyngeal arches and the **lower limb buds** are visible by the end of the fourth week (see Fig. *6-5E*). Rudiments of many organ systems, especially the *cardiovascular system*, are established.

Fifth Week

Changes in body form are minor during the fifth week compared with those that occurred during the fourth week. Growth of the head exceeds that of other regions (Fig. *6-10A* and *B*). Enlargement of the head is caused mainly by the rapid development of the brain and the facial prominences. The face soon contacts the heart prominence. The *mesonephric ridges* indicate the site of the mesonephric kidneys, which are interim excretory organs in humans (see Fig. *6-10A* and *B*).

Sixth Week

By the sixth week, embryos show reflex responses to touch. The primordia of the digits—the **digital rays**—begin to develop, indicating the formation of digits (fingers) (Fig. *6-11A* and *B*). It has been reported that embryos in the sixth week show spontaneous movements, such as twitching of the trunk and limbs. Development of the lower limbs occurs 4 to 5 days later than that of the upper limbs. Several small swellings—**auricular hillocks**—develop and contribute to the formation of the *auricle*, the shell-shaped part of the external ear. Largely because retinal pigment has formed, the eyes are now obvious. The head is much larger relative to the trunk and is bent over the large **heart prominence**. This head position results from bending in the cervical (neck) region. By this time, the trunk and neck have begun to straighten. During the sixth week, the *intestines enter the extraembryonic coelom in the proximal part of the umbilical cord*. This **umbilical herniation** is a normal event in the embryo, occurring because the abdominal cavity is too small at this stage to accommodate the rapidly growing intestines.

FIGURE 6-8. **A,** Lateral view of a 27-somite embryo at Carnegie stage 12, approximately 26 days. The embryo is very curved, especially its long, tail-like caudal eminence. The lens placode is the primordium of the lens of the eye. The otic pit indicates early development of the internal ear. **B,** Illustration of the structures shown in **A.** The rostral neuropore is closed, and three pairs of pharyngeal arches are present. (**A,** From Nishimura H, Semba H, Tanimura T, Tanaka O: Prenatal Development of the Human with Special Reference to Craniofacial Structures: An Atlas. Washington, DC, National Institutes of Health, 1977.)

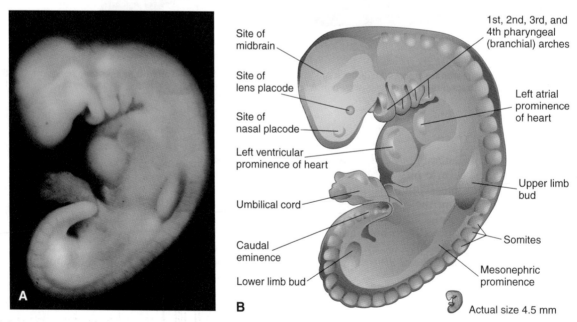

FIGURE 6-9. **A,** Lateral view of an embryo at Carnegie stage 13, approximately 28 days. The primordial heart is large and is divided into a primordial atrium and a ventricle. The rostral and caudal neuropores are closed. **B,** Illustration of the structures shown in **A.** The embryo has a characteristic C-shaped curvature, four pharyngeal arches, and upper and lower limb buds. (**A,** From Nishimura H, Semba H, Tanimura T, Tanaka O: Prenatal Development of the Human with Special Reference to Craniofacial Structures: An Atlas. Washington, DC, National Institutes of Health, 1977.)

Seventh Week

The limbs undergo considerable change during the seventh week. Notches appear between the digital rays in the **handplates,** partially separating the future digits. Communication between the primordial gut and the umbilical vesicle is now reduced to a relatively slender duct, the *omphaloenteric duct.*

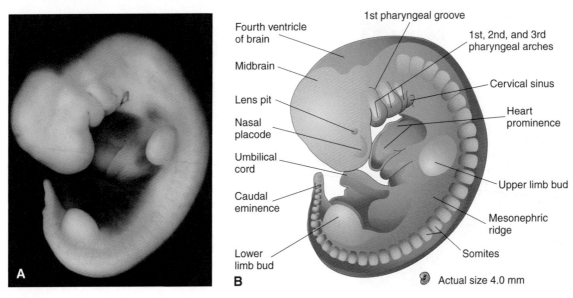

FIGURE 6-10. **A,** Lateral view of an embryo at Carnegie stage 14, approximately 32 days. The second pharyngeal arch has overgrown the third arch, forming a depression known as the *cervical sinus*. The mesonephric ridge indicates the site of the mesonephric kidney, an interim functional kidney. **B,** Illustration of the structures shown in **A**. The upper limb buds are paddle-shaped, whereas the lower limb buds are flipper-like. (**A,** From Nishimura H, Semba H, Tanimura T, Tanaka O: Prenatal Development of the Human with Special Reference to Craniofacial Structures: An Atlas. Washington, DC, National Institutes of Health, 1977.)

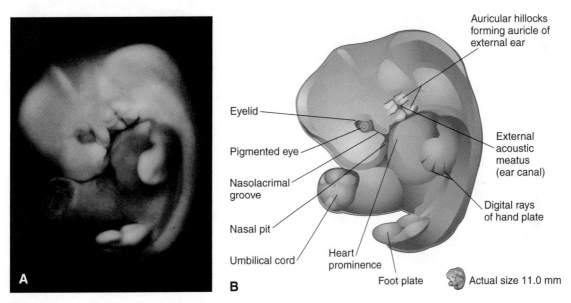

FIGURE 6-11. **A,** Lateral view of an embryo at Carnegie stage 17, approximately 42 days. Digital rays are visible in the handplate, indicating the future site of the digits (fingers). **B,** Illustration of the structures shown in **A**. The eye, auricular hillocks, and external acoustic meatus are now clearly discernible.

Eighth Week

At the beginning of this final week of the embryonic period, the digits of the hand are separated, but noticeably webbed. Notches are now clearly visible between the digital rays of the feet. The **scalp vascular plexus** has appeared and forms a characteristic band around the head. By the end of the eighth week, all regions of the limbs are apparent, and the digits have lengthened and are completely separated (Fig. 6-12*A* and *B*). *Purposeful limb movements first occur during this week*. Ossification begins in the femur. All evidence of the tail-like caudal eminence has disappeared by the end of

the eighth week. The hands and feet each approach each other ventrally. At the end of the eighth week, the embryo has distinct human characteristics; however, the head is still disproportionately large, constituting almost one half of the embryo. The neck region is established, and the eyelids are more obvious. The eyelids are closing, and by the end of the eighth week, they begin to unite by epithelial fusion. The intestines are still in the proximal portion of the umbilical cord. The auricles of the external ears begin to assume their final shape, but are still low-set on the head. Although sex differences exist in the appearance of the external genitalia, they are not distinctive enough to permit accurate sex

Scalp vascular plexus

Eyelid

Eye

Nose

Mouth

Wrist

Umbilical cord

Toes separated

Sole of foot

Knee

Auricle of external ear

Shoulder

Lower jaw

Arm

Elbow

Actual size 30.0 mm

FIGURE 6-12. **A,** Lateral view of an embryo at Carnegie stage 23, approximately 56 days. The embryo now has a distinctly human appearance. **B,** Illustration of the structures shown in **A**. The scalp vascular plexus is reduced, and the caudal eminence has disappeared. (**A,** From Nishimura H, Semba H, Tanimura T, Tanaka O: Prenatal Development of the Human with Special Reference to Craniofacial Structures: An Atlas. Washington, DC, National Institutes of Health, 1977.)

Chorionic cavity

Embryo

Umbilical vesicle

CC

A

FIGURE 6-13. Ultrasonographic images of embryos. **A,** Crown-rump length (CRL), 4.8 mm. The 4.5-week embryo is indicated by the measurement cursors (+). Ventral to the embryo is the umbilical vesicle. The chorionic cavity appears black. **B,** Coronal scan of a 6.5-week embryo (CRL, 2.09 cm). The upper limbs are visible. The embryo is surrounded by a thin amnion. A, site of amnion; CC, chorionic cavity. (Courtesy of E.A. Lyons, MD, Professor of Radiology and Obstetrics and Gynecology, Health Sciences Centre, University of Manitoba, Winnipeg, Manitoba, Canada.)

identification. The external genitalia are not recognizable as male or female until the 12th week.

■ ESTIMATION OF EMBRYONIC AGE

Estimates of the age of recovered embryos (e.g., after spontaneous abortion) are determined from their external characteristics and measurements of their length (see Table 6-1). Size alone may be an unreliable criterion because some embryos undergo a progressively slower rate of growth before death. The appearance of the developing limbs is a very helpful criterion for estimating embryonic age. Because embryos are straight in the third and early fourth weeks (Fig. 6-13*A*), their measurements indicate the greatest length. The sitting height, or *crown-rump length*, is

FIGURE 6-14. Methods used to measure the length of embryos. **A,** Greatest length (GL). **B** and **C,** Crown-rump length (CRL). **D,** Crown-heel length (CHL).

ULTRASONOGRAPHIC EXAMINATION OF EMBRYOS

Most women seeking obstetric care have at least one ultrasonographic examination during their pregnancy for one or more of the following reasons:

- Estimation of gestational age for confirmation of clinical dating
- Evaluation of embryonic growth when intrauterine growth restriction (IUGR) is suspected
- Guidance during chorionic villus or amniotic fluid sampling
- Suspected ectopic pregnancy
- Possible uterine abnormality
- Detection of congenital anomalies

The size of an embryo in a pregnant woman can be estimated using ultrasonographic measurements. *Transvaginal or endovaginal sonography* permits accurate measurement of crown-rump length in early pregnancy (Fig. 6-13).

used to estimate the age of older embryos (see Fig. 6-13*B* and *C*). Standing height, or *crown-heel length*, is sometimes measured in 8-week embryos (see Fig. 6-13*D*). The *Carnegie Embryonic Staging System* is used internationally (see Table 6-1) for comparison.

CLINICALLY ORIENTED QUESTIONS

1. There is little apparent difference between an 8-week embryo and a 9-week fetus. Why do embryologists give them different names?
2. When does the embryo become a human being? What guidelines can be used to distinguish this stage?
3. Can the sex of embryos be determined by ultrasonographic study? What other methods can be used to diagnose sex?

The answers to these questions are at the back of the book.

THE FETAL PERIOD: THE NINTH WEEK TO BIRTH

The transformation of an embryo to a fetus is gradual. Development during the fetal period is concerned primarily with body growth and differentiation of tissues, organs, and systems. The rate of body growth during the fetal period is rapid, and fetal weight gain is phenomenal during the terminal weeks (Table 7-1).

TABLE 7-2. Comparison of Gestational Time Units

REFERENCE POINT	CALENDAR			LUNAR
	Days	Weeks	Months	Months
Fertilization	266	38	8¾	9½
Last normal menstrual period	280	40	9¼	10

■ ESTIMATION OF FETAL AGE

Ultrasonographic measurements of the crown-rump length (CRL) can be used to determine fetal size and probable age, and to provide a reliable prediction of the *expected date of delivery*. Fetal head measurements and femur length may also be used to evaluate the age of the fetus. The intrauterine period may be divided into days, weeks, or months (Table 7-2), but confusion arises if it is not stated whether the age is calculated from the last normal menstrual period (LNMP) or from the *fertilization age*. Unless otherwise stated, fetal age in this book is calculated from the estimated time of fertilization, and months refer to calendar months. Clinically, the gestational period is divided into three **trimesters,** each lasting 3 months.

Various measurements and external characteristics are useful for estimating fetal age (see Table 7-1). Measurement of the CRL is the method of choice for estimating fetal age until the end of the *first trimester*. In the *second and third trimesters*, several structures can be identified and measured ultrasonographically, but the basic measurements used for age estimation are **biparietal diameter**—the diameter of the head measured between the two parietal eminences—head circumference, abdominal circumference, and femur length.

Neonatal weight is often a useful criterion for estimating age, but a discrepancy may exist between the age and the weight of a fetus, particularly if the mother had experienced metabolic disturbances, such as diabetes mellitus, during pregnancy. Determination of the size of a fetus, especially of its head, is of great value to the obstetrician for the management of certain patients, such as women with small pelves or fetuses with intrauterine growth restriction (IUGR), congenital anomalies, or both.

TABLE 7-1. Criteria for Estimating Fertilization Age During the Fetal Period

AGE (WEEKS)	CROWN-RUMP LENGTH (MM)*	FOOT LENGTH (MM)*	FETAL WEIGHT (G)†	MAIN EXTERNAL CHARACTERISTICS
Previable Fetus				
9	50	7	8	Eyelids are closing or have closed. Head is round. External genitalia are still not distinguishable as male or female. Intestine is in the umbilical cord.
10	61	9	14	Intestine is in the abdomen. Early fingernail development.
12	87	14	45	Sex is distinguishable externally. Well-defined neck.
14	120	20	110	Head is erect. Lower limbs are well developed. Early toenail development.
16	140	27	200	Ears stand out from the head.
18	160	33	320	Vernix caseosa covers the skin. Quickening (fetal movement) is felt by the mother.
20	190	39	460	Head and body hair (lanugo) are visible.
Viable Fetus‡				
22	210	45	630	Skin is wrinkled and red.
24	230	50	820	Fingernails are present. Lean body.
26	250	55	1000	Eyes are partially open. Eyelashes are present.
28	270	59	1300	Eyes are open. Most fetuses have a good head of hair. Skin is slightly wrinkled.
30	280	63	1700	Toenails are present. Body is filling out. Testes are descending.
32	300	68	2100	Fingernails extend to fingertips. Skin is smooth.
36	340	79	2900	Body is usually plump. Lanugo is almost absent. Toenails extend to the toe tips. Flexed limb; firm grasp.
38	360	83	3400	Prominent chest; breasts protrude. Testes in the scrotum or palpable in the inguinal canals. Fingernails extend beyond fingertips.

*These measurements are averages and so may not apply to specific cases; dimensional variations increase with age.
†These weights refer to fetuses that have been fixed for approximately 2 weeks in 10% formalin. Fresh specimens usually weigh approximately 5% less.
‡There is no sharp limit of development, age, or weight at which a fetus automatically becomes viable or beyond which survival is ensured, but experience has shown that it is uncommon for an infant to survive if its weight is less than 500 g or if its fertilization age or developmental age is less than 22 weeks. Even fetuses born during the 26- to 28-week period have difficulty surviving, mainly because the respiratory and central nervous systems are not completely differentiated. The term *abortion* refers to all pregnancies that terminate before the period of viability.

■ HIGHLIGHTS OF THE FETAL PERIOD

There is not a formal staging system for the fetal period; however, it is helpful to consider the main changes that occur in terms of periods of 4 to 5 weeks.

Nine to Twelve Weeks

At the beginning of the ninth week, *the head constitutes half of the CRL of the fetus* (Fig. 7-1). Subsequently, growth in body length accelerates rapidly, and by the end of 12 weeks, the CRL has more than doubled (see Table 7-1). At 9 weeks, the face is broad, the eyes are widely separated, the ears are low set, and the eyelids are fused. Early in the ninth week, the legs are short and the thighs are relatively small. By the end of 12 weeks, the upper limbs have almost reached their final relative lengths, but the lower limbs are still slightly shorter than their final relative lengths. The *external genitalia* of males and females are not in their mature fetal form until the 12th week. Intestinal coils are clearly visible in the proximal end of the umbilical cord until the middle of the 10th week. By the 11th week, *the intestines have returned to the abdomen* (Fig. 7-2).

At the beginning of the fetal period, the liver is the major site of *erythropoiesis* (formation of red blood cells). By the end of the 12th week, this activity has decreased in the liver and has begun in the spleen. *Urine formation* begins between the 9th and 12th weeks, and urine is discharged through the urethra into the amniotic fluid. The fetus reabsorbs some of this fluid after swallowing it. Fetal waste products are transferred to the maternal circulation by passing across the placental membrane (see Chapter 8).

FIGURE 7-2. An 11-week fetus with its chorionic and amniotic sacs removed (×1.5). Note that the head is relatively large. (Courtesy of Professor Jean Hay [Retired], Department of Human Anatomy and Cell Science, University of Manitoba, Winnipeg, Manitoba, Canada.)

Thirteen to Sixteen Weeks

Growth is very rapid during the 13th to 16th weeks (Figs. 7-3 and 7-4; see Table 7-1). By 16 weeks, the head is relatively small compared with that of the 12-week fetus, and the lower limbs have lengthened. *Limb movements*, which first occur at the end of the embryonic period, become coordinated by the 14th week, but are too slight to be felt by the mother. However, these movements are visible during ultrasonographic examinations. By the beginning of the 16th week, the bones are clearly visible on ultrasound images. *Slow eye movements* occur at 14 weeks. Scalp hair patterning is also determined during this period. By 16 weeks, the ovaries are differentiated and contain primordial follicles that have oogonia. By 16 weeks, the eyes face anteriorly rather than anterolaterally.

Seventeen to Twenty Weeks

Growth slows down during weeks 17 to 20, but the fetus still increases its CRL by approximately 50 mm (Figs. 7-3 and 7-5; see Table 7-1). Fetal movements—**quickening**—are commonly felt by the mother. The skin is now covered with a greasy material, called **vernix caseosa**, which consists of dead epidermal cells and a fatty secretion

FIGURE 7-1. Transvaginal ultrasonographic scan of a fetus (1) early in the ninth week. The relationship of the fetus to the amniotic cavity (2), the chorionic cavity (3), and the amnion (4) is shown. (From Wathen NC, Cass PL, Kitan MJ, Chard T: Human chorionic gonadotrophin and alpha-fetoprotein levels in matched samples of amniotic fluid, extra-embryonic coelomic fluid, and maternal serum in the first trimester of pregnancy. Prenat Diagn 11:145, 1991.)

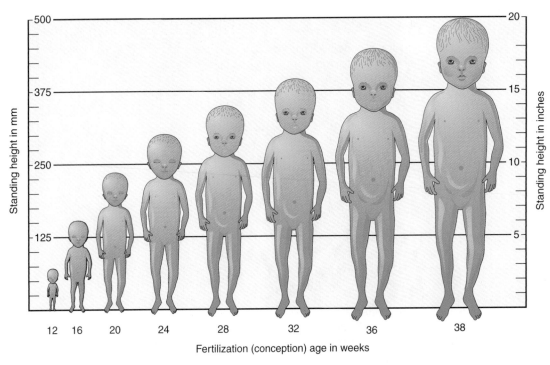

FIGURE 7-3. Diagram, drawn to scale, showing the progressive changes in the size of the human fetus.

FIGURE 7-4. A 13-week fetus. **A,** An enlarged photograph of the head and shoulders (×2). **B,** Actual size. (Courtesy of Professor Jean Hay [Retired], Department of Human Anatomy and Cell Science, University of Manitoba, Winnipeg, Manitoba, Canada.)

from the fetal sebaceous glands. The vernix caseosa protects the delicate fetal skin from abrasions, chapping, and hardening that could result from exposure to the amniotic fluid. Fetuses are usually completely covered with fine, downy hair called *lanugo*, which helps to hold the vernix caseosa on the skin. Eyebrows and head hair are also visible. *Brown fat* forms during weeks 17 through 20 and is the site of heat production, particularly in the newborn. This specialized adipose tissue produces heat by oxidizing fatty acids. By 18 weeks, the uterus is formed

A

Figure 7-5. **A,** A 17-week fetus (actual size). Fetuses at this age are unable to survive if born prematurely, mainly because the respiratory system is immature. (From Moore KL, Persaud TVN, Shiota K: Color Atlas of Clinical Embryology, 2nd ed. Philadelphia, WB Saunders, 2000).

in female fetuses and canalization of the vagina has begun. By this time, many *primordial ovarian follicles* containing oogonia have formed. In male 20-week fetuses, the testes have begun to descend, but they are still located on the posterior abdominal wall.

Twenty-One to Twenty-Five Weeks

Substantial weight gain occurs during weeks 21 to 25, and the fetus is better proportioned. At 21 weeks, rapid eye movements begin; *blink-startle responses* have been reported at 22 to 23 weeks. By 24 weeks, the secretory epithelial cells (type II pneumocytes) in the interalveolar walls of the lung have begun to secrete *surfactant,* a surface-active lipid that maintains the patency of the developing alveoli of the lungs. *Fingernails* are also present by 24 weeks. Although a 22- to 25-week fetus born prematurely may survive initially if given intensive care support, the fetus may die because its respiratory system is still immature.

Twenty-Six to Twenty-Nine Weeks

At 26 to 29 weeks, a fetus often survives if born because the *lungs* have developed sufficiently to provide adequate gas exchange. In addition, the central nervous system has matured to the stage at which it can direct rhythmic breathing movements and control body temperature. The greatest neonatal deaths occur in low–birth weight infants (weighing 2500 g or less) and very low–birth weight infants (weighing 1500 g or less). *The eyelids are open at 26 weeks,* and lanugo and head hair are well developed. Toenails are visible, and considerable subcutaneous fat is now present, smoothing out many of the wrinkles. Formation of red blood cells—*erythropoiesis*—in the spleen ends by 28 weeks, by which time the bone marrow has become the major site of this process.

Thirty to Thirty-Four Weeks

The *pupillary light reflex of the eyes* can be elicited by 30 weeks. Usually, by the end of this period, the skin is pink

FIGURE 7-5. CONT'D **B,** Magnetic resonance imaging scan of an 18-week old normal fetus (20 weeks' gestational age). (Courtesy of Dr. Deborah Levine, Director of Obstetric and Gynecologic Ultrasound, Beth Israel Deaconess Medical Center, Boston, MA).

FIGURE 7-6. A healthy male newborn infant at 36 weeks' gestational age. (Courtesy of Michael and Michele Rice).

and smooth, and the upper and lower limbs have a chubby appearance. Fetuses 32 weeks and older usually survive if born.

Thirty-Five to Thirty-Eight Weeks

Fetuses at 35 weeks have a firm grasp and exhibit a spontaneous orientation to light. As term approaches (37–38 weeks), the nervous system is sufficiently mature to carry out some integrative functions. Most fetuses during this "finishing period" are plump (Fig. 7-6). By 36 weeks, the circumferences of the head and the abdomen are approximately equal. Growth slows as the time of birth approaches (Fig. 7-7). Most fetuses have a CRL of 360 mm and weigh approximately 3400 g. A fetus adds approximately 14 g of fat daily during the last weeks of gestation. The chest is prominent, and the breasts protrude slightly in both sexes. The testes are usually in the scrotum in full-term infants; premature infants commonly have undescended testes.

Expected Date of Delivery

The expected date of delivery of a fetus is 266 days, or 38 weeks, after fertilization (i.e., 280 days, or 40 weeks, after the LNMP) [see Table 7-1]. Approximately 12% of

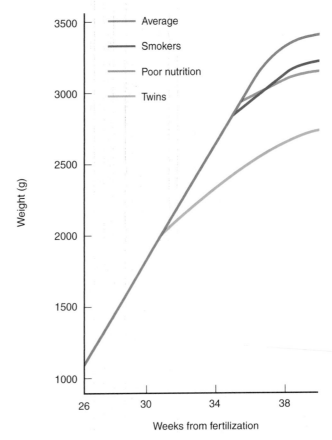

FIGURE 7-7. Graph showing the rate of fetal growth during the last trimester. *Average* refers to the rate of growth of infants born in the United States. After 36 weeks, the growth rate deviates from the straight line. The decline, particularly after full term (38 weeks), probably reflects inadequate fetal nutrition caused by placental changes. (Adapted from Gruenwald P: Growth of the human fetus. I. Normal growth and its variation. Am J Obstet Gynecol 94:1112, 1966.)

babies are born 1 to 2 weeks after the expected time of birth. The common delivery date method (Nägele's rule) for determining the expected date of delivery is to count back 3 months from the first day of the LNMP and add 1 year and 7 days.

■ FACTORS INFLUENCING FETAL GROWTH

The fetus requires substrates for growth and the production of energy. Gases and nutrients pass freely to the fetus from the mother through the placental membrane (see Chapter 8). **Glucose** is a primary source of energy for fetal metabolism and growth; **amino acids** are also required. These substances pass from the mother's blood to the fetus through the placental membrane. **Insulin**, which is required for the metabolism of glucose, is secreted by the fetal pancreas. Insulin, human growth hormone, and some small polypeptides (e.g., insulin-like growth factor I) are believed to stimulate fetal growth.

Many factors—maternal, fetal, and environmental—may affect prenatal growth. In general, factors operating throughout pregnancy, such as *cigarette smoking* and *consumption of alcohol*, tend to produce IUGR and small infants, whereas factors operating during the last trimester (e.g., maternal malnutrition) usually produce underweight infants with normal length and head size. IUGR is usually defined as infant weight within the lowest 10th percentile for gestational age. Severe maternal malnutrition resulting from a poor-quality diet is known to cause reduced fetal growth (see Fig. 7-7). Poor nutrition and faulty food habits are common during pregnancy and are not restricted to mothers living in poverty.

Cigarette Smoking

Smoking is a well-established cause of IUGR. The growth rate for fetuses of mothers who smoke cigarettes is less than normal during the last 6 to 8 weeks of pregnancy (see Fig. 7-7). On average, the birth weight of infants whose mothers smoke heavily during pregnancy is 200 g less than normal.

Multiple Pregnancies

Neonates resulting from twin, triplet, and other multiple pregnancies usually weigh considerably less than infants resulting from a single pregnancy (see Fig. 7-7). It is evident that the total requirements of two or more fetuses exceed the nutritional supply available from the placenta during the third trimester.

Social Drugs

Infants born to mothers with alcoholism often exhibit *IUGR* as part of *fetal alcohol syndrome*. Similarly, the use of marijuana and other illicit drugs (e.g., cocaine) can cause IUGR and other obstetric complications.

Impaired Uteroplacental Blood Flow

Maternal-placental circulation may be reduced by conditions that decrease uterine blood flow (e.g., small chorionic or umbilical vessels, severe hypotension, renal disease). Chronic reduction of uterine blood flow can cause fetal starvation that results in IUGR. Placental dysfunction or defects (e.g., infarction; see Chapter 8) can also cause IUGR.

Genetic Factors and Growth Restriction

Genetic factors can cause intrauterine growth restriction (IUGR). Repeated cases of IUGR in one family indicate that recessive genes may be the cause of the abnormal growth. In recent years, structural and numeric chromosomal aberrations have also been shown to be associated with cases of retarded fetal growth. IUGR is pronounced in infants with trisomy 21 (Down syndrome) and is also characteristic of fetuses with trisomy 18 syndrome (see Chapter 19).

■ PROCEDURES FOR ASSESSING FETAL STATUS

Perinatology is the branch of medicine that is concerned with the well-being of the fetus and newborn infant, generally encompassing the period from approximately 26 weeks after fertilization to 4 weeks after birth. Many new procedures for assessing the status of the fetus have been developed in the last two decades. It is now possible to treat many fetuses whose lives are in jeopardy.

Ultrasonography

Ultrasonography is the primary imaging modality in the evaluation of the fetus because of its wide availability, low cost, and lack of known adverse effects (Fig. 7-8). Placental and fetal size, multiple births, abnormalities of placental shape, and abnormal presentations can also be determined. Some developmental defects can also be detected prenatally by ultrasonography.

Diagnostic Amniocentesis

Diagnostic amniocentesis is a common invasive prenatal diagnostic procedure (Fig. 7-9A). For prenatal diagnosis, amniotic fluid is sampled by insertion of a hollow needle through the mother's anterior abdominal and uterine walls and into the amniotic sac. A syringe is then attached to the needle, and amniotic fluid is withdrawn. The procedure is relatively devoid of risk, especially when performed by an experienced physician using ultrasonography as a guide for outlining the position of the fetus and the placenta.

FIGURE 7-8. Sonogram (axial scan) of a 22-week fetus showing the facial profile. The nose, lips, and mandible are visible. (Courtesy of E.A. Lyons, MD, Professor of Radiology and Obstetrics and Gynecology, University of Manitoba, Health Sciences Centre, Winnipeg, Manitoba, Canada. From Moore KL, Persaud TVN, Shiota K: Color Atlas of Clinical Embryology, 2nd ed. Philadelphia, WB Saunders, 2000.)

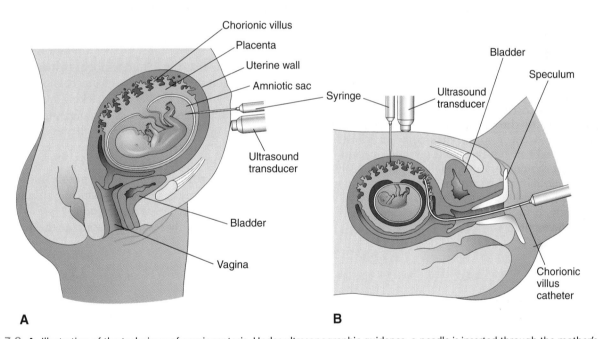

A   B

FIGURE 7-9. **A,** Illustration of the technique of amniocentesis. Under ultrasonographic guidance, a needle is inserted through the mother's abdominal and uterine walls into the amniotic sac. A syringe is attached, and amniotic fluid is withdrawn for diagnostic purposes. **B,** Illustration of chorionic villus sampling. This technique is usually performed at approximately the ninth week after the last normal menstrual period. Two sampling approaches are shown, one through the maternal anterior abdominal wall using a needle, and one through the vagina and cervical canal using a malleable catheter.

Cell Cultures

Fetal sex and chromosomal aberrations can also be determined by studying the sex chromosomes in cultured fetal cells obtained during amniocentesis. These cultures are commonly performed when an autosomal abnormality, such as occurs in Down syndrome, is suspected. Inborn errors of metabolism and enzyme deficiencies in fetuses can also be detected by studying cell cultures.

Percutaneous Umbilical Cord Blood Sampling

For chromosomal analysis, blood samples may be obtained from the umbilical vessels by **percutaneous umbilical cord blood sampling**. Ultrasonographic scanning is used to outline the location of the vessels. Percutaneous umbilical cord blood sampling is often performed approximately 20 weeks after the LNMP to obtain samples for chromosomal analysis when ultrasonographic or other examinations have shown characteristics of fetal anomalies, such as trisomy 13 (see Chapter 19).

Computed Tomography and Magnetic Resonance Imaging

When fetal treatment, such as surgery, is planned, computed tomography and magnetic resonance imaging may be used. Magnetic resonance imaging has the advantage of not using ionizing radiation to produce images. These studies can provide additional information about a fetal abnormality detected ultrasonographically.

Fetal Monitoring

Continuous fetal heart rate monitoring in high-risk pregnancies is routine and provides information about the oxygenation of the fetus. *Fetal distress*, as indicated by an abnormal heart rate or rhythm, suggests that the fetus is in jeopardy.

Intrauterine Fetal Transfusion

Some fetuses with *hemolytic disease of the newborn* can be saved through intrauterine blood transfusions. The blood is injected into the fetal peritoneal cavity. Over a period of 5 to 6 days, most of the injected blood cells pass into the fetal circulation through the diaphragmatic lymphatics. With recent advances in percutaneous umbilical cord puncture, blood can be transfused directly into the fetal cardiovascular system. The need for fetal blood transfusions has been reduced by the treatment of Rh-negative mothers of Rh-positive fetuses with anti-Rh immunoglobulin. Consequently, hemolytic disease of the newborn is now relatively uncommon.

Alpha Fetoprotein Assay

Alpha fetoprotein, a glycoprotein that is synthesized in the fetal liver and umbilical vesicle, escapes from the fetal circulation into the amniotic fluid in fetuses with open neural tube defects, such as spina bifida with myeloschisis (see Chapter 19). Open neural tube defects refer to lesions that are not covered with skin. Alpha fetoprotein can also enter the amniotic fluid from open ventral wall defects, as occurs with gastroschisis and omphalocele (see Chapter 13). Alpha fetoprotein can also be measured in maternal serum.

Chorionic Villus Sampling

Biopsy of chorionic villi (see Fig. 7-9*B*) is performed to detect chromosomal abnormalities, inborn errors of metabolism, and X-linked disorders. Chorionic villus sampling can be performed as early as 7 weeks after fertilization. The rate of fetal loss is approximately 1%, slightly more than the risk associated with amniocentesis. The major advantage of chorionic villus sampling over amniocentesis is that it allows fetal chromosomal sampling to be performed several weeks earlier.

CLINICALLY ORIENTED QUESTIONS

1. Some say that the mature embryo twitches and that a first-trimester fetus moves its limbs. Is this true? If so, can the mother feel her baby kicking at this time?
2. Some reports suggest that vitamin supplementation around the time of conception will prevent neural tube defects, such as spina bifida. Is there scientific proof to support this statement?
3. Can the fetus be injured by the needle during amniocentesis? Is there a risk of inducing an abortion or causing maternal or fetal infection?

The answers to these questions are at the back of the book.

THE PLACENTA AND THE FETAL MEMBRANES

The fetal part of the placenta and the fetal membranes separate the embryo or fetus from the endometrium. An interchange of substances (e.g., nutrients and oxygen) occurs between the maternal and fetal blood through the placenta. The vessels in the umbilical cord connect the placental circulation with the fetal circulation. The chorion, amnion, umbilical vesicle (yolk sac), and allantois constitute the fetal membranes.

■ THE PLACENTA

The placenta is a **fetomaternal organ** that has two components:
- A **fetal part** that develops from part of the chorionic sac
- A **maternal part** that is derived from the endometrium

The placenta and the umbilical cord function as a *transport system* for substances passing between the mother and the fetus. Nutrients and oxygen pass from the maternal blood through the placenta to the fetal blood, and waste materials and carbon dioxide pass from the fetal blood through the placenta to the maternal blood. The placenta and the fetal membranes perform the following functions and activities: protection, nutrition, respiration, excretion, and hormone production. Shortly after birth, the placenta and the fetal membranes are expelled from the uterus as the *afterbirth*.

Decidua

The *decidua* is the gravid endometrium, the functional layer of the endometrium in a pregnant woman that separates from the remainder of the uterus after *parturition* (childbirth).

Three regions of the decidua are named according to their relation to the implantation site (Fig. 8-1):
- **Decidua basalis**—the part of the decidua deep to the conceptus that forms the maternal part of the placenta
- **Decidua capsularis**—the superficial part of the decidua overlying the conceptus
- **Decidua parietalis**—all of the remaining parts of the decidua

In response to increasing progesterone levels in the maternal blood, the connective tissue cells of the decidua enlarge to form pale-staining **decidual cells**. These cells enlarge as glycogen and lipid accumulate in their cytoplasm. The cellular and vascular changes in the decidua that result from pregnancy are referred to as the **decidual reaction**. Many decidual cells degenerate near the chorionic sac in the region of the syncytiotrophoblast and, together with maternal blood and uterine secretions, provide a rich source of nutrition for the embryo. Decidual regions, clearly recognizable during ultrasonography, are important in diagnosing early pregnancy.

Development of the Placenta

Early placental development is characterized by the rapid proliferation of the trophoblast and development of the chorionic sac and chorionic villi. By the end of the third week, the anatomic arrangements necessary for physiologic exchanges between the mother and the embryo have been established. By the end of the fourth week, a complex vascular network develops in the placenta, allowing maternal-embryonic exchanges of gases, nutrients, and metabolic waste products. Chorionic villi cover the entire chorionic sac until the beginning of the eighth week (Figs. 8-1C and 8-2). As this sac grows, the villi associated with the decidua capsularis are compressed, reducing the blood supply to them. These villi soon degenerate (see Fig. 8-1D), producing a relatively avascular, bare area, the **smooth chorion**. As the villi disappear, those associated with the decidua basalis rapidly increase in number, branch profusely, and enlarge (Fig. 8-3). This bushy part of the chorionic sac is known as the **villous chorion**.

ULTRASONOGRAPHY OF THE CHORIONIC SAC

The size of the chorionic sac is useful in determining the gestational age of embryos in pregnant women with uncertain menstrual histories. Growth of the chorionic sac is extremely rapid between the 5th and 10th weeks of development. Modern ultrasound devices permit detection of the chorionic sac when it has a median diameter of 2 to 3 mm (Fig. 8-4). Chorionic sacs with this diameter indicate a gestational age of approximately 18 days.

Fetomaternal Junction

The fetal part of the placenta (villous chorion) is attached to the maternal part of the placenta (decidua basalis) by the **cytotrophoblastic shell**, the external layer of trophoblastic cells on the maternal surface of the placenta (Fig. 8-5). The chorionic villi, which are attached firmly to the decidua basalis through the cytotrophoblastic shell, anchor the chorionic sac to the decidua basalis. Endometrial arteries and veins pass freely through gaps in the cytotrophoblastic shell and open into the intervillous space. The **shape of the placenta** is determined by the shape of the persistent area of chorionic villi (see Fig. 8-1F). Usually, this is a circular area, giving the placenta a discoid shape. As the chorionic villi invade the decidua basalis during placental formation, decidual tissue is eroded to enlarge the intervillous space. This erosion produces several wedge-shaped areas of decidua—**placental septa**—that project toward the **chorionic plate** (see Fig. 8-5). The placental septa divide the fetal part of the placenta into irregular convex areas called **cotyledons** (see Fig. 8-3). Each cotyledon consists of two or more stem villi and their many branch villi.

The **decidua capsularis**, the layer overlying the implanted chorionic sac, forms a capsule over the external surface of the sac (see Fig. 8-1A to D). As the conceptus enlarges, the decidua capsularis bulges into the uterine cavity and becomes greatly attenuated. Eventually, parts of the decidua capsularis make contact and fuse with

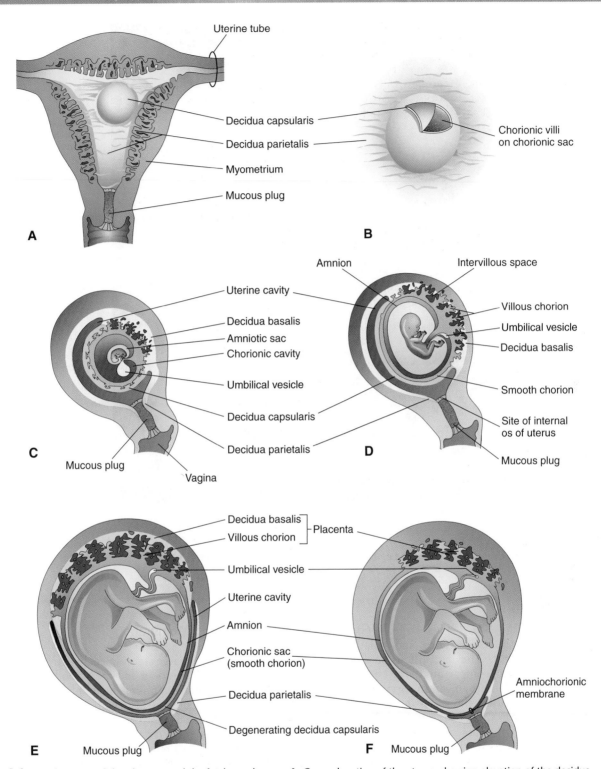

FIGURE 8-1. Development of the placenta and the fetal membranes. **A,** Coronal section of the uterus, showing elevation of the decidua capsularis by the expanding chorionic sac at 4 weeks. **B,** Enlarged illustration of the implantation site. The chorionic villi were exposed by cutting an opening in the decidua capsularis. **C** to **F,** Sagittal sections of the gravid uterus from the 5th to 22nd weeks, showing the changing relationship of the fetal membranes to the decidua. In **F,** the amnion and the chorion are fused with each other and with the decidua parietalis, thereby obliterating the uterine cavity.

the **decidua parietalis**, thereby slowly obliterating the uterine cavity (see Fig. 8-1*E* and *F*). By 22 to 24 weeks, reduced blood supply to the decidua capsularis causes it to degenerate and disappear, after which the smooth part of the chorionic sac fuses with the decidua parietalis.

Intervillous Space

The intervillous space of the placenta contains maternal blood, which is derived from the lacunae that developed in the syncytiotrophoblast during the second week of

Chorionic villi of villous chorion

Smooth chorion

Chorionic vessels

Umbilical cord

Amnion covering chorionic vessels

FIGURE 8-2. Lateral view of a spontaneously aborted embryo at Carnegie stage 14, approximately 32 days. The chorionic and amniotic sacs have been opened to show the embryo.

development (see Fig. 4-1*C*). This large, blood-filled space results from the coalescence and enlargement of the lacunar networks. The intervillous space of the placenta is divided into compartments by the *placental septa;* however, free communication occurs between the compartments because the septa do not reach the **chorionic plate** (see Fig. 8-5)—the part of the chorion associated with the placenta. Maternal blood enters the intervillous space from the **spiral arteries** in the decidua basalis; these arteries pass through gaps in the cytotrophoblastic shell and discharge blood into the intervillous space (see Fig. 8-5). This large space is drained by endometrial veins that also penetrate the cytotrophoblastic shell. The numerous **branch villi**, arising from stem chorionic villi, are continuously showered with maternal blood as it circulates through the intervillous space. The blood in this space carries oxygen and nutritional materials that are necessary for fetal growth and development. The maternal blood also contains fetal waste products, such as carbon dioxide, salts, and products of protein metabolism.

Amniochorionic Membrane

The amniotic sac enlarges more quickly than the chorionic sac. As a result, the amnion and the smooth chorion soon fuse to form the amniochorionic membrane (see Fig. 8-1*F*). This composite membrane fuses with the decidua capsularis and, after disappearance of this part of the decidua, adheres to the decidua parietalis. *It is the amniochorionic membrane that ruptures during labor.* Preterm rupture of this membrane is the most common event leading to premature labor. When the amniochorionic membrane ruptures, the amniotic fluid escapes through the cervix and vagina.

Placental Circulation

The many *branch chorionic villi* provide a large surface area where materials may be exchanged across the very thin **placental membrane** interposed between the fetal and the maternal circulations (Figs. 8-6*B* and *C*). It is through the branch villi that the main exchange of material between

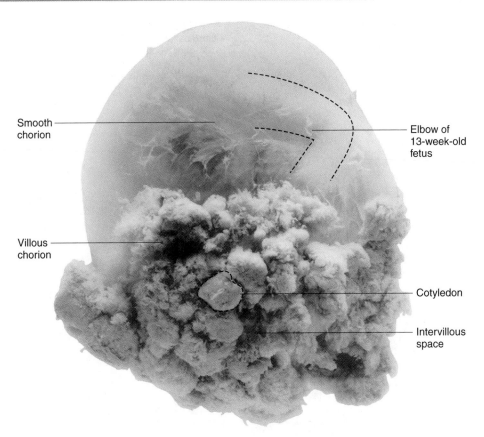

FIGURE 8-3. A human chorionic sac containing a 13-week fetus. The villous chorion is where chorionic villi persist and form the fetal part of the placenta. In situ, the cotyledons were attached to the decidua basalis and the intervillous space was filled with maternal blood.

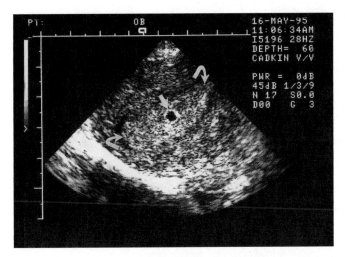

FIGURE 8-4. Transverse endovaginal scan of an early intrauterine chorionic sac. A cross-section of the chorionic sac (*straight arrow*) shows a thick, bright (echogenic) ring of chorionic villi surrounding the black chorionic fluid. The ring is surrounded by the less echogenic decidua parietalis (lateral borders indicated by *curved arrows*). (Courtesy of Dr. Alan V. Cadkin, MD, Fort Myers, FL.)

the mother and the fetus takes place. The placental membrane consists of extrafetal tissues.

Fetoplacental Circulation

Poorly oxygenated blood leaves the fetus via the **umbilical arteries** (Figs. 8-5 and 8-7). At the attachment of the umbilical cord to the placenta, these arteries divide into a number of radially disposed **chorionic arteries** that branch freely in the chorionic plate before entering the chorionic villi (see Fig. 8-5). The blood vessels form an extensive **arteriocapillary venous system** within the chorionic villi (see Fig. 8-6*A*) that brings the fetal blood extremely close to the maternal blood (see Fig. 8-7). This system provides a very large surface area for the exchange of metabolic and gaseous products between the maternal and fetal blood. Normally, no intermingling of fetal and maternal blood occurs. The well-oxygenated fetal blood in the fetal capillaries passes into thin-walled veins that follow the chorionic arteries to the site of attachment of the umbilical cord, where they converge to form the **umbilical vein**. This large vessel carries oxygen-rich blood to the fetus.

Maternal-Placental Circulation

The maternal blood enters the intervillous space through 80 to 100 **spiral arteries** in the decidua basalis. The entering blood is at considerably higher pressure than that in the intervillous space, so it spurts toward the **chorionic plate** (see Fig. 8-5). As the pressure dissipates, the blood flows slowly around the branch villi, allowing an exchange of metabolic and gaseous products with the fetal blood. The blood eventually returns through the endometrial veins to the maternal circulation (see Fig. 8-7). Reductions of uteroplacental circulation result in **fetal hypoxia** (decreased level of oxygen) and intrauterine growth restriction.

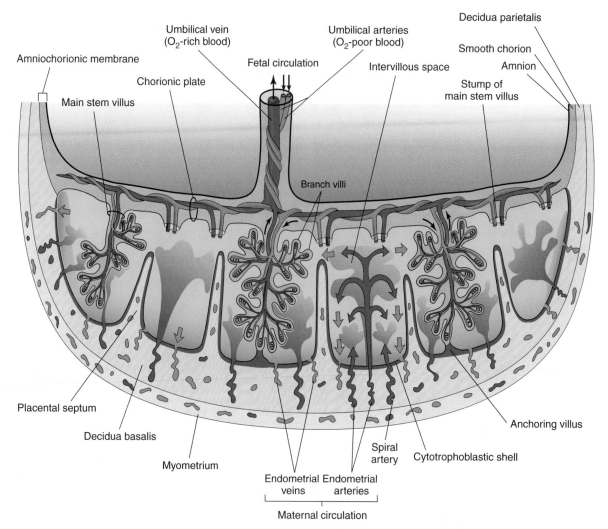

FIGURE 8-5. Illustration of a transverse section through a full-term placenta, showing (1) the relation of the villous chorion (fetal part of the placenta) to the decidua basalis (maternal part of the placenta); (2) the fetal placental circulation; and (3) the maternal placental circulation. Maternal blood flows into the intervillous spaces in funnel-shaped spurts from the spiral arteries, and exchanges occur with the fetal blood as the maternal blood flows around the branch villi. The inflowing arterial blood pushes venous blood out of the intervillous space and into the endometrial veins. Note that the umbilical arteries carry poorly oxygenated fetal blood (shown in *blue*) to the placenta and that the umbilical vein carries oxygenated blood (shown in *red*) to the fetus. Only one stem villus is shown in each cotyledon, but the stumps of those that have been removed are indicated. *Arrows* indicate direction of maternal (red and blue) and fetal (black) blood flow.

The intervillous space of the mature placenta contains approximately 150 mL of blood that is replenished three or four times each minute.

Placental Membrane

The **placental membrane** consists of the extrafetal tissues that separate the maternal and the fetal blood. Until approximately 20 weeks, *the placental membrane consists of four layers* (see Fig. 8-6B): syncytiotrophoblast, cytotrophoblast, connective tissue of the villus, and endothelium of the fetal capillaries.

After the 20th week, histologic changes occur in the branch villi that result in the cytotrophoblast becoming attenuated in many villi. Eventually, cytotrophoblastic cells disappear over large areas of the villi, leaving only thin patches of syncytiotrophoblast. As a result, the placental membrane at full term consists of only three layers in

most places (see Fig. 8-6C). In some areas, the placental membrane becomes markedly thinned and attenuated. At these sites, the syncytiotrophoblast comes in direct contact with the endothelium of the fetal capillaries to form a *vasculosyncytial placental membrane*.

Only a few substances, endogenous or exogenous, are unable to pass through the placental membrane. The membrane acts as a true barrier only when the molecule or organism has a certain size, configuration, and charge. *Most drugs and other substances in the maternal plasma pass through the placental membrane and are found in the fetal plasma* (see Fig. 8-7).

During the third trimester, numerous nuclei in the syncytiotrophoblast of the villi aggregate to form **syncytial knots** (see Fig. 8-6C). These *nuclear aggregations* continually break off and are carried from the intervillous space into the maternal circulation. Some knots may lodge in capillaries of the maternal lung, where they are

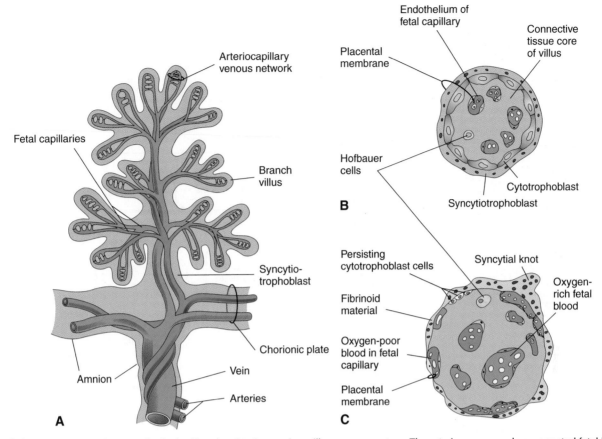

FIGURE 8-6. **A,** Illustration of a stem chorionic villus showing its arteriocapillary-venous system. The arteries carry poorly oxygenated fetal blood and waste products from the fetus, whereas the vein carries oxygenated blood and nutrients to the fetus. **B** and **C,** Sections through a branch villus at 10 weeks' gestation and at full term, respectively. The placental membrane, composed of extrafetal tissues, separates the maternal blood in the intervillous space from the fetal blood in the capillaries in the villi. Note that the placental membrane becomes very thin at full term. Hofbauer cells are believed to be phagocytic cells.

rapidly destroyed by local enzyme action. Toward the end of pregnancy, **fibrinoid material** forms on the surfaces of the villi.

The placenta has three main functions:
● Metabolism (e.g., synthesis of glycogen)
● Transport of gases and nutrients
● Endocrine secretion (e.g., hCG)

Placental Metabolism

The placenta synthesizes glycogen, cholesterol, and fatty acids, which serve as sources of nutrients and energy for the embryo or fetus. Many of the metabolic activities of the placenta are critical for its other two major activities: transport and endocrine secretion.

Placental Transfer

The transport of substances in both directions between the placenta and the maternal blood is facilitated by the great surface area of the placental membrane. Almost all materials are transported across the placental membrane by one of the following four main **transport mechanisms**: simple diffusion, facilitated diffusion, active transport, and pinocytosis.

Passive transport by simple diffusion is usually characteristic of substances moving from areas of higher to lower concentration until equilibrium is established. In *facilitated diffusion*, transport occurs through electrical gradients. *Active transport* against a concentration gradient requires energy. This mechanism of transport may involve carrier molecules that temporarily combine with the substances to be transported. *Pinocytosis* is a form of endocytosis in which the material being engulfed is a small amount of extracellular fluid. Some proteins are transferred very slowly through the placenta by pinocytosis.

TRANSFER OF GASES

Gases, such as oxygen, carbon dioxide, and carbon monoxide, cross the placental membrane by simple diffusion. *Interruption of oxygen transport for several minutes endangers the survival of the embryo or fetus.* The efficiency of the placental membrane approaches that of the lungs for gas exchange. The quantity of oxygen reaching the fetus is generally flow-limited, rather than diffusion-limited; hence, fetal hypoxia results primarily from factors that diminish either uterine blood flow or fetal blood flow through the placenta. Nitrous oxide, an inhalation anesthetic, also readily crosses the placenta.

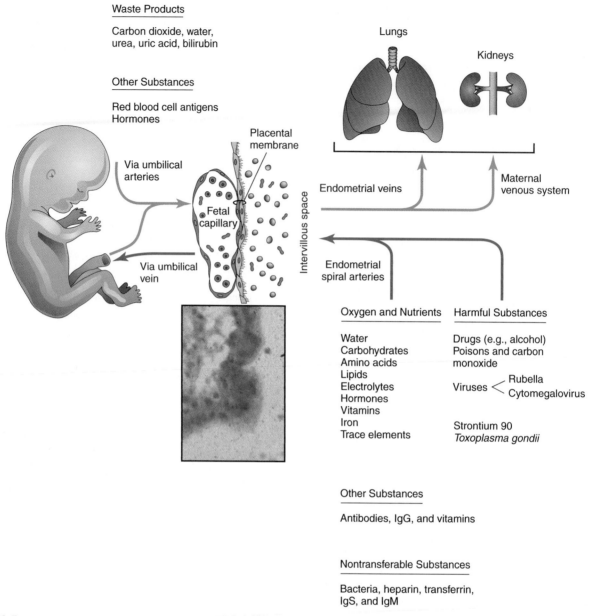

Waste Products

Carbon dioxide, water, urea, uric acid, bilirubin

Other Substances

Red blood cell antigens
Hormones

Via umbilical arteries

Via umbilical vein

Placental membrane

Fetal capillary

Intervillous space

Lungs

Kidneys

Endometrial veins

Maternal venous system

Endometrial spiral arteries

Oxygen and Nutrients

Water
Carbohydrates
Amino acids
Lipids
Electrolytes
Hormones
Vitamins
Iron
Trace elements

Harmful Substances

Drugs (e.g., alcohol)
Poisons and carbon monoxide

Viruses < Rubella
Cytomegalovirus

Strontium 90
Toxoplasma gondii

Other Substances

Antibodies, IgG, and vitamins

Nontransferable Substances

Bacteria, heparin, transferrin, IgS, and IgM

FIGURE 8-7. Transfer across the placental membrane. The extrafetal tissues, across which transport of substances between the mother and the fetus occurs, collectively constitute the placental membrane. IgG, immunoglobulin G; IgM, immunoglobulin M; IgS, immunoglobulin S.

NUTRITIONAL SUBSTANCES

Nutrients constitute the bulk of substances transferred from the mother to the fetus. *Water* is rapidly exchanged by simple diffusion and in increasing amounts as pregnancy advances. *Glucose* produced by the mother and the placenta is quickly transferred to the embryo or fetus by facilitated diffusion. Very small amounts of maternal cholesterol, triglycerides, and phospholipids are transferred. Although free fatty acids are transported, the amount transferred appears to be relatively small. *Amino acids* cross the placenta to the fetus in high concentrations by active transport. *Vitamins* cross the placental membrane and are essential for normal development. A maternal protein, *transferrin*, crosses the placental membrane and carries iron to the embryo or fetus. The placental surface contains special receptors for this protein.

HORMONES

Protein hormones do not reach the embryo or fetus in significant amounts, except for a slow transfer of thyroxine and triiodothyronine. Unconjugated *steroid hormones* cross the placental membrane relatively freely. Testosterone and certain synthetic progestins also cross the placenta.

ELECTROLYTES

Electrolytes are freely exchanged in significant quantities, each at its own rate. When a mother receives intravenous fluids with electrolytes, they also pass to the fetus and affect the fetal water and electrolyte status.

MATERNAL ANTIBODIES

The fetus produces only small amounts of antibodies because of its immature immune system. Some passive immunity is conferred on the fetus by placental transfer of maternal antibodies. Only immunoglobulin G is transferred across the placenta (receptor-mediated transcytosis). *Maternal antibodies confer fetal immunity* for diseases such as diphtheria, smallpox, and measles; however, no immunity is acquired to pertussis (whooping cough) or chickenpox.

WASTE PRODUCTS

Urea and uric acid pass through the placental membrane by simple diffusion. Conjugated bilirubin (which is fat soluble) is easily transported by the placenta and is quickly cleared.

DRUGS AND DRUG METABOLITES

Most drugs and drug metabolites cross the placenta by simple diffusion. Some drugs cause major congenital anomalies (see Chapter 19). *Fetal drug addiction* may occur after maternal use of drugs such as heroin, and newborn infants may experience withdrawal symptoms. Most drugs used for the management of labor readily cross the placental membrane. Depending on their dose and timing in relation to delivery, these drugs may cause respiratory depression of the newborn infant. Neuromuscular blocking agents, such as succinylcholine, that might be used during operative obstetrics, cross the placenta in only very small amounts. All sedatives and analgesics affect the fetus to some degree. Drugs taken by the mother can affect the embryo or fetus, directly or indirectly, by interfering with maternal or placental metabolism. Inhaled anesthetics can also cross the placental membrane and affect fetal breathing if used during parturition.

INFECTIOUS AGENTS

Cytomegalovirus, rubella, and coxsackie viruses, as well as viruses associated with variola, varicella, measles, and poliomyelitis, may pass through the placental membrane and cause *fetal infection*. In some cases, as with the **rubella** virus, severe congenital anomalies may result (see Chapter 19). Microorganisms, such as *Treponema pallidum*, cause syphilis, and *Toxoplasma gondii* produces destructive changes in the brain and eyes of the fetus.

Placental Endocrine Synthesis and Secretion

Using precursors derived from the fetus, the mother, or both, the *syncytiotrophoblast* of the placenta synthesizes protein and steroid hormones. **Protein hormones** synthesized by the placenta include the following:
● Human chorionic gonadotropin (hCG)
● Human chorionic somatomammotropin, or human placental lactogen
● Human chorionic thyrotropin
● Human chorionic corticotropin

The glycoprotein hCG, similar to luteinizing hormone, is first secreted by the syncytiotrophoblast during the second week. The *hCG maintains the corpus luteum*, preventing the onset of menstrual periods. The concentration of hCG in the maternal blood and urine rises to a maximum by the eighth week and then declines. The placenta also plays a major role in the production of **steroid hormones** (i.e., progesterone and

estrogens). Progesterone is essential for the maintenance of pregnancy.

Uterine Growth during Pregnancy

The uterus of a nonpregnant woman lies in the pelvis. It increases in size during pregnancy to accommodate the growing fetus. As the uterus enlarges, it increases in weight and its walls become thinner. During the first trimester, the uterus expands out of the pelvic cavity, and by 20 weeks, it usually reaches the level of the umbilicus. By 28 to 30 weeks, the uterine fundus reaches the epigastric region, the area between the xiphoid process of the sternum and the umbilicus.

■ PARTURITION

Parturition (childbirth) is the process during which the fetus, placenta, and fetal membranes are expelled from the mother (Fig. 8-8). **Labor** is the *sequence of uterine contractions* that results in dilation of the cervix and delivery of the fetus and placenta from the uterus. The factors that trigger labor are not completely understood, but several hormones are related to the initiation of contractions. The fetal hypothalamus secretes **corticotropin-releasing hormone**, which stimulates the pituitary gland to produce **adrenocorticotrophic hormone**, which causes the secretion of cortisol from the suprarenal (adrenal) cortex. **Cortisol** is involved in the synthesis of estrogens.

Peristaltic contractions of the uterine smooth muscle are elicited by **oxytocin**, which is released by the mother's neurohypophysis of the pituitary gland. This hormone is administered clinically when it is necessary to induce labor. Oxytocin also stimulates the release of **prostaglandins** that, in turn, stimulate myometrial contractility by sensitizing the myometrial cells to oxytocin. Estrogens also increase

HEMOLYTIC DISEASE OF THE NEWBORN

Small amounts of fetal blood may pass to the maternal blood through microscopic breaks in the placental membrane. If the fetus is Rh positive and the mother is Rh negative, the fetal cells may stimulate the formation of anti-Rh antibody by the mother's immune system. This antibody passes to the fetal blood and causes hemolysis of fetal Rh-positive blood cells and anemia in the fetus. Some fetuses with hemolytic disease of the newborn, or fetal erythroblastosis, do not make a satisfactory intrauterine adjustment. They may die unless delivered early or given intrauterine, intraperitoneal, or intravenous transfusions of packed Rh-negative blood cells to maintain the fetus until after birth. Hemolytic disease of the newborn is relatively uncommon now because Rh immunoglobulin given to the mother usually prevents development of this disease in the fetus.

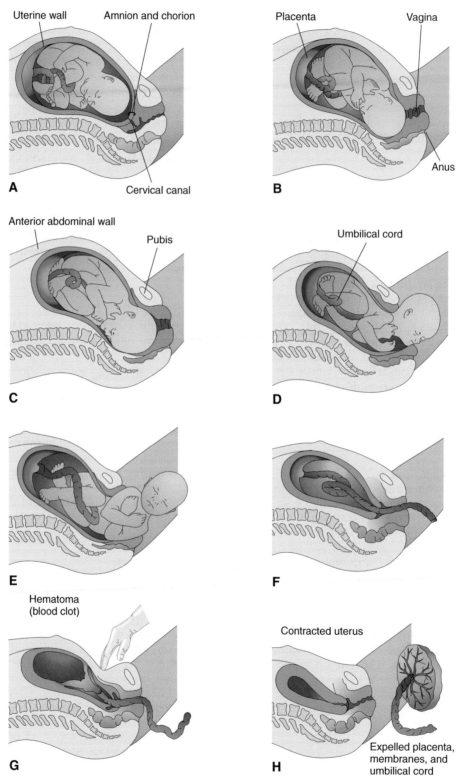

FIGURE 8-8. Illustrations of parturition. **A** and **B,** The cervix is dilating during the first stage of labor. **C** to **E,** The fetus is passing through the cervix and the vagina during the second stage of labor. **F** and **G,** As the uterus contracts during the third stage of labor, the placenta folds and pulls away from the uterine wall. Separation of the placenta results in bleeding and the formation of a large hematoma (mass of blood). Pressure on the abdomen facilitates placental separation. **H,** The placenta is expelled and the uterus contracts.

myometrial contractile activity and stimulate the release of oxytocin and prostaglandins.

Stages of Labor

Labor is a continuous process, but clinically it is divided into three stages:

- **Dilation** begins with *progressive dilation of the cervix* (see Fig. 8-8A and B), and ends with complete dilation of the cervix. During this phase, regular contractions of the uterus occur less than 10 minutes apart. The average duration of the first stage is approximately 12 hours for first pregnancies (primigravidas) and approximately 7 hours for women who have had a child previously (multigravidas).
- **Expulsion** begins when the cervix is fully dilated and ends with delivery of the infant (see Fig. 8-8C to E). During this stage, the *fetus descends through the cervix and the vagina.* As soon as the fetus is outside the mother, it is called a *newborn infant, or neonate.* The average duration of this stage is 50 minutes for primigravidas and 20 minutes for multigravidas.
- **Placental separation** begins as soon as the infant is born and *ends with the expulsion of the placenta and the fetal membranes* (see Fig. 8-8F to H). A hematoma forms deep to the placenta, separating it from the uterine wall. The placenta and the fetal membranes are then expelled. Contractions of the uterus constrict the spiral arteries, preventing excessive uterine bleeding. The duration of this stage is approximately 15 minutes. A retained or **adherent placenta**—one not expelled within 1 hour of delivery—is a cause of postpartum bleeding.

GESTATIONAL CHORIOCARCINOMA

Abnormal proliferation of the trophoblast results in gestational trophoblastic disease, which encompasses a spectrum of lesions, including highly malignant tumors (choriocarcinomas). The cells invade the decidua basalis, penetrate its blood vessels and lymphatics, and metastasize to the maternal lungs, bone marrow, liver, and other organs.

The Placenta and the Fetal Membranes after Birth

The placenta is commonly discoid, with a diameter of 15 to 20 cm and a thickness of 2 to 3 cm (Fig. 8-9). The margins of the placenta are continuous with the ruptured amniotic and chorionic sacs.

Variations in Placental Shape

As the placenta develops, chorionic villi usually persist only where the villous chorion is in contact with the decidua basalis. When villi persist elsewhere, several variations in placental shape occur, such as **accessory placenta** (Fig. 8-10). Examination of the placenta, prenatally by ultrasonography or postnatally by gross and microscopic study, may provide clinical information about the causes of placental dysfunction, intrauterine growth restriction, fetal distress and death, and neonatal illness. Postnatal placental studies can also determine whether the placenta is complete. Retention of a cotyledon or an accessory placenta in the uterus causes postpartum uterine hemorrhage.

FIGURE 8-9. Placentas and fetal membranes after birth, shown approximately one third their actual size. **A,** Maternal surface, showing cotyledons and the grooves around them. Each convex cotyledon consists of a number of main stem villi with their many branch villi. The grooves were occupied by the placental septa when the maternal and fetal parts of the placenta were together (see Fig. 8-5). **B,** Fetal surface, showing blood vessels running in the chorionic plate deep to the amnion and converging to form the umbilical vessels at the attachment of the umbilical cord.

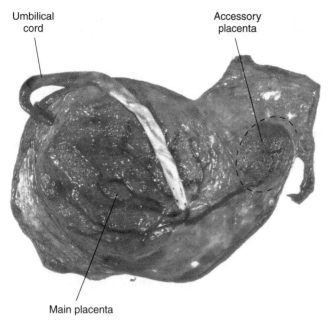

Umbilical cord

Accessory placenta

Main placenta

FIGURE 8-10. The maternal surface of a full-term placenta and an accessory placenta, shown approximately one fourth its actual size.

THE PLACENTA AS AN ALLOGRAFT

The placenta, a part of the conceptus that inherits both paternal and maternal genes, can be regarded as an allograft with respect to the mother. What protects the placenta from rejection by the mother's immune system? This question remains a major biologic enigma. The syncytiotrophoblastic layer of the chorionic villi, although exposed to maternal immune cells within the blood sinusoids, lacks immune antigens (major histocompatibility complex antigens), and thus does not evoke rejection responses. However, extravillous trophoblastic cells that invade the uterus do express major histocompatibility complex antigens. In addition to averting T cells, trophoblastic cells must also shield themselves from potential attack by natural killer lymphocytes and from injury inflicted by the activation of complement. Multiple mechanisms appear to be in place to guard the placenta.

PLACENTAL ABNORMALITIES

Abnormal adherence of the chorionic villi to the myometrium of the uterine wall is called *placenta accreta* (Fig. 8-11). When chorionic villi penetrate the myometrium all the way to the perimetrium (peritoneal covering), the abnormality is called *placenta percreta*. Third-trimester bleeding is the most common presenting sign of these placental abnormalities. After birth, the placenta does not separate from the uterine wall, and attempts to remove it may cause severe hemorrhage that is difficult to control. When the blastocyst implants close to or overlying the internal os of the uterus, the abnormality is called *placenta previa*. Late-pregnancy bleeding can result from this placental abnormality. In such cases, the fetus is delivered by cesarean section because the placenta blocks the cervical canal.

Maternal Surface of the Placenta

The *cobblestone appearance* of the maternal surface of the placenta is produced by slightly bulging villous areas—the **cotyledons**—which are separated by grooves formerly occupied by **placental septa** (see Fig. 8-9*A*).

Fetal Surface of the Placenta

The umbilical cord usually attaches to the fetal surface, and its epithelium is continuous with the amnion adhering to the chorionic plate of the placenta (see Fig. 8-9*B*). The chorionic vessels radiating to and from the umbilical cord

are visible through the smooth, transparent amnion. The **umbilical vessels** branch on the fetal surface, forming the **chorionic vessels**, which enter the chorionic villi (see Fig. 8-5).

Umbilical Cord

The attachment of the umbilical cord, which connects the embryo or fetus to the placenta, is usually near the center of the fetal surface (see Fig. 8-9*B*). However, it may be found at any point. *Doppler ultrasonography* may be used for prenatal diagnosis of the position and structural abnormalities of the umbilical cord. The umbilical cord is usually 1 to 2 cm in diameter and 30 to 90 cm in length (average, 55 cm). Long cords have a tendency to prolapse or coil around the fetus. Prompt recognition of *prolapse of the cord* is important because, during delivery, it may be compressed between the presenting body part of the fetus and the mother's bony pelvis, causing fetal anoxia. If the deficiency of oxygen persists for more than 5 minutes, the infant's brain may be damaged.

The umbilical cord usually has *two arteries and one vein* surrounded by mucoid connective tissue (*Wharton jelly*). Because the umbilical vessels are longer than the cord, twisting and bending of the vessels is common. They frequently form loops, producing *false knots* that are of no significance; however, in approximately 1% of pregnancies, *true knots* form in the umbilical cord. These may tighten and cause fetal death secondary to fetal anoxia. In most cases, the knots form during labor as a result of the fetus passing through a loop of the cord. Because these knots are usually loose, they have no clinical significance. Simple looping of the cord around the fetus occasionally occurs (Fig. 8-12*B*). In approximately one fifth of all deliveries, the cord is loosely *looped around the neck* without causing increased fetal risk.

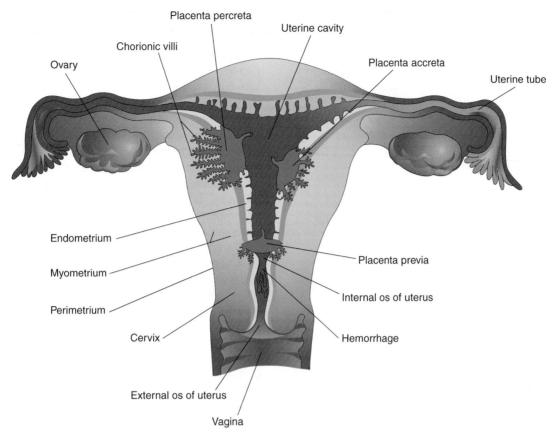

FIGURE 8-11. Placental abnormalities. In placenta accreta, there is abnormal adherence of the placenta to the myometrium. In placenta percreta, the placenta has penetrated the full thickness of the myometrium (muscle layer). In placenta previa, the placenta overlies the internal os of the uterus and blocks the cervical canal.

FIGURE 8-12. **A** and **B,** A 12-week fetus within its amniotic sac (shown actual size). The fetus and its membranes aborted spontaneously. It was removed from its chorionic sac with the amniotic sac intact.

In approximately 1 in 200 newborn infants, only one umbilical artery is present (Fig. 8-13), a condition that may be associated with chromosomal and fetal abnormalities. Absence of an umbilical artery is accompanied by a 15% to 20% incidence of cardiovascular anomalies in the fetus. Absence of an artery results from either agenesis or degeneration of this vessel early in development.

Amnion
Mucous connective tissue
Umbilical artery
Umbilical vein

FIGURE 8-13. Transverse section of the umbilical cord from a newborn infant. Note that the cord is covered by a single-layered epithelium derived from the enveloping amnion. It has a core of mucous connective tissue. Observe also that the cord has one umbilical artery and one vein. Usually, there are two arteries. (Courtesy of Professor V. Becker, Pathologisches Institut der Universität, Erlangen, Germany.)

■ THE AMNION AND THE AMNIOTIC FLUID

The **amnion** forms a fluid-filled, membranous *amniotic sac* that surrounds the embryo and fetus (Figs. 8-14*A* and *B* and 8-12*A*). As the amnion enlarges, it gradually obliterates the chorionic cavity and forms the epithelial covering of the umbilical cord (see Fig. 8-14*C* and *D*). **Amniotic fluid** plays a major role in fetal growth and development. Initially, most amniotic fluid is derived from *maternal tissue fluid* by diffusion across the amniochorionic membrane from the decidua parietalis (see Fig. 8-5). Some fluid is secreted by amniotic cells. Later, there is diffusion of fluid through the chorionic plate from blood in the intervillous space of the placenta. Before keratinization of the skin occurs, a major pathway for passage of water and solutes in tissue fluid from the fetus to the amniotic cavity is through the skin; thus, amniotic fluid is similar to fetal interstitial fluid. Fluid is also secreted by the fetal respiratory and gastrointestinal tracts and enters the amniotic cavity. Beginning in the 11th week, the fetus contributes to the amniotic fluid by expelling urine into the amniotic cavity. Normally, the *volume of amniotic fluid* increases slowly, reaching approximately 30 mL at 10 weeks, 350 mL at 20 weeks, and 700 to 1000 mL by 37 weeks.

The water content of amniotic fluid changes every 3 hours. Large amounts of water pass through the amnio-

A low volume of amniotic fluid—*oligohydramnios*—results, in many cases, from placental insufficiency, with diminished placental blood flow. Preterm rupture of the amniochorionic membrane occurs in approximately 10% of pregnancies and is the most common cause of oligohydramnios. In the presence of renal agenesis (failure of kidney formation), the lack of fetal urine in the amniotic fluid is the main cause of oligohydramnios. A similar decrease in amniotic fluid occurs with obstructive uropathy (urinary tract obstruction). Complications of oligohydramnios include fetal abnormalities (pulmonary hypoplasia, facial defects, and limb defects) caused by fetal compression by the uterine wall.

A high volume of amniotic fluid is termed *polyhydramnios*. Most cases of polyhydramnios (60%) are idiopathic (of unknown cause); 20% of cases are caused by maternal factors, whereas 20% are fetal in origin. Polyhydramnios may be associated with severe anomalies of the central nervous system, such as meroencephaly or anencephaly (see Chapter 16). With other anomalies, such as esophageal atresia, amniotic fluid accumulates because it cannot pass to the fetal stomach and the intestines for absorption.

chorionic membrane into the maternal tissue fluid and into the uterine capillaries. An exchange of fluid with fetal blood also occurs through the umbilical cord and at the site where the amnion adheres to the chorionic plate on the fetal surface of the placenta (see Figs. 8-5 and 8-9*B*); thus, amniotic fluid is in balance with the fetal circulation.

Amniotic fluid is swallowed by the fetus and absorbed by the fetus's respiratory and digestive tracts. It has been estimated that during the final stages of pregnancy, the fetus swallows up to 400 mL of amniotic fluid daily. The fluid passes into the fetal bloodstream, and the waste products in it cross the placental membrane and enter the maternal blood in the intervillous space. Excess water in the fetal blood is excreted by the fetal kidneys and returned to the amniotic sac through the fetal urinary tract.

Virtually all of the fluid in the amniotic cavity is water, in which undissolved material (such as desquamated fetal epithelial cells) is suspended. Amniotic fluid contains approximately equal portions of dissolved organic and inorganic salts. Half of the organic constituents are protein; the other half is composed of carbohydrates, fats, enzymes, hormones, and pigments. As pregnancy advances, the composition of the amniotic fluid changes as fetal excreta (*meconium* and urine) are added. Because fetal urine enters the amniotic fluid, fetal enzyme systems, amino acids, hormones, and other substances can be studied by examining fluid removed by **amniocentesis**. Studies of cells in the amniotic fluid permit the detection of chromosomal abnormalities.

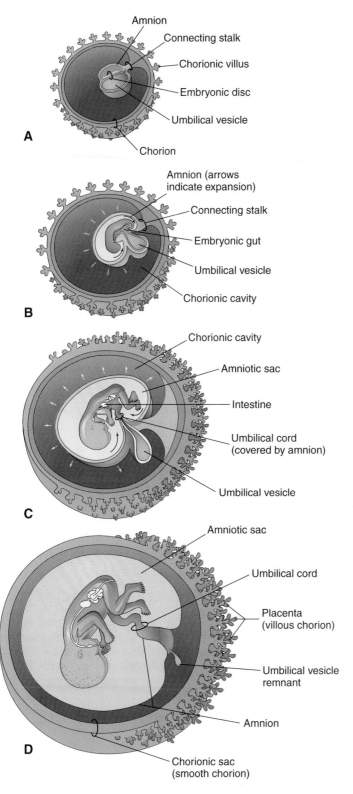

A

B

C

D

FIGURE 8-14. Illustrations of how the amnion enlarges, fills the chorionic sac, and envelops the umbilical cord. Observe that part of the umbilical vesicle (yolk sac) is incorporated into the embryo as the primordial gut. Formation of the fetal part of the placenta and degeneration of the chorionic villi are also shown. **A,** At 3 weeks. **B,** At 4 weeks. **C,** At 10 weeks. **D,** At 20 weeks.

Significance of the Amniotic Fluid

The amniotic fluid:
- Permits symmetrical external growth of the embryo
- Acts as a barrier to infection
- Permits fetal lung development
- Prevents adherence of the amnion to the embryo
- Cushions the embryo against injuries by distributing impacts that the mother may receive
- Helps to control embryonic body temperature by maintaining a relatively constant temperature
- Enables the fetus to move freely, thereby aiding muscular development (e.g., in the limbs)
- Assists in maintaining homeostasis of fluid and electrolytes

FIGURE 8-15. **A,** A fetus with amniotic band syndrome, showing amniotic bands constricting the left arm. **B,** Illustrations of the structures shown in **A.** (**A,** Courtesy of Professor V. Becker, Pathologisches Institut der Universität, Erlangen, Germany.)

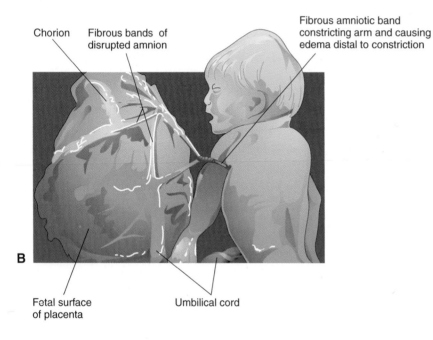

Chorion   Fibrous bands of disrupted amnion

Fibrous amniotic band constricting arm and causing edema distal to constriction

Fetal surface of placenta   Umbilical cord

PREMATURE RUPTURE OF THE FETAL MEMBRANES

Premature rupture of the amniochorionic membrane is the most common event leading to premature labor and delivery and the most common complication resulting in oligohydramnios. Loss of amniotic fluid removes the major protection the fetus has against infection. Rupture of the membrane may cause various fetal anomalies that constitute amniotic band syndrome, or amniotic band disruption complex. These anomalies are associated with a variety of abnormalities, ranging from digital constriction to major scalp, craniofacial, and visceral defects. The cause of these anomalies is probably related to constriction by encircling amniotic bands (Fig. 8-15). The incidence of amniotic band syndrome is approximately 1 in 1200 live births. Prenatal ultrasound diagnosis of amniotic band syndrome is possible.

■ THE UMBILICAL VESICLE (YOLK SAC)

The umbilical vesicle (yolk sac) can be observed sonographically early in the fifth week. Early development of the umbilical vesicle was described in Chapter 4. At 32 days, the umbilical vesicle is large (see Fig. 8-1C). By 10 weeks, the umbilical vesicle has shrunk to a pear-shaped remnant approximately 5 mm in diameter (see Fig. 8-14C). By 20 weeks, the umbilical vesicle is very small (see Fig. 8-14D).

Significance of the Umbilical Vesicle

The umbilical vesicle is nonfunctional as far as yolk storage is concerned (hence the name change), but its presence is essential for several reasons:
● It has a role in the *transfer of nutrients* to the embryo during the second and third weeks before the uteroplacental circulation is established.
● *Blood* first develops in the well-vascularized, extraembryonic mesoderm covering the wall of the umbilical vesicle beginning in the third week (see

Chapter 5), and it continues to develop there until hematopoietic activity begins in the liver during the sixth week.
● During the fourth week, the dorsal part of the umbilical vesicle is incorporated into the embryo as the *primordial gut* (see Fig. 6-1). Its endoderm, derived from the epiblast, gives rise to the epithelium of the trachea, bronchi, lungs, and alimentary tract.
● *Primordial germ cells* appear in the endodermal lining of the wall of the umbilical vesicle in the third week and subsequently migrate to the developing gonads (see Chapter 13). They differentiate into the spermatogonia in males and the oogonia in females.

■ THE ALLANTOIS

Although the allantois is not functional in human embryos, it is important for three reasons:
● Blood formation occurs in its wall during the third to fifth weeks of development.
● Its blood vessels become the umbilical vein and arteries (Fig. 8-16*A* and *B*).

● The intraembryonic portion of the allantois runs from the umbilicus to the urinary bladder, with which it is continuous (see Fig. 8-16*B*). As the bladder enlarges, the allantois involutes to form a thick tube, the *urachus* (see Fig. 8-16*C*). After birth, the urachus becomes a fibrous cord, the *median umbilical ligament*, which extends from the apex of the urinary bladder to the umbilicus (see Fig. 8-16*D*).

■ FETAL MEMBRANES IN MULTIPLE PREGNANCIES

Multiple gestations are associated with higher risks of fetal morbidity and mortality than single gestations. The risks are progressively greater as the number of fetuses increases. In North America, *twins* normally occur approximately once in every 85 pregnancies, *triplets* approximately once in every 90^2 pregnancies, *quadruplets* approximately once in every 90^3 pregnancies, and *quintuplets* approximately once in every 90^4 pregnancies.

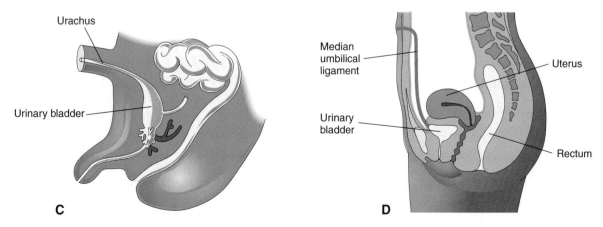

FIGURE 8-16. Development and the usual fate of the allantois. **A,** A 3-week embryo. **B,** A 9-week fetus. **C,** A 3-month male fetus. **D,** Adult female. The nonfunctional allantois forms the urachus in the fetus and the median umbilical ligament in the adult.

FIGURE 8-17. Dizygotic twins developing from two zygotes. The relationship of the fetal membranes and placentas are shown for instances in which the blastocysts implant separately (**A**) and the blastocysts implant close together (**B**). In both cases, there are two amnions and two chorions. The placentas are usually fused when they implant close together.

Twins and Fetal Membranes

Twins that originate from two zygotes are **dizygotic (DZ) twins**, or fraternal twins (Fig. 8-17), whereas twins that originate from one zygote are **monozygotic (MZ) twins**, or identical twins (Fig. 8-18). The fetal membranes and placentas vary according to the origin of the twins. *Approximately two thirds of twins are dizygotic, and the rate of DZ twinning increases with maternal age.*

The study of twins is important in human genetics because it is useful for comparing the effects of genes and environment on development. If an abnormal condition

ANASTOMOSIS OF THE PLACENTAL BLOOD VESSELS

Anastomoses between the blood vessels of the fused placentas of DZ twins occur and may result in *erythrocytic mosaicism*. In such cases, the DZ twins have red blood cells of two different types because of the exchange of red blood cells between the two circulations.

FIGURE 8-18. Illustrations of how approximately 65% of monozygotic twins develop from one zygote by division of the inner cell mass. These twins always have separate amnions, a single chorionic sac, and a common placenta. If there is anastomosis of the placental vessels, one twin may receive most of the nutrition from the placenta (see Fig. 8-19).

TWIN TRANSFUSION SYNDROME

Twin transfusion syndrome occurs in 15% to 30% of monochorionic-diamniotic MZ twins. Arterial blood may be preferentially shunted from one twin through arteriovenous anastomoses in the placenta into the venous circulation of the other twin. The donor twin is small, pale, and anemic (Fig. 8-19), whereas the recipient twin is large and polycythemic (i.e., having a higher than normal red blood cell count). The placenta shows similar abnormalities; the part of the placenta supplying the anemic twin is pale, whereas the part supplying the polycythemic twin is dark red. In lethal cases, death results from anemia in the donor twin and from congestive heart failure in the recipient twin.

does not show a simple genetic pattern, comparison of its incidence in MZ and DZ twins may show that heredity is involved.

Dizygotic Twins

Because they result from the fertilization of two oocytes by two sperms, DZ twins may be of the same sex or different

FIGURE 8-19. Monozygotic, monochorionic-diamniotic twins. Note the wide discrepancy in size resulting from an uncompensated arteriovenous anastomosis of the placental vessels. Blood was shunted from the smaller twin to the larger one, producing twin transfusion syndrome.

Separate chorionic sacs

Diamniotic dichorionic separate placentas

Two blastocysts

Two morulas

Two-cell stage

Zygote

Two chorions   Two amnions

Separate placentas

Fused chorions   Two amnions

Diamniotic dichorionic fused placentas

Fused chorionic sacs

Fused placentas

FIGURE 8-20. Illustrations of how approximately 35% of monozygotic twins develop from one zygote. Separation of the blastomeres may occur at any point from the two-cell stage to the morula stage, producing two identical blastocysts. Each embryo subsequently develops its own amniotic and chorionic sacs. The placentas may be separate or fused. In most cases, there is a single placenta resulting from secondary fusion, whereas in fewer cases, there are two placentas. In the latter cases, examination of the placenta suggests that they are dizygotic twins. This explains why some monozygotic twins are incorrectly classified as dizygotic twins at birth.

sexes. For the same reason, they are no more alike genetically than brothers or sisters born at different times. *DZ twins always have two amnions and two chorions* (see Fig. 8-17*A*), but the chorions and placentas may be fused (see Fig. 8-17*B*). DZ twinning shows a hereditary tendency. The recurrence risk in families with one set of DZ twins is approximately triple that of the general population. The incidence of DZ twinning shows considerable racial variation, ranging from 1 in 500 in Asian populations, to 1 in 125 in white populations, to as high as 1 in 20 in some African populations.

Monozygotic Twins

Because they result from the fertilization of one oocyte and develop from one zygote (see Fig. 8-18), *MZ twins are of the same sex, are genetically identical, and are similar in physical appearance.* Physical differences between MZ twins are environmentally induced, such as by anastomosis of the placental vessels, resulting in differences in blood supply from the placenta (see Fig. 8-19). MZ twinning usually begins in the blastocyst stage, approximately at the end of the first week, and results from division of the embryoblast

into two embryonic primordia (see Fig. 8-18). Subsequently, two embryos, each in its own amniotic sac, develop within one chorionic sac and share a common placenta, a monochorionic-diamniotic twin placenta. Uncommonly, early separation of the embryonic blastomeres (e.g., during the two- to eight-cell stage) results in MZ twins with two amnions, two chorions, and two placentas that may or may not be fused (Fig. 8-20). In such cases, it is impossible to determine, from the membranes alone, whether the twins are monozygotic or dizygotic.

Other Types of Multiple Births

Triplets may be derived from:
● One zygote and be identical
● Two zygotes and consist of identical twins and a singleton
● Three zygotes and be of the same sex or of different sexes, in which case the infants are no more similar than infants from three separate pregnancies

Similar combinations occur in quadruplets, quintuplets, sextuplets, and septuplets.

ESTABLISHING THE ZYGOSITY OF TWINS

Establishment of the zygosity of twins has become important, particularly because of the introduction of tissue and organ transplantation (e.g., bone marrow transplants). Twin zygosity is now determined by molecular testing. Any two people who are not MZ twins are virtually certain to show differences in some of the large number of DNA markers that can be studied.

Late division of the early embryonic cells (i.e., division of the embryonic disc during the second week) results in MZ twins with one amniotic sac and one chorionic sac. A monochorionic-monoamniotic twin placenta is associated with a fetal mortality rate approaching 50%. The umbilical cords are frequently so entangled that circulation of the blood through their vessels ceases, and one or both fetuses die. Ultrasonography plays an important role in the diagnosis of twin pregnancies and the management of various conditions that may complicate MZ twinning, such as intrauterine growth restriction, intrauterine fetal distress, and premature labor.

CLINICALLY ORIENTED QUESTIONS

1. What is meant by the term *stillbirth*? Do older women have more stillborn infants?
2. An infant was born dead, reportedly because of a "cord accident." What does this mean? Do these accidents always kill the infant? If not, what defects may be present?
3. What is the scientific basis of the home pregnancy tests that are sold in drugstores?
4. What is the proper name for what laypeople sometimes refer to as the *bag of waters*? What is meant by a *dry birth*? Does premature rupture of this "bag" induce the birth of the infant?

EARLY DEATH OF A TWIN

Because ultrasonographic studies are a common part of prenatal care, it is known that early death with resorption of one member of a twin pair is fairly common. This possibility must be considered when discrepancies occur between prenatal cytogenetic findings and the karyotype of an infant. Errors in the prenatal cytogenetic diagnosis may occur if extra-embryonic tissues (e.g., part of a chorionic villus) from the resorbed twin are examined.

CONJOINED TWINS

If the embryonic disc does not divide completely, various types of conjoined (MZ) twins may form. These twins are named according to the regions of the body that are attached; for example, *thoracopagus* indicates anterior union of the thoracic regions. In some cases, the twins are connected to each other by skin only or by cutaneous and other tissues, such as fused livers. Some conjoined twins can be separated successfully by surgery. The incidence of conjoined twins is 1 in 50,000 to 1 in 100,000 births.

5. What does the term *fetal distress* mean? How is the condition recognized? What causes fetal distress?
6. Some say that twins are born more commonly to older mothers. Is this true? Others maintain that twinning is hereditary. Is this correct?

The answers to these questions are at the back of the book.

BODY CAVITIES AND MESENTERIES

Early in the fourth week, the **intraembryonic coelom**—the primordium of the embryonic body cavity—appears as a horseshoe-shaped cavity in the cardiogenic and lateral mesoderm (Fig. 9-1*A*). The bend in this cavity at the cranial end of the embryo represents the future *pericardial cavity*, and its limbs indicate the future *pleural and peritoneal cavities*. The distal part of each limb of the intraembryonic coelom is continuous with the **extraembryonic coelom** at the lateral edges of the embryonic disc (see Fig. 9-1*B*). This communication is important because most of the midgut normally herniates through this communication into the umbilical cord. The intraembryonic coelom provides room for the organs to develop and move. During embryonic lateral folding, the limbs of the coelom are brought together on the ventral aspect of the embryo (Fig. 9-2*A* to *F*).

■ **THE EMBRYONIC BODY CAVITY**

The intraembryonic coelom gives rise to three well-defined body cavities during the fourth week (see Figs. 9-2 and 9-4): a *pericardial cavity*, two *pericardioperitoneal canals* connecting the pericardial and the peritoneal cavities, and a large *peritoneal cavity*.

These body cavities are lined by the mesothelium—a parietal wall derived from the somatic mesoderm and a visceral wall derived from the splanchnic mesoderm (Fig. 9-3*E*). The mesothelium forms the major portion of the peritoneum. The **peritoneal cavity** is connected to the extraembryonic coelom at the umbilicus (see Fig. 9-4*C* and *D*). The peritoneal cavity loses its connection with the extraembryonic coelom during the 10th week, after the intestines return to the abdomen from the umbilical cord (see Chapter 12). During the formation of the head fold, the heart and the **pericardial cavity** move ventrocaudally, anterior to the foregut (see Fig. 9-2*A*, *B*, *D*, and *E*). As a result, the pericardial cavity opens into the **pericardioperitoneal canals**, which pass dorsal to the

foregut (see Fig. 9-4*B* and *D*). After embryonic folding, the caudal parts of the foregut, midgut, and hindgut are suspended in the peritoneal cavity from the dorsal abdominal wall by the **dorsal mesentery** (see Figs. 9-2F and 9-3*B* to *E*).

Mesenteries

A mesentery is a double layer of peritoneum that begins as an extension of the visceral peritoneum that covers an organ; it connects the organ to the body wall and conveys its vessels and nerves. Transiently, the dorsal and ventral mesenteries divide the peritoneal cavity into right and left halves (see Fig. 9-3*C*). However, the ventral mesentery soon disappears (see Fig. 9-3*E*), except where it is attached to the caudal part of the foregut. The peritoneal cavity then becomes a continuous space (see Figs. 9-3*A* and 9-4*D*). The arteries that supply the primordial gut—the *celiac arterial trunk* (foregut), the *superior mesenteric artery* (midgut), and the *inferior mesenteric artery* (hindgut)—pass between the layers of the dorsal mesentery (see Fig. 9-3*C*).

Division of the Embryonic Body Cavity

Each pericardioperitoneal canal lies lateral to the foregut and dorsal to the **septum transversum**—a thick plate of mesoderm that occupies the space between the thoracic cavity and the omphaloenteric duct (see Fig. 9-4*A* and *B*). The septum transversum is the primordium of the **central tendon of the diaphragm**. Partitions form in each pericardioperitoneal canal, separating the pericardial cavity from the pleural cavities and the pleural cavities from the peritoneal cavity (see Fig. 9-3*A*). Because of the growth of the **bronchial buds** (primordia of the bronchi and lungs) into the pericardioperitoneal canals (Fig. 9-5*A*), a pair of membranous ridges is produced in the lateral wall of each

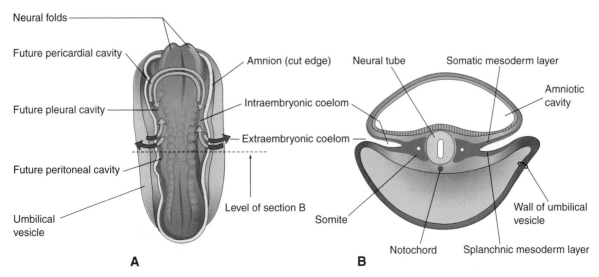

FIGURE 9-1. **A,** Dorsal view of a 22-day embryo, showing the outline of the horseshoe-shaped intraembryonic coelom. The amnion has been removed, and the coelom is shown as if the embryo were translucent. The continuity of the intraembryonic coelom, as well as the communication of its right and left limbs with the extraembryonic coelom, is indicated by *arrows*. **B,** Transverse section through the embryo at the level shown in **A**.

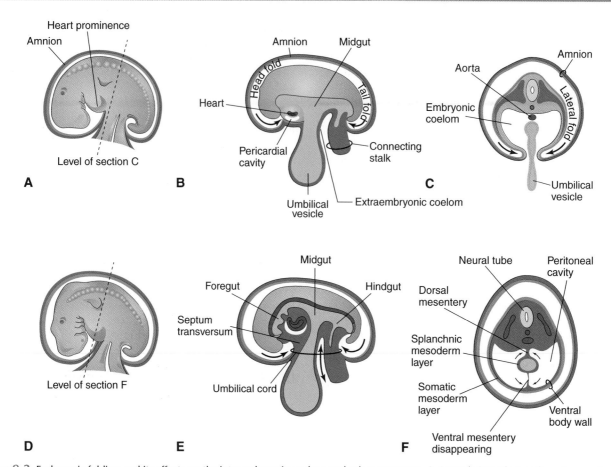

FIGURE 9-2. Embryonic folding and its effects on the intraembryonic coelom and other structures. **A,** Lateral view of an embryo (approximately 26 days). **B,** Schematic sagittal section of the embryo, showing the head and tail folds. **C,** Transverse section at the level shown in **A,** indicating how fusion of the lateral folds gives the embryo a cylindric form. **D,** Lateral view of an embryo (approximately 28 days). **E,** Schematic sagittal section of the embryo, showing the reduced communication between the intraembryonic and extraembryonic coeloms (*double-headed arrow*). **F,** Transverse section, as indicated in **D,** showing the formation of the ventral body wall and the disappearance of the ventral mesentery. The *arrows* indicate the junction of the somatic and the splanchnic layers of the mesoderm. The somatic mesoderm will become the parietal peritoneum lining the abdominal wall, and the splanchnic mesoderm will become the visceral peritoneum covering the organs (e.g., stomach).

canal. The cranial ridges—the *pleuropericardial folds*—are located superior to the developing lungs. The caudal ridges—the *pleuroperitoneal folds*—are located inferior to the lungs.

As the **pleuropericardial folds** enlarge, they form partitions that separate the pericardial cavity from the pleural cavities. These partitions—**pleuropericardial membranes**—contain the **common cardinal veins** (see Fig. 9-5*A* and *B*). These large veins drain the primordial venous system into the sinus venosus of the primordial heart (see Chapter 14). Initially, the **bronchial buds** are small relative to the heart and the pericardial cavity (see Fig. 9-5*A*). Subsequently, they grow laterally from the caudal end of the trachea into the pericardioperitoneal canals (future pleural canals). As the **primordial pleural cavities** expand ventrally around the heart, they extend into the body wall, splitting the mesenchyme into two layers: (1) an outer layer that becomes the thoracic wall and (2) an inner layer (the pleuropericardial membrane) that becomes the fibrous pericardium, the outer layer of the pericardial sac that encloses the heart (see Fig. 9-5*C* and *D*).

The *pleuropericardial membranes* project into the cranial ends of the **pericardioperitoneal canals** (see Fig. 9-5*B*). With subsequent growth of the common cardinal veins,

descent of the heart, and expansion of the pleural cavities, the pleuropericardial membranes become mesentery-like folds that extend from the lateral thoracic wall. By the seventh week, the pleuropericardial membranes fuse with the mesenchyme ventral to the esophagus, forming the **primordial mediastinum** and separating the pericardial cavity from the pleural cavities (see Fig. 9-5*C*). The right pleuropericardial opening closes slightly earlier than the left one.

As the **pleuroperitoneal folds** enlarge, they project into the pericardioperitoneal canals. Gradually, the folds become membranous, forming the **pleuroperitoneal membranes** (Fig. 9-6*B* and *C*). Eventually, these membranes separate the pleural cavities from the peritoneal cavity. The *pleuroperitoneal membranes* are produced as the developing lungs and pleural cavities expand and invade the body wall. They are attached dorsolaterally to the abdominal wall and, initially, their crescentic free edges project into the caudal ends of the **pericardioperitoneal canals**. They become relatively more prominent as the lungs enlarge cranially and the liver expands caudally. During the sixth week, the pleuroperitoneal membranes extend ventromedially until their free edges fuse with the dorsal mesentery of the esophagus and the septum transversum (see Fig.

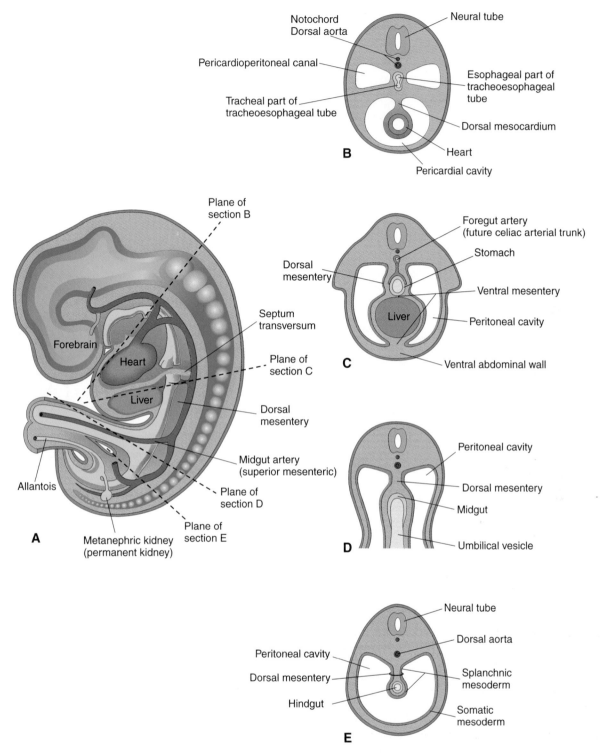

FIGURE 9-3. Mesenteries and body cavities at the beginning of the fifth week. **A,** Schematic sagittal section. Note that the dorsal mesentery serves as a pathway for the arteries that supply the developing gut. Nerves and lymphatics also pass between the layers of this mesentery. **B** to **E,** Transverse sections through the embryo at the levels shown in **A.** The ventral mesentery disappears, except in the region of the terminal esophagus, stomach, and first part of the duodenum. Note that the right and left parts of the peritoneal cavity, which are separate in **C,** are continuous in **E.**

9-6C). This membrane separates the pleural cavities from the peritoneal cavity. *Closure of the pleuroperitoneal openings* is assisted by the migration of myoblasts (primordial muscle cells) into the pleuroperitoneal membranes. The pleuroperitoneal opening on the right side closes slightly before the left one.

■ DEVELOPMENT OF THE DIAPHRAGM

The diaphragm is a dome-shaped, musculotendinous partition that separates the thoracic and abdominal cavities. It is a composite structure that develops from four embryonic components (see Fig. 9-6):

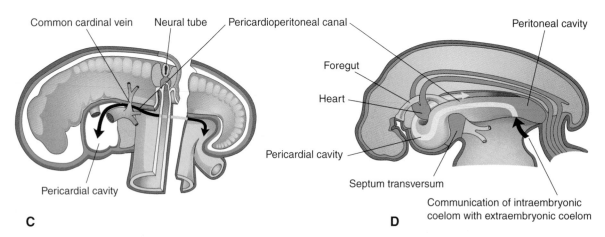

FIGURE 9-4. Illustration of an embryo (approximately 24 days). **A,** The lateral wall of the pericardial cavity has been removed to show the primordial heart. **B,** Transverse section of the embryo, showing the relationship of the pericardioperitoneal canals to the septum transversum and the foregut. **C,** Lateral view of the embryo, with the heart removed. The embryo has also been sectioned transversely to show the continuity of the intraembryonic and extraembryonic coeloms *(black arrow).* **D,** Illustration of the pericardioperitoneal canals that arise from the dorsal wall of the pericardial cavity and pass on each side of the foregut to join the peritoneal cavity. The *arrow* shows the communication of the extraembryonic coelom with the intraembryonic coelom and the continuity of the intraembryonic coelom at this stage.

● The septum transversum
● The pleuroperitoneal membranes
● The dorsal mesentery of the esophagus
● The lateral body walls

Septum Transversum

The transverse septum, which is composed of mesodermal tissue, is the **primordium of the central tendon of the diaphragm** (see Fig. 9-6*D* and *E*). The septum transversum grows dorsally from the ventrolateral body wall and forms a semicircular shelf that separates the heart from the liver. A large part of the liver is embedded in the septum transversum during its early development. The septum transversum is located caudal to the pericardial cavity and partially separates it from the developing peritoneal cavity. After the head folds ventrally during the fourth week, the septum transversum forms a thick, but incomplete partition between the pericardial and abdominal cavities (Fig. 9-4). The septum transversum expands and fuses with the mesenchyme ventral to the

esophagus and the pleuroperitoneal membranes (see Fig. 9-6*C*).

Pleuroperitoneal Membranes

The pleuroperitoneal membranes fuse with the dorsal mesentery of the esophagus and the septum transversum (see Fig. 9-6*C*). This fusion completes the partition between the thoracic and abdominal cavities and forms the **primordial diaphragm.** Although the pleuroperitoneal membranes form large portions of the fetal diaphragm, they represent relatively small parts of the newborn infant's diaphragm (see Fig. 9-6*E*).

Dorsal Mesentery of the Esophagus

The septum transversum and the pleuroperitoneal membranes fuse with the dorsal mesentery of the esophagus. This mesentery becomes the median portion of the diaphragm. The **crura of the diaphragm**—a pair of

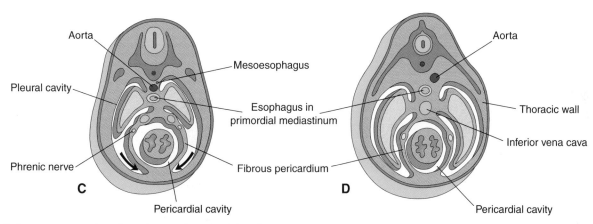

FIGURE 9-5. Transverse sections through an embryo cranial to the septum transversum, showing successive stages in the separation of the pleural cavities from the pericardial cavity. Growth and development of the lungs, expansion of the pleural cavities, and formation of the fibrous pericardium are also shown. **A,** At 5 weeks. The *arrows* indicate the communications between the pericardioperitoneal canals and the pericardial cavity. **B,** At 6 weeks. The *arrows* indicate the development of the pleural cavities as they expand into the body wall. **C,** At 7 weeks. Expansion of the pleural cavities ventrally *(arrows)* around the heart is evident. The pleuropericardial membranes are now fused in the median plane with each other and with the mesoderm ventral to the esophagus. **D,** At 8 weeks. Continued expansion of the lungs and the pleural cavities and formation of the fibrous pericardium and the thoracic wall are shown.

diverging muscle bundles that cross in the median plane anterior to the aorta (see Fig. 9-6*E*)—develop from myoblasts that grow into the dorsal mesentery of the esophagus.

Lateral Body Walls

During the 9th to 12th weeks, the lungs and pleural cavities enlarge, "burrowing" into the lateral body walls (see Fig. 9-5). During this process, the tissue of the body wall is split into two layers:

- An external layer that becomes part of the definitive thoracic and abdominal wall
- An internal layer that contributes muscle to the peripheral portions of the diaphragm, external to the parts derived from the pleuroperitoneal membranes (see Fig. 9-6*D* and *E*)

Further extension of the developing pleural cavities into the lateral body walls forms the right and left **costodia-phragmatic recesses** (Fig. 9-7), establishing the characteristic dome-shaped configuration of the diaphragm.

Positional Changes and Innervation of the Diaphragm

During the fourth week of development, the septum transversum lies opposite the third to fifth cervical somites (Fig. 9-8*A*). During the fifth week, myoblasts (primordial muscle cells that differentiate into skeletal muscle) from these somites migrate into the developing diaphragm, bringing their nerve fibers with them. Consequently, the **phrenic nerves** that supply motor innervation to the diaphragm arise from the ventral primary rami of the third, fourth, and fifth cervical spinal nerves, which join together on each side to form a phrenic nerve. The phrenic nerves also supply sensory fibers to the superior and inferior surfaces of the right and left domes of the diaphragm.

Rapid growth of the dorsal part of the embryo's body results in an *apparent descent of the diaphragm*. By the sixth week, the developing diaphragm is at the level of the thoracic somites (see Fig. 9-8*B*). The phrenic nerves now have a descending course. By the beginning of the eighth week, the dorsal part of the diaphragm lies at the level of the first lumbar vertebra (see Fig. 9-8*C*). The

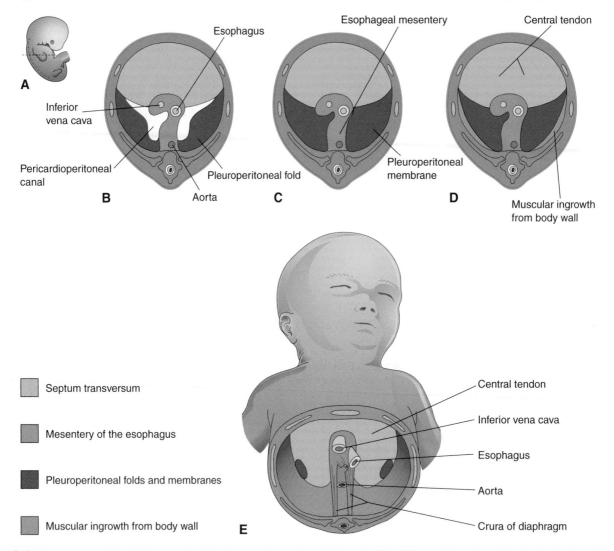

FIGURE 9-6. Development of the diaphragm. **A,** Lateral view of an embryo at the end of the fifth week (actual size), indicating the level of sections in **B** to **D**. **B** to **E** show the developing diaphragm as viewed inferiorly. **B,** Transverse section, showing the unfused pleuroperitoneal membranes. **C,** Similar section at the end of the sixth week, after fusion of the pleuroperitoneal membranes with the other two diaphragmatic components. **D,** Transverse section of a 12-week embryo, after ingrowth of the fourth diaphragmatic component from the body wall. **E,** View of the diaphragm of a newborn infant, indicating the embryologic origin of its components.

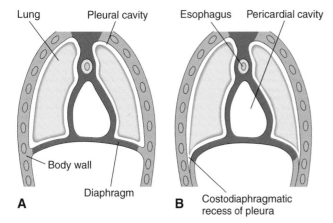

FIGURE 9-7. Extension of the pleural cavities into the body walls to form the peripheral parts of the diaphragm, the costodiaphragmatic recesses, and the characteristic dome-shaped configuration of the diaphragm.

phrenic nerves in the embryo enter the diaphragm by passing through the pleuropericardial membranes. For this reason, the phrenic nerves subsequently lie on the fibrous pericardium, which is derived from the pleuropericardial membranes (see Fig. 9-5C and D).

The costal border of the diaphragm receives sensory fibers from the lower intercostal nerves because of the origin of the peripheral part of the diaphragm from the lateral body walls (Fig. 9-6D and E).

CONGENITAL DIAPHRAGMATIC HERNIA

A posterolateral defect of the diaphragm is the only relatively common congenital anomaly involving the diaphragm (Fig. 9-9A). This diaphragmatic defect occurs in approximately 1 in 2200 newborn infants and is associated with **congenital diaphragmatic hernia**

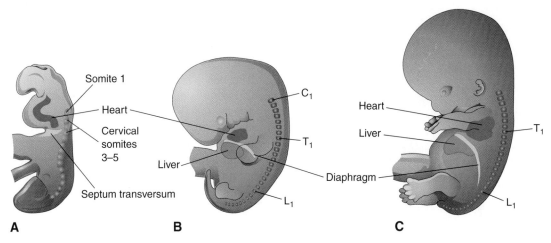

FIGURE 9-8. Positional changes of the developing diaphragm. **A,** At approximately 24 days. The septum transversum is at the level of the third, fourth, and fifth cervical segments. **B,** At approximately 41 days. **C,** At approximately 52 days. C, cervical; T, thoracic; L, lumbar.

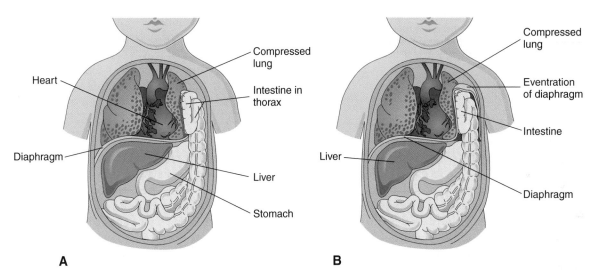

FIGURE 9-9. **A,** A "window view" overlooking the thorax and the abdomen shows the herniation of the intestine into the thorax through a posterolateral defect in the left side of the diaphragm. Note that the left lung is compressed and hypoplastic. **B,** Eventration of the diaphragm resulting from defective muscular development in the diaphragm. The abdominal viscera are displaced into the thorax, along with a pouch of diaphragmatic tissue.

(CDH) [herniation of the abdominal contents into the thoracic cavity].

The *most common cause of pulmonary hypoplasia*, CDH can lead to life-threatening respiratory difficulties. If severe lung hypoplasia is present, some primordial alveoli may rupture, causing air to enter the pleural cavity (*pneumothorax*). Usually unilateral, CDH results from defective formation or fusion of the pleuroperitoneal membrane with the other three parts of the diaphragm (see Fig. 9-6*B*). This defect produces a large opening in the posterolateral region of the diaphragm. If a pleuroperitoneal canal is still open when the intestines return to the abdomen from the umbilical cord in the 10th week, some intestine and other viscera may pass into the thorax. The abdominal viscera in the thorax push the lungs and the heart anteriorly, compressing the lungs. Often the stomach, spleen, and most of the intestines herniate (Figs. 9-9*A* and 9-10). The defect usually occurs on the left side, and it is likely related to the earlier closure of the right pleuroperitoneal opening. Ultrasonographic and magnetic resonance imaging can provide a *prenatal diagnosis* of CDH.

FIGURE 9-10. Diaphragmatic hernia. Note the herniation of the stomach and the small intestine into the thorax through a posterolateral defect in the left side of the diaphragm, similar to that shown in Figure 9-9A. Note that the heart is pushed to the right side of the thorax. (Courtesy of Dr. Nathan E. Wiseman, Professor of Surgery, Children's Hospital, University of Manitoba, Winnipeg, Manitoba, Canada.)

EVENTRATION OF THE DIAPHRAGM

In the uncommon condition of **diaphragmatic eventration,** part of the diaphragm has defective musculature, causing it to balloon into the thoracic cavity as an aponeurotic (membranous) sheet, forming a large diaphragmatic pouch (see Fig. 9-9B). Consequently, the abdominal viscera are displaced superiorly into the pocket-like outpouching of the diaphragm. This congenital anomaly results mainly from failure of the muscular tissue from the body wall to extend into the pleuroperitoneal membrane on the affected side.

RETROSTERNAL (PARASTERNAL) HERNIA

Herniations may occur through the sternocostal hiatus, the opening for the superior epigastric vessels in the retrosternal area. This hiatus is located between the sternal and the costal parts of the diaphragm. Herniation of the intestine into the pericardial sac may occur or, conversely, part of the heart may descend into the peritoneal cavity in the epigastric region. Large defects are commonly associated with body wall defects in the umbilical region (e.g., omphalocele; see Chapter 12).

CLINICALLY ORIENTED QUESTIONS

1. There have been reports of an infant who was born with its stomach and liver in its chest. Is this possible?
2. Can an infant with most of its abdominal viscera in the chest survive? Some say that diaphragmatic defects can be operated on before birth. Is this true?
3. Do the lungs develop normally in infants who are born with a congenital diaphragmatic hernia?
4. A man underwent routine chest radiography approximately 1 year ago and was told that a small part of his small intestine was in his chest. Is it possible for him to have a congenital diaphragmatic hernia without being aware of it? Would his lung on the affected side be normal?

The answers to these questions are at the back of the book.

10

PHARYNGEAL APPARATUS

The **pharyngeal (branchial) apparatus** (Fig. 10-1) consists of the following: *pharyngeal arches, pharyngeal pouches, pharyngeal grooves,* and *pharyngeal membranes.*

These embryonic structures contribute to the formation of the head and neck. Most congenital anomalies in these regions originate during transformation of the pharyngeal apparatus into its adult derivatives.

■ PHARYNGEAL ARCHES

The pharyngeal arches begin to develop early in the fourth week as **neural crest cells** migrate from the hindbrain into the future head and neck regions. Initially, each pharyngeal arch consists of a core of mesenchyme (embryonic connective tissue) and is covered externally by ectoderm and internally by endoderm (see Fig. 10-1*D* and *E*). The first pair of arches, the primordia of the jaws, appears as surface elevations lateral to the developing pharynx (see Fig. 10-1*A* and *B*). Other arches soon appear as obliquely disposed, rounded ridges on each side of the future head and neck regions (see Fig. 10-1*C*). By the end of the fourth week, four well-defined pairs of arches are visible (Fig. 10-1*A*).

The pharyngeal arches support the lateral walls of the primordial pharynx, which is derived from the cranial part of the foregut. The primordial mouth, or **stomodeum,**

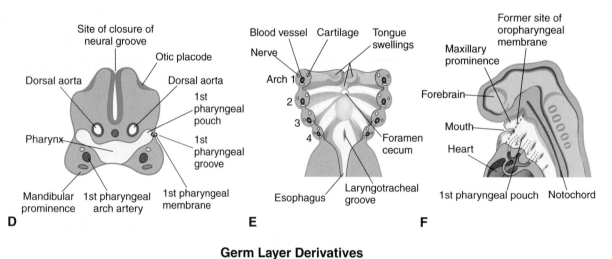

Germ Layer Derivatives

Ectoderm   Endoderm   Mesoderm

FIGURE 10-1. Illustrations of the human pharyngeal apparatus. **A,** Lateral view showing the development of four pharyngeal arches. **B** and **C,** Ventral or facial views showing the relationship of the pharyngeal arches to the stomodeum. **D,** Frontal section through the cranial region of an embryo. **E,** Horizontal section showing the arch components and the floor of the primordial pharynx. **F,** Sagittal section of the cranial region of an embryo, showing the openings of the pharyngeal pouches in the lateral wall of the primordial pharynx.

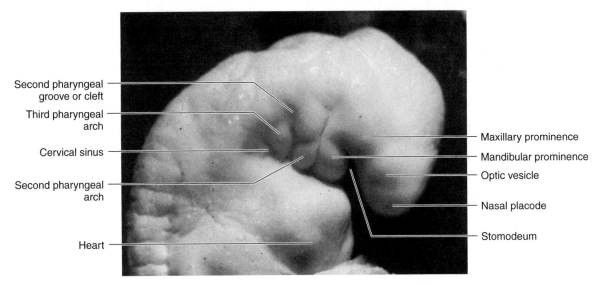

Second pharyngeal groove or cleft

Third pharyngeal arch

Cervical sinus

Second pharyngeal arch

Heart

Maxillary prominence

Mandibular prominence

Optic vesicle

Nasal placode

Stomodeum

FIGURE 10-2. A Carnegie stage 13, 4¹/₂-week human embryo. (Courtesy of the late Professor Emeritus Dr. K.V. Hinrichsen, Medizinische Fakultät, Institut für Anatomie, Ruhr-Universität Bochum, Bochum, Germany.)

initially appears as a slight depression of the surface ectoderm (see Fig. 10-1B). It is separated from the cavity of the primordial pharynx by a bilaminar membrane—the **oropharyngeal membrane**—composed of ectoderm externally and endoderm internally. The oropharyngeal membrane ruptures at approximately 26 days, bringing the primordial pharynx and foregut into communication with the amniotic cavity (see Fig. 10-1B and C). The pharyngeal arches contribute extensively to the formation of the face, nasal cavities, mouth, larynx, pharynx, and neck (Figs. 10-2, 10-3 and 10-4). During the fifth week of development, the second pharyngeal arch enlarges and overgrows the third and fourth arches, forming an ectodermal depression known as the **cervical sinus** (see Fig. 10-4A to D). By the end of the seventh week, the second to fourth pharyngeal grooves and the cervical sinus have disappeared, giving the neck a smooth contour.

The **first pharyngeal arch** develops two prominences (see Figs. 10-1B and 10-2):
● The smaller **maxillary prominence** gives rise to the maxilla (upper jaw), the zygomatic bone, and the squamous part of the temporal bone.
● The larger **mandibular prominence** forms the mandible (lower jaw).

The **second pharyngeal arch** makes a major contribution to the formation of the hyoid bone (Fig. 10-5B).

Pharyngeal Arch Components

A typical pharyngeal arch has the following components (see Fig. 10-3A and B):
● A **pharyngeal arch artery** (aortic arch artery) that arises from the truncus arteriosus of the primordial heart and runs around the primordial pharynx to enter the dorsal aorta
● A **cartilaginous rod** that forms the skeleton of the arch
● A **muscular component** that is the primordium of the muscles in the head and neck

● A **nerve** that supplies the mucosa and muscles derived from the arch

Derivatives of the Pharyngeal Arch Arteries

The transformation of the pharyngeal arch arteries into the adult arterial pattern of the head and neck is described in the section on the pharyngeal arch artery derivatives in Chapter 14. Blood in the pharyngeal arch arteries supplies the pharyngeal arches and then enters the **dorsal aorta** (see Fig. 10-3A).

Derivatives of the Pharyngeal Arch Cartilages

Refer to Figure 10-5 and Table 10-1. The dorsal end of the **first pharyngeal arch cartilage** (Meckel cartilage) becomes ossified to form two middle ear bones, the **malleus** and the **incus**. The middle section of the cartilage regresses, but its *perichondrium* forms the **anterior ligament of the malleus** and the **sphenomandibular ligament**. Ventral parts of the first arch cartilages form the primordium of the mandible. Each half of the mandible forms lateral to and in close association with its cartilage. The cartilage disappears as the mandible develops around it by *intramembranous ossification*.

The dorsal end of the **second pharyngeal arch cartilage** ossifies to form the **stapes** of the middle ear and the styloid process of the temporal bone. The part of the cartilage between the **styloid process** and the hyoid bone regresses; its perichondrium forms the **stylohyoid ligament**. The ventral end of the second arch cartilage ossifies to form the lesser cornu and the superior part of the body of the **hyoid bone**.

The **third pharyngeal arch cartilage** ossifies to form the greater cornu and the inferior part of the body of the hyoid bone. The **fourth and sixth pharyngeal arch cartilages** fuse to form the laryngeal cartilages, except for the epiglottis. The cartilage of the epiglottis develops from the mesenchyme in the **hypopharyngeal eminence** (see Fig. 10-22A to C).

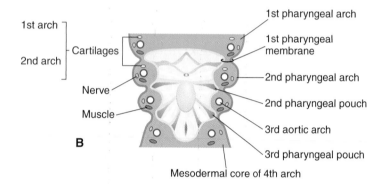

FIGURE 10-3. **A,** Illustration of the pharyngeal pouches and pharyngeal arch arteries (aortic arches). **B,** Horizontal section through the embryo showing the floor of the primordial pharynx and illustrating the germ layer origin of the pharyngeal arch components.

Germ Layer Derivatives

Ectoderm   Endoderm   Mesoderm

TABLE 10-1. Structures Derived from Pharyngeal Arch Components*				
ARCH	**NERVE**	**MUSCLES**	**SKELETAL STRUCTURES**	**LIGAMENTS**
First (mandibular)	Trigeminal[†] (CN V)	Muscles of mastication[‡] Mylohyoid and anterior belly of digastric Tensor tympani Tensor veli palatini	Malleus Incus	Anterior ligament of malleus Sphenomandibular ligament
Second (hyoid)	Facial (CN VII)	Muscles of facial expression[§] Stapedius Stylohyoid Posterior belly of digastric	Stapes Styloid process Lesser cornu of hyoid bone Upper part of body of hyoid bone	Stylohyoid ligament
Third	Glossopharyngeal (CN IX)	Stylopharyngeus	Greater cornu of hyoid bone Lower part of body of hyoid bone	
Fourth and sixth[‖]	Superior laryngeal branch of vagus (CN X) Recurrent laryngeal branch of vagus (CN X)	Cricothyroid Levator veli palatini Constrictors of pharynx Intrinsic muscles of larynx Striated muscles of esophagus	Thyroid cartilage Cricoid cartilage Arytenoid cartilage Corniculate cartilage Cuneiform cartilage	

*The derivatives of the pharyngeal arch arteries are described in Chapter 14.
[†]The ophthalmic division of the fifth cranial nerve (CN V) does not supply any pharyngeal arch components.
[‡]Temporalis, masseter, medial, and lateral pterygoids.
[§]Buccinator, auricularis, frontalis, platysma, and orbicularis oris and oculi.
[‖]The fifth pharyngeal arch regresses. The cartilaginous components of the fourth and sixth arches fuse to form the cartilages of the larynx.

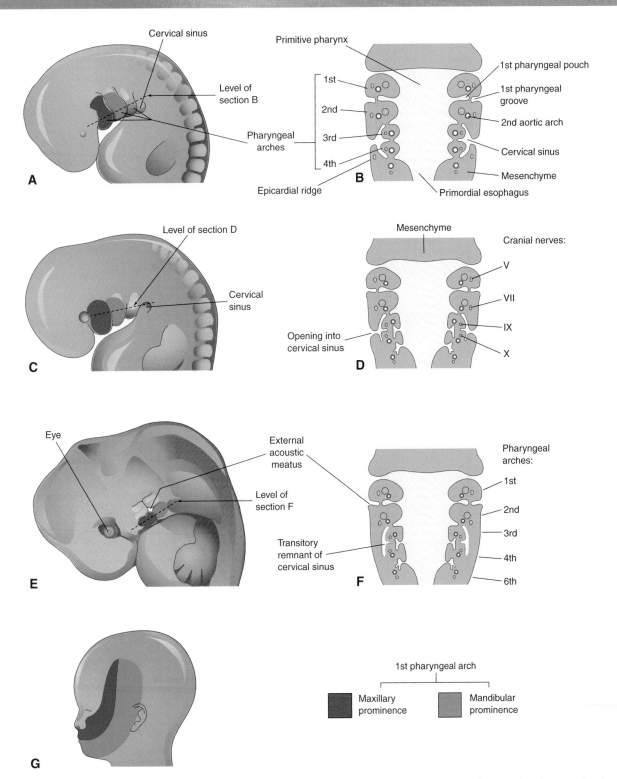

FIGURE 10-4. **A,** Lateral view of the head, neck, and thoracic regions of an embryo (approximately 32 days), showing the pharyngeal arches and the cervical sinus. **B,** Diagrammatic section through the embryo at the level shown in **A,** showing growth of the second arch over the third and fourth arches. **C,** An embryo of approximately 33 days. **D,** Section of the embryo at the level shown in **C,** showing early closure of the cervical sinus. **E,** An embryo of approximately 41 days. **F,** Section of the embryo at the level shown in **E,** showing the transitory cystic remnant of the cervical sinus. **G,** Illustration of a 20-week fetus, showing the area of the face derived from the first pair of pharyngeal arches.

Derivatives of the Pharyngeal Arch Muscles

The muscular components of the arches form various muscles in the head and neck; for example, the musculature of the first pharyngeal arch forms the **muscles of mastication** and others (Fig. 10-6*A* and *B*; see Table 10-1).

Derivatives of the Pharyngeal Arch Nerves

Each arch is supplied by its own cranial nerve (CN). The *special visceral efferent (branchial) components* of the cranial nerves supply muscles derived from the pharyngeal arches (Fig. 10-7*A*; see Table 10-1). Because the mesenchyme

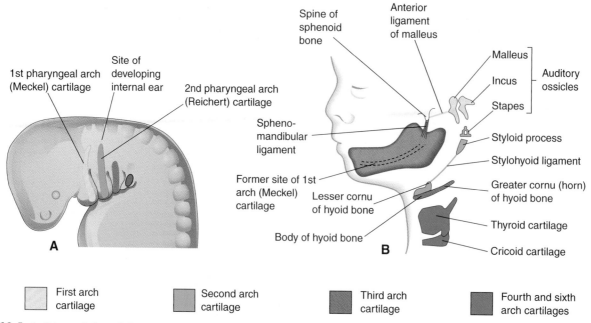

FIGURE 10-5. **A,** Schematic lateral view of the head, neck, and thoracic regions of a 4-week embryo, showing the location of the cartilages in the pharyngeal arches. **B,** Similar view of a 24-week fetus, showing the adult derivatives of the arch cartilages. Note that the mandible is formed by intramembranous ossification of the mesenchymal tissue surrounding the first arch cartilage.

FIGURE 10-6. **A,** Lateral view of the head, neck, and thoracic regions of a 4-week embryo showing the muscles derived from the pharyngeal arches. The *arrow* shows the pathway taken by myoblasts from the occipital myotomes to form the tongue musculature. **B,** The head and neck regions of a 20-week fetus, dissected to show the muscles derived from the pharyngeal arches. Parts of the platysma and sternocleidomastoid muscles have been removed to show the deeper muscles. Note that myoblasts from the second arch migrate from the neck to the head, where they give rise to the muscles of facial expression. These muscles are supplied by the facial nerve (cranial nerve VII), the nerve of the second pharyngeal arch.

from the pharyngeal arches contributes to the dermis and the mucous membranes of the head and neck, these areas are supplied with the *special visceral afferent nerves.* The facial skin is supplied by the fifth cranial nerve (CN V, or **trigeminal nerve**); however, only the caudal two branches (*maxillary* and *mandibular*) supply derivatives of the first pharyngeal arch (see Fig. 10-7*B*). CN V is the principal sensory nerve of the head and neck and is the motor nerve for the muscles of mastication (see Table 10-1). Its sensory branches innervate the face, the teeth, and the mucous membranes of the nasal cavities, palate, mouth, and tongue (see Fig. 10-7*C*). The seventh cranial

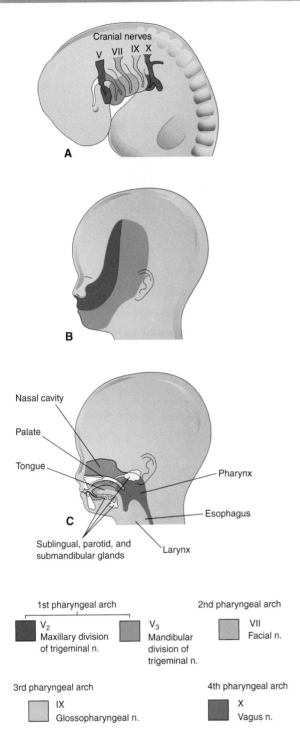

FIGURE 10-7. **A,** Lateral view of the head, neck, and thoracic regions of a 4-week embryo, showing the cranial nerves that supply the pharyngeal arches. **B,** The head and neck regions of a 20-week fetus, showing the superficial distribution of the two caudal branches of the first arch nerve (cranial nerve V). **C,** Sagittal section of the fetal head and neck, showing the deep distribution of the sensory fibers of the nerves to the teeth and mucosa of the tongue, pharynx, nasal cavity, palate, and larynx.

nerve (CN VII, or **facial nerve**), the ninth cranial nerve (CN IX, or **glossopharyngeal nerve**), and the 10th cranial nerve (CN X, or **vagus nerve**) supply the second, third, and caudal (fourth to sixth) arches, respectively. The fourth arch is supplied by the superior laryngeal branch of

the vagus nerve, whereas the sixth arch is supplied by its recurrent laryngeal branch. The nerves of the second to sixth pharyngeal arches have little cutaneous distribution (see Fig. 10-7C); however, they innervate the mucous membranes of the tongue, pharynx, and larynx.

■ PHARYNGEAL POUCHES

The primordial pharynx widens cranially where it joins the primordial mouth, or *stomodeum*, and narrows caudally, where it joins the *esophagus* (see Figs. 10-3A and 10-4B). The endoderm of the pharynx lines the internal aspects of the pharyngeal arches and passes into diverticula known as the **pharyngeal pouches** (see Figs. 10-1D to F and 10-3A and B). These pairs of pouches develop in a craniocaudal sequence between the arches. The first pair of pouches, for example, lies between the first and second pharyngeal arches. Four pairs of pharyngeal pouches are well defined; the fifth pair is absent or rudimentary. The endoderm of the pouches contacts the ectoderm of the pharyngeal grooves, and together they form the double-layered **pharyngeal membranes** (see Fig. 10-3B).

Derivatives of the Pharyngeal Pouches

The endodermal epithelial lining of the pharyngeal pouches (Fig. 10-8A) gives rise to important organs in the head and neck.

The **first pharyngeal pouch** gives rise to the **tubotympanic recess** (see Fig. 10-8B). The first pharyngeal membrane contributes to the formation of the **tympanic membrane** (eardrum) (see Fig. 10-8C). The cavity of the tubotympanic recess gives rise to the **tympanic cavity** and the **mastoid antrum**. The connection of the tubotympanic recess with the pharynx forms the **pharyngotympanic tube** (auditory tube).

The **second pharyngeal pouch** is largely obliterated as the **palatine tonsil** develops (Figs. 10-8C and 10-9). A part of this pouch remains as the **tonsillar sinus, or fossa**. The endoderm of the second pouch proliferates and grows into the underlying mesenchyme. The central parts of these buds break down, forming **tonsillar crypts**. The pouch endoderm forms the surface epithelium and the lining of the crypts. The mesenchyme around the crypts differentiates into lymphoid tissue, which soon organizes into the lymphatic nodules of the palatine tonsil.

The **third pharyngeal pouch** expands and develops a solid, bulbar, dorsal part and a hollow, elongated, ventral part (see Fig. 10-8B). The connection between the pouch and the pharynx is reduced to a narrow duct that soon degenerates. By the sixth week of development, the epithelium of each bulbar dorsal part begins to differentiate into an **inferior parathyroid gland**. The epithelium of the elongated ventral parts of the third pair of pouches proliferates, obliterating their cavities. These parts come together in the median plane to form the **thymus**. The primordia of the thymus and parathyroid glands lose their connections with the pharynx. Later, the parathyroid glands separate from the thymus and lie on the dorsal surface of the thyroid gland, whereas the thymus descends

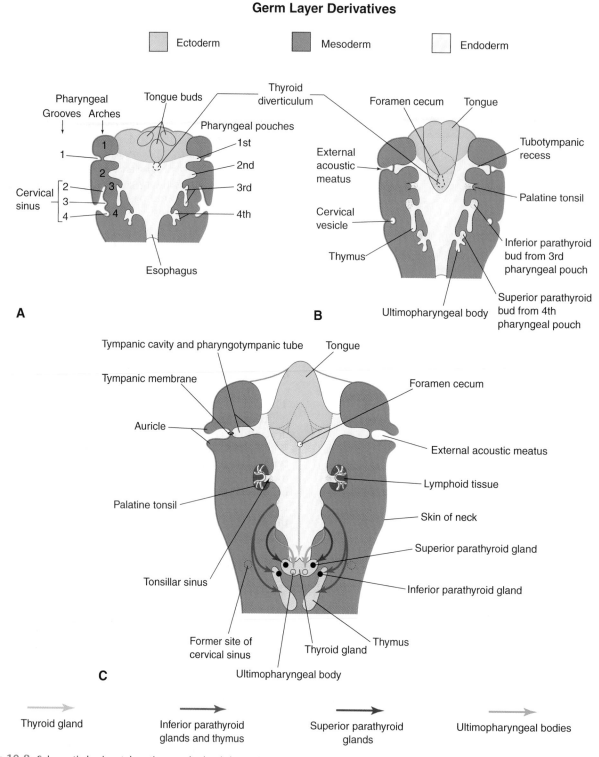

Germ Layer Derivatives

Ectoderm Mesoderm Endoderm

FIGURE 10-8. Schematic horizontal sections at the level shown in Figure 10-4A, showing the adult derivatives of the pharyngeal pouches. **A,** At 5 weeks. Note that the second pharyngeal arch grows over the third and fourth arches, burying the second to fourth pharyngeal grooves in the cervical sinus. **B,** At 6 weeks. **C,** At 7 weeks. Note the migration of the developing thymus, parathyroid, and thyroid glands into the neck.

into the superior mediastinum (see Figs. 10-8C and 10-9). The mesenchyme surrounding the thymic primordium and certain epithelial cells in the thymus are derived from *neural crest cells*.

The dorsal part of each **fourth pharyngeal pouch** develops into a **superior parathyroid gland**, which

lies on the dorsal surface of the thyroid gland (see Fig. 10-8B). The parathyroid glands derived from the third pouches descend with the thymus and are carried to a more inferior position than the parathyroid glands that are derived from the fourth pouches. This difference explains why the parathyroid glands derived from the third pair

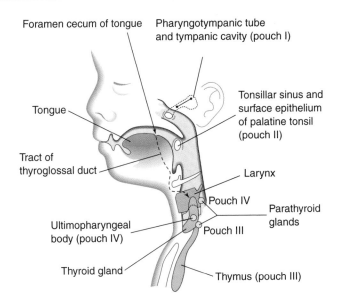

Figure 10-9. A sagittal section of the head, neck, and upper thoracic regions of a 20-week fetus, showing the adult derivatives of the pharyngeal pouches and the descent of the thyroid gland into the neck.

Labels in figure: Foramen cecum of tongue; Pharyngotympanic tube and tympanic cavity (pouch I); Tongue; Tonsillar sinus and surface epithelium of palatine tonsil (pouch II); Tract of thyroglossal duct; Larynx; Pouch IV; Parathyroid glands; Ultimopharyngeal body (pouch IV); Pouch III; Thyroid gland; Thymus (pouch III)

of pouches are located inferior to those derived from the fourth pouches (see Fig. 10-9). The elongated ventral part of each fourth pouch develops into the **ultimopharyngeal body**, which fuses with the thyroid gland, giving rise to the **parafollicular cells (C cells)** of the thyroid gland. These cells produce calcitonin, a hormone involved in the regulation of calcium. C cells differentiate from the **neural crest cells** that migrate from the pharyngeal arches into the fourth pair of pharyngeal pouches.

If the **fifth pharyngeal pouch** develops, it is rudimentary and becomes part of the fourth pharyngeal pouch.

■ PHARYNGEAL GROOVES

The head and neck regions of the human embryo exhibit four pharyngeal grooves on each side during the fourth and fifth weeks (see Fig. 10-1A). These grooves separate the pharyngeal arches externally. Only one pair of grooves contributes to the adult structures; the first pair persists as the **external acoustic meatus** or ear canals (see Fig. 10-8C). The other grooves lie in a slitlike depression—the **cervical sinus**—and are usually obliterated with it as the neck develops (see Fig. 10-4B to F).

■ PHARYNGEAL MEMBRANES

The pharyngeal membranes appear in the floors of the pharyngeal grooves during the fourth week (Fig. 10-1B and D). These membranes form where the epithelia of a groove and a pouch approach each other. The endoderm of the pouches and the ectoderm of the grooves are separated by a mesenchyme. Only the first pair contributes to the formation of the adult structures; it becomes the **tympanic membrane** (Fig. 10-8C).

Small auricular sinuses (pits) and cysts are usually located in a triangular area of skin anterior to the auricle of the external ear (Fig. 10-10D); however, they may occur in other sites around the auricle or in its lobule (earlobe). Although some sinuses and cysts are remnants of the first pharyngeal groove, others represent ectodermal folds sequestered during formation of the auricle from the auricular hillocks (swellings that contribute to the auricle). These small sinuses and cysts are classified as minor anomalies that are of no serious medical consequence.

BRANCHIAL (CERVICAL) SINUSES

Branchial sinuses are uncommon, and almost all that open externally on the side of the neck result from failure of the second pharyngeal groove and the cervical sinus to obliterate (Figs. 10-10B and 10-11A). The sinus typically opens along the anterior border of the sternocleidomastoid muscle in the inferior third of the neck. Anomalies of the other pharyngeal grooves occur in approximately 5% of cases. **External branchial sinuses** are commonly detected during infancy because of the discharge of mucous material from their orifices in the neck. These *lateral cervical sinuses* are bilateral in approximately 10% of cases and are commonly associated with auricular sinuses. **Internal branchial sinuses** open into the pharynx and are very rare. Because they usually open into the tonsillar sinus or near the palatopharyngeal arch (see Fig. 10-10B and D), almost all of these sinuses result from persistence of the proximal part of the second pharyngeal pouch. Normally, this pouch disappears as the palatine tonsil develops; its normal remnant is the tonsillar sinus.

BRANCHIAL FISTULA

An abnormal canal that opens internally into the tonsillar sinus and externally on the side of the neck is a *branchial fistula*. This rare anomaly results from persistence of parts of the second pharyngeal groove and the second pharyngeal pouch (see Figs. 10-10C and D and 10-11B). The fistula ascends from its opening in the neck, through the subcutaneous tissue and the platysma muscle, to reach the tonsillar sinus.

■ DEVELOPMENT OF THE THYROID GLAND

The thyroid gland is the first endocrine gland to develop. It begins to form at approximately 24 days from a median endodermal thickening in the floor of the primordial

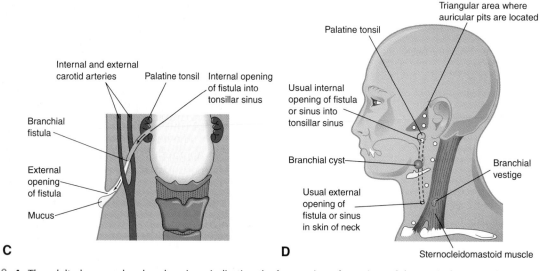

FIGURE 10-10. **A,** The adult pharyngeal and neck regions, indicating the former sites of openings of the cervical sinus and the pharyngeal pouches (2 and 3). The *broken lines* indicate possible courses of branchial fistulas. **B,** The embryologic basis for various types of branchial sinus. **C,** Illustration of a branchial fistula resulting from the persistence of parts of the second pharyngeal groove and the second pharyngeal pouch. **D,** Possible sites of branchial cysts and openings of the branchial sinuses and fistulas. A branchial vestige is also shown.

BRANCHIAL CYSTS

The third and fourth pharyngeal arches are buried in the cervical sinus (see Fig. 10-8A). Remnants of parts of the cervical sinus, the second pharyngeal groove, or both may persist and form a spherical or elongated cyst (see Fig. 10-10A and D). Branchial cysts often do not become apparent until late childhood or early adulthood, when they produce a slowly enlarging, painless swelling in the neck (Fig. 10-12). The cysts enlarge because of the accumulation of fluid and cellular debris derived from desquamation of their epithelial linings (Fig. 10-13).

BRANCHIAL VESTIGES

Normally, the pharyngeal cartilages disappear, except for the parts that form ligaments or bones; however, in unusual cases, cartilaginous or bony remnants of the pharyngeal arch cartilages appear under the skin on the side of the neck. These are usually found anterior to the inferior third of the sternocleidomastoid muscle (see Fig. 10-10D).

---

pharynx (Fig. 10-16A). This thickening soon forms a small outpouching known as the **thyroid primordium**. As the embryo and the tongue grow, the developing thyroid gland descends in the neck, passing ventral to the developing hyoid bone and the laryngeal cartilages. For a short time,

it is connected to the tongue by the **thyroglossal duct** (see Fig. 10-16B and C). As a result of rapid cell proliferation, the lumen of the thyroid diverticulum soon obliterates, and then it divides into right and left lobes connected by the **thyroid isthmus**. By 7 weeks, the thyroid gland has assumed its definitive shape and has usually reached its final site in the neck (see Fig. 10-16D). By this time, the thyroglossal duct has usually degenerated and disappeared. The proximal opening of the thyroglossal duct persists as a small, blind

FIGURE 10-11. **A,** A child's neck, showing a catheter inserted into the external opening of a branchial sinus. The catheter allows definition of the length of the tract, which facilitates surgical excision. **B,** A fistulogram of a complete branchial fistula. The radiograph was taken after injection of a contrast medium to show the course of the fistula through the neck. (Courtesy of Dr. Pierre Soucy, Division of Paediatric Surgery, Children's Hospital of Eastern Ontario, Ottawa, Ontario, Canada.)

FIRST ARCH SYNDROME

Abnormal development of the first pharyngeal arch results in various congenital anomalies of the eyes, ears, mandible, and palate that together constitute first arch syndrome (Fig. 10-14). This syndrome is believed to result from insufficient migration of neural crest cells into the first arch during the fourth week. There are *two main manifestations of first arch syndrome*:

• **Treacher Collins syndrome** (mandibulofacial dysostosis), which is caused by an autosomal dominant gene, results in underdevelopment of the zygomatic bones of the face—malar hypoplasia. Characteristic features of the syndrome include down-slanting palpebral fissures, defects of the lower eyelids, deformed external ears, and sometimes abnormalities of the middle and internal ears.

• **Pierre Robin syndrome** consists of hypoplasia of the mandible, cleft palate, and defects of the eye and ear. Many cases of this syndrome are sporadic; however, some appear to have a genetic basis. In *Robin morphogenetic complex*, the initiating defect is a small mandible (micrognathia), which results in posterior displacement of the tongue and obstruction to full closure of the palatine processes, resulting in bilateral cleft palate.

FIGURE 10-12. A boy with swelling in the neck produced by a branchial cyst. Branchial cysts often lie free in the neck, just inferior to the angle of the mandible, or they may be found anywhere along the anterior border of the sternocleidomastoid muscle. (Courtesy of Dr. Pierre Soucy, Division of Paediatric Surgery, Children's Hospital of Eastern Ontario, Ottawa, Ontario, Canada.)

FIGURE 10-13. Branchial (cleft) cyst (B) shown by computed tomography of the neck region of a woman who had a "lump" in the neck, similar to that shown in Figure 10-12. The low-density cyst is anterior to the right sternocleidomastoid muscle (s) at the level of the hyoid bone (h). The normal appearance of the carotid sheath (c) is shown for comparison with the compressed sheath on the right side. (From McNab T, McLennan MK, Margolis M: Radiology rounds. Can Fam Physician 41:1673, 1995.)

FIGURE 10-14. An infant with first arch syndrome, a pattern of anomalies resulting from insufficient migration of the neural crest cells into the first pharyngeal arch. Note the following characteristics: deformed auricle of the external ear, preauricular appendage, defect in the cheek between the auricle and the mouth, hypoplasia of the mandible, and macrostomia (large mouth).

pit—the **foramen cecum** of the tongue. A **pyramidal lobe** extends superiorly from the isthmus in approximately 50% of individuals. This lobe may be attached to the hyoid bone by fibrous tissue, smooth muscle, or both.

At 11 weeks, colloid begins to appear in the **thyroid follicles**; thereafter, iodine concentration and the synthesis of thyroid hormones can be demonstrated.

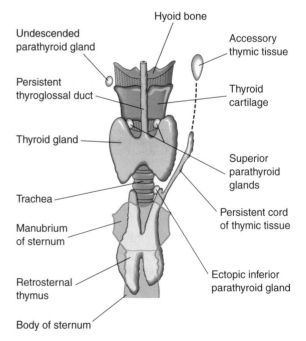

FIGURE 10-15. Anterior view of the thyroid gland, thymus, and parathyroid glands, showing various possible congenital anomalies.

Infants with DiGeorge syndrome are born without a thymus and parathyroid glands, although in some cases, ectopic glandular tissue has been found. The disease is characterized by *congenital hypoparathyroidism*; increased susceptibility to infections (from immune deficiency—specifically, defective T-cell function); anomalies of the mouth (shortened philtrum of the lip [fish-mouth deformity]); low-set, notched ears; nasal clefts; *thyroid hypoplasia*; and cardiac abnormalities

(defects of the arch of the aorta and the heart). *DiGeorge syndrome* occurs when the third and fourth pharyngeal pouches do not differentiate into the thymus and parathyroid glands. The facial abnormalities result primarily from abnormal development of the first arch components during formation of the face and ears. *DiGeorge syndrome involves a microdeletion (22q11.2 region), mutation of the* HIRA *and* UFDIL *genes, and neural crest cell defects.*

ECTOPIC PARATHYROID GLANDS

The parathyroids are highly variable in number and location. They may be found anywhere near or within the thyroid gland or the thymus (Fig. 10-15). The superior glands are more constant in position than the inferior ones. Occasionally, an inferior parathyroid gland does not descend and remains near the bifurcation of the common carotid artery. In other cases, it may accompany the thymus into the thorax.

ABNORMAL NUMBER OF PARATHYROID GLANDS

In unusual cases, there may be more than four parathyroid glands. Supernumerary parathyroid glands probably result from division of the primordia of the original glands. Absence of a parathyroid gland results from failure of one of the primordia to differentiate or from atrophy of a gland early in development.

■ DEVELOPMENT OF THE TONGUE

Near the end of the fourth week, a median triangular elevation appears in the floor of the primordial pharynx, just rostral to the foramen cecum (Fig. 10-22*A*). This swelling—the **median lingual swelling**—is the first indication of tongue development. Two oval **lateral lingual swellings** soon develop on each side of the median swelling. The swellings result from the proliferation of the mesenchyme in the ventromedial parts of the first pair of pharyngeal arches. The lateral swellings rapidly increase in size, merge, and overgrow the median tongue bud. The merged lateral swellings form the anterior two thirds, or the oral part, of the tongue (see Fig. 10-22*C*). The plane of fusion of the lateral swellings is indicated superficially by the midline groove of the tongue and internally by the fibrous lingual septum. The median lingual swelling forms no recognizable part of the adult tongue.

Formation of the posterior third, or the pharyngeal part, of the tongue is indicated by two elevations that develop caudal to the foramen cecum (see Fig. 10-22*A*):

● The copula forms by fusion of the ventromedial parts of the second pair of pharyngeal arches.

● The hypopharyngeal eminence develops caudal to the copula from the mesenchyme in the ventromedial parts of the third and fourth pairs of arches.

The copula is gradually overgrown by the hypopharyngeal eminence and disappears (see Fig. 10-22*B* and *C*). As a result, the pharyngeal part of the tongue develops from the rostral part of the hypopharyngeal eminence. The line of fusion of the anterior and posterior parts of the tongue is roughly indicated by

THYROGLOSSAL DUCT CYSTS AND SINUSES

A remnant of the thyroglossal duct may persist and form a cyst in the tongue or in the anterior part of the neck, usually just inferior to the hyoid bone (Fig. 10-17). The swelling produced by a *thyroglossal duct cyst* usually develops as a painless, progressively enlarging, movable median mass (Fig. 10-18). The cyst may contain some thyroid tissue. After infection of a cyst, perforation of the skin occurs in some cases, forming a **thyroglossal duct sinus** that usually opens in the median plane of the neck, anterior to the laryngeal cartilages (Fig. 10-19*A*).

ECTOPIC THYROID GLAND

Infrequently, an ectopic thyroid gland is located along the normal route of its descent from the tongue (see Fig. 10-16*C*). **Lingual thyroid glandular tissue** is the most common type. Incomplete descent of the thyroid gland results in a **sublingual thyroid gland** that appears high in the neck, at or just inferior to the hyoid bone (Figs. 10-20 and 10-21). As a rule, an ectopic sublingual thyroid gland is the only thyroid tissue present. It is clinically important to differentiate an ectopic thyroid gland from a thyroglossal duct cyst or from accessory thyroid tissue to prevent *inadvertent surgical removal of the thyroid gland* because this may be the only thyroid tissue present. Failure to recognize the thyroid gland may leave the person permanently dependent on thyroid medication.

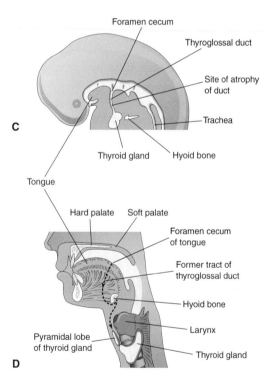

FIGURE 10-16. Development of the thyroid gland. **A** to **C**, Schematic sagittal sections of the head and neck regions of 4-week, 5-week, and 6-week embryos, showing successive stages in the development of the thyroid gland. **D**, Similar section of an adult head and neck, showing the path taken by the thyroid gland during its embryonic descent (indicated by the former tract of the thyroglossal duct)

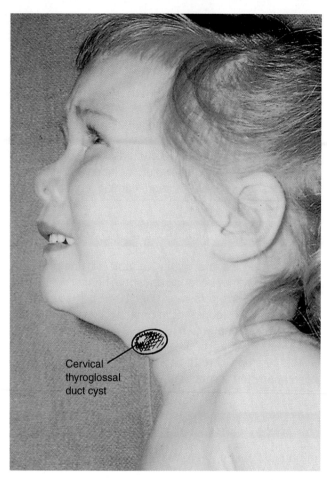

FIGURE 10-17. A typical thyroglossal duct cyst in a girl. The round, firm mass (indicated by the sketch) produced a swelling in the median plane of the neck, just inferior to the hyoid bone.

myoblasts during their migration and innervates the tongue muscles as they develop.

Papillae and Taste Buds of the Tongue

The **lingual papillae** appear by the end of the eighth week. The vallate and foliate papillae appear first, close to the terminal branches of the glossopharyngeal nerve. The fungiform papillae appear later, near the terminations of the chorda tympani branch of the facial nerve. Filiform papillae, the most common papillae, develop during the early fetal period (10–11 weeks). They contain afferent nerve endings that are sensitive to touch. Taste buds develop during weeks 11 to 13 by inductive interaction between the epithelial cells of the tongue and invading gustatory nerve cells from the chorda tympani, glossopharyngeal, and vagus nerves. Facial responses in the fetus can be induced by bitter-tasting substances at 26 to 28 weeks, indicating that reflex pathways between taste buds and facial muscles are established by this stage.

Nerve Supply of the Tongue

The sensory supply to the mucosa of almost the entire anterior tongue (oral part) is from the lingual branch of

a V-shaped groove called the *terminal sulcus* (see Fig. 10-22C). The pharyngeal arch mesenchyme forms the connective tissue and vasculature of the tongue. The tongue muscles are derived from myoblasts that migrate from the occipital somites (see Fig. 10-6A). The hypoglossal nerve (CN XII) accompanies the

FIGURE 10-18. Computed tomography scans. **A,** The level of the thyrohyoid membrane and the base of the epiglottis. **B,** The level of the thyroid cartilage, which is calcified. The thyroglossal duct cyst extends cranially to the margin of the hyoid bone. (Courtesy of Dr. Gerald S. Smyser, Altru Health System, Grand Forks, ND.)

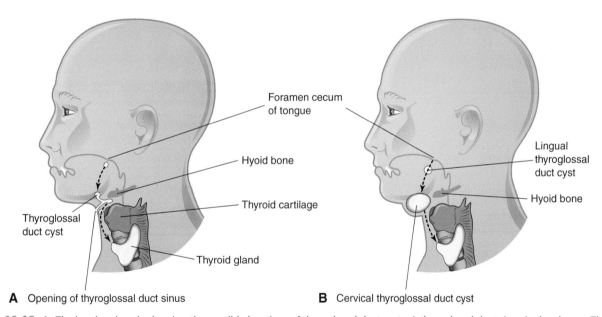

FIGURE 10-19. **A,** The head and neck, showing the possible locations of thyroglossal duct cysts. A thyroglossal duct sinus is also shown. The *broken line* indicates the course taken by the thyroglossal duct during the descent of the developing thyroid gland from the foramen cecum to its final position in the anterior part of the neck. **B,** Similar sketch showing lingual and cervical thyroglossal duct cysts. Most thyroglossal duct cysts are located just inferior to the hyoid bone.

the mandibular division of the trigeminal nerve (CN V), the nerve of the first pharyngeal arch (see Fig. 10-22C). Although the facial nerve is the nerve of the second pharyngeal arch, its chorda tympani branch supplies the taste buds in the anterior tongue, except for the vallate papillae. Because the second arch component, the copula, is overgrown by the third arch component (the hypopharyngeal eminence), the facial nerve does not supply any of the tongue mucosa, except for the taste buds. The vallate papillae in the anterior tongue are innervated by the glossopharyngeal nerve of the third pharyngeal arch (see Fig. 10-22C). The posterior tongue (pharyngeal part) is innervated mainly by the glossopharyngeal nerve (CN IX). The superior laryngeal branch of the vagus nerve of the fourth arch supplies a small area of the tongue anterior to the epiglottis (see Fig. 10-22C). All muscles of the tongue are supplied by the hypoglossal nerve (CN XII), except for the palatoglossus, which is supplied from the pharyngeal plexus by fibers arising from the vagus nerve.

■ DEVELOPMENT OF THE SALIVARY GLANDS

During the sixth and seventh weeks, the salivary glands begin as solid epithelial buds from the primordial oral cavity (see Fig. 10-7C). The ends of the buds grow into the underlying mesenchyme. The connective tissue in the glands is derived from neural crest cells. All secretory

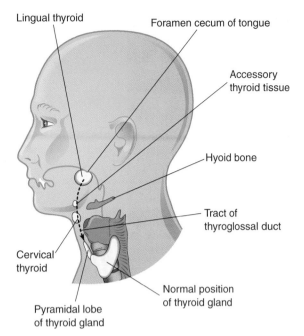

FIGURE 10-20. The head and neck, showing the usual sites of ectopic thyroid tissue. The *broken line* indicates the path followed by the thyroid gland during its descent, as well as the former tract of the thyroglossal duct.

(parenchymal) tissue arises by proliferation of the oral epithelium.

The **parotid glands** are the first to appear (early in the sixth week). They develop from the oral ectodermal lining near the angles of the stomodeum. The buds grow toward the ears and branch to form solid cords with rounded ends. Later, the cords canalize—(i.e., develop lumina) —and become ducts by approximately 10 weeks. The rounded ends of the cords differentiate into acini, which begin to secrete at 18 weeks. The capsule and the connective tissue develop from the surrounding mesenchyme.

The **submandibular glands** appear late in the sixth week. They develop from endodermal buds in the floor of the stomodeum. Solid cellular processes grow posteriorly, lateral to the developing tongue. Later, they branch and differentiate. Acini begin to form at 12 weeks, and secretory

---

CONGENITAL LINGUAL CYSTS AND FISTULAS

Cysts in the tongue may be derived from remnants of the thyroglossal duct (see Fig. 10-17B). They may enlarge and produce pharyngeal pain, dysphagia (difficulty in swallowing), or both. Fistulas may also arise as a result of persistence of the lingual parts of the thyroglossal duct; such fistulas open through the *foramen cecum* into the oral cavity.

ANKYLOGLOSSIA (TONGUE-TIE)

The lingual frenulum normally connects the inferior surface of the tongue to the floor of the mouth (Fig. 10-23). Ankyloglossia occurs in approximately 1 in 300 North American infants, but is usually of no functional significance. A short frenulum usually stretches with time, making surgical correction of the anomaly unnecessary.

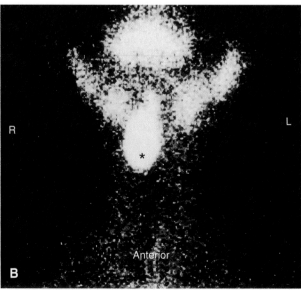

FIGURE 10-21. **A,** A sublingual thyroid mass in a 5-year-old girl. **B,** Technetium 99m pertechnetate scan showing an ectopic sublingual thyroid gland (*) without evidence of functioning thyroid tissue in the lower neck. (From Leung AKC, Wong AL, Robson WLLM: Ectopic thyroid gland simulating a thyroglossal duct cyst: A case report. Can J Surg 38:87, 1995.)

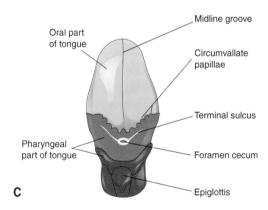

Arch Derivatives of Tongue

☐ 1st pharyngeal arch (CN V-mandibular division)   ☐ 2nd pharyngeal arch (CN VII-chorda tympani)

☐ 3rd pharyngeal arch (CN IX-glossopharyngeal)   ☐ 4th pharyngeal arch (CN X-vagus)

FIGURE 10-22. **A** and **B,** Schematic horizontal sections through the pharynx at the level shown in Figure 10-4A, showing successive stages in the development of the tongue during the fourth and fifth weeks. **C,** The adult tongue, showing the pharyngeal arch derivation of the nerve supply of its mucosa.

activity begins at 16 weeks. Growth of the submandibular glands continues after birth, with the formation of mucous acini. Lateral to the developing tongue, a linear groove forms that soon closes over to form the *submandibular duct*.

The **sublingual glands** appear in the eighth week, approximately 2 weeks later than the other salivary glands.

FIGURE 10-23. An infant with ankyloglossia, or tongue-tie. Note the short frenulum, which extends to the tip of the tongue. Tongue-tie interferes with protrusion of the tongue and may make breast-feeding difficult. (Courtesy of Dr. Evelyn Jain, Lakeview Breastfeeding Clinic, Calgary, Alberta, Canada.)

They develop from multiple endodermal epithelial buds in the **paralingual sulcus** (see Fig. 10-7C). These buds branch and canalize to form 10 to 12 ducts that open independently into the floor of the mouth.

■ DEVELOPMENT OF THE FACE

The facial primordia begin to appear around the large **primordial stomodeum** early in the fourth week (Fig. 10-24A). Facial development depends on the inductive influence of organizing centers. The **prosencephalic organizing center**, derived from the prechordal mesoderm that migrates from the primitive streak, is located rostral to the notochord and ventral to the prosencephalon, or forebrain (see Chapter 6). The **rhombencephalic organizing center** is ventral to the rhombencephalon (hindbrain).

The **five facial primordia**, which appear around the *stomodeum* (primordium of the mouth), are:

● The single frontonasal prominence
● The paired maxillary prominences
● The paired mandibular prominences

Both paired prominences are derivatives of the first pair of pharyngeal arches. The prominences are produced by mesenchyme derived from **neural crest cells** that migrate into the arches during the fourth week of development. These cells are the major source of connective tissue components, including cartilage, bone, and ligaments in the facial and oral regions.

The **frontonasal prominence** surrounds the ventrolateral part of the forebrain, which gives rise to the optic vesicles that form the eyes (Figs. 10-24A and 10-25). The frontal part of the frontonasal prominence forms the forehead; the nasal part of the frontonasal prominence forms the rostral boundary of the stomodeum and the nose. The **maxillary prominences** form the lateral boundaries of the stomodeum, whereas **mandibular prominences** constitute the caudal boundary of the primordial mouth (see Figs. 10-24A and 10-25). The lower jaw and the lower lip are the first parts of the face to

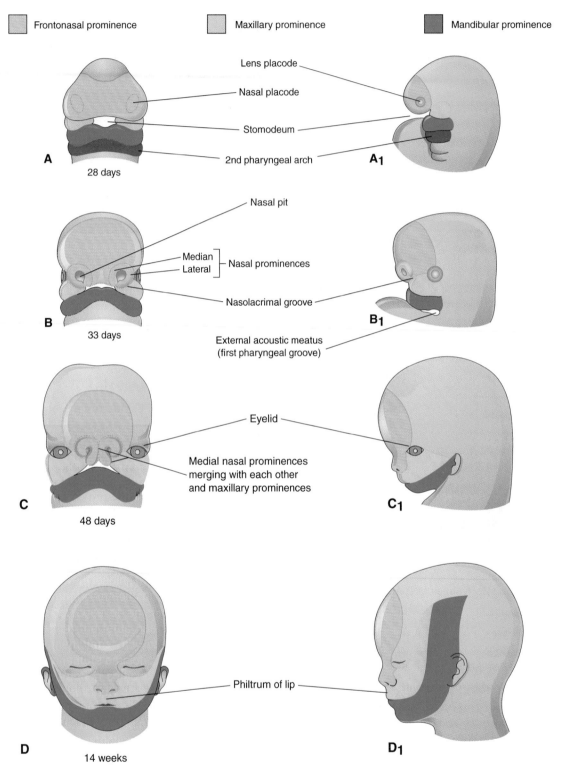

Frontonasal prominence   Maxillary prominence   Mandibular prominence

Lens placode
Nasal placode
Stomodeum
A   **A₁**
28 days
2nd pharyngeal arch

Nasal pit
Median ⎤ Nasal prominences
Lateral ⎦
Nasolacrimal groove
B   **B₁**
33 days
External acoustic meatus
(first pharyngeal groove)

Eyelid
Medial nasal prominences
merging with each other
and maxillary prominences
C   **C₁**
48 days

Philtrum of lip
D   **D₁**
14 weeks

FIGURE **10-24.** Illustrations of the progressive stages in the development of the human face.

form. They result from merging of the medial ends of the mandibular prominences.

By the end of the fourth week, bilateral oval thickenings of the surface ectoderm—**nasal placodes**—have developed on the inferolateral parts of the frontonasal prominence (Figs. 10-25 and 10-26*A* and *B*). Initially, these placodes are convex, but later, they are stretched to produce a flat depression in each placode. The mesenchyme in the margins of the placodes proliferates, producing horseshoe-shaped elevations—the medial and lateral **nasal prominences** (see Figs. 10-24*B* and 10-26*D* and *E*). As a result, the nasal placodes lie in depressions, called **nasal pits** (see Figs. 10-24*B* and 10-26*C* and *D*). These pits are the primordia of the anterior nares (nostrils) and nasal cavities (see Fig. 10-26*E*). Proliferation of the mesenchyme in the maxillary prominences causes them to enlarge and grow medially toward each other and the nasal prominences (see Figs. 10-24*B* and *C* and 10-25).

The medial migration of the maxillary prominences moves the medial nasal prominences toward the median plane and each other. Each lateral nasal prominence is separated from the maxillary prominence by a cleft called the **nasolacrimal groove** (see Fig. 10-24*B*).

FIGURE 10-26. Progressive stages in the development of a human nasal sac (primordial nasal cavity). **A,** Ventral view of an embryo at approximately 28 days. **B** to **E,** Transverse sections through the left side of the developing nasal sac.

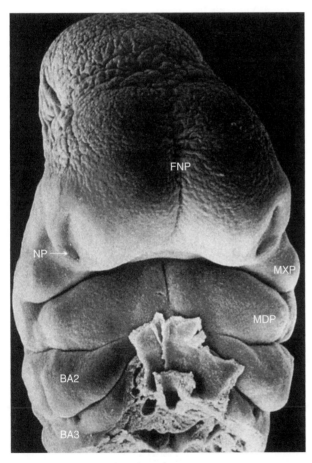

FIGURE 10-25. Scanning electron micrograph showing a ventral view of a human embryo at approximately 33 days (stage 15; crown-rump length [CRL], 8 mm). Observe the prominent frontonasal prominence (FNP) surrounding the telencephalon (forebrain). Also observe the nasal pits (NP) located in the ventrolateral regions of the frontonasal prominence. Medial and lateral nasal prominences surround these pits. The wedge-shaped maxillary prominences (MXP) form the lateral boundaries of the stomodeum. The fusing mandibular prominences (MDP) are located just caudal to the stomodeum. The second pharyngeal (branchial) arch (BA2) is clearly visible and shows overhanging margins (opercula). The third pharyngeal (branchial) arch (BA3) is also clearly visible. (From Hinrichsen K: The early development of morphology and patterns of the face in the human embryo. Adv Anat Embryol Cell Biol 98:1, 1985.)

By the end of the fifth week, **six auricular hillocks** (mesenchymal swellings) form around the first pharyngeal groove (three on each side), the *primordia of the auricle*, and the external acoustic meatus (canal). Initially, the external ears are located in the neck region; however, as the mandible develops, they ascend to the side of the head at the level of the eyes (see Fig. 10-24*B* and C). By the end of the sixth week, each maxillary prominence has begun to merge with the lateral nasal prominence along the line of the nasolacrimal groove (Fig. 10-27*A* and *B*). This establishes continuity between the side of the nose, formed by the lateral nasal prominence, and the cheek region, formed by the maxillary prominence.

The **nasolacrimal duct** develops from a rodlike thickening of the ectoderm in the floor of the *nasolacrimal groove*. This thickening gives rise to a solid epithelial cord that separates from the ectoderm and sinks into the mesenchyme. Later, as a result of cell apoptosis, the cord canalizes to form the nasolacrimal duct. The cranial end of this duct expands to form the *lacrimal sac*. By the late fetal period, the nasolacrimal duct drains into the inferior meatus in the lateral wall of the nasal cavity. The duct usually becomes completely patent only after birth.

Between weeks 7 and 10, the medial nasal prominences merge with each other and with the maxillary and lateral nasal prominences (see Fig. 10-24*C*), resulting in disintegration of their contacting surface epithelia. This causes inter-

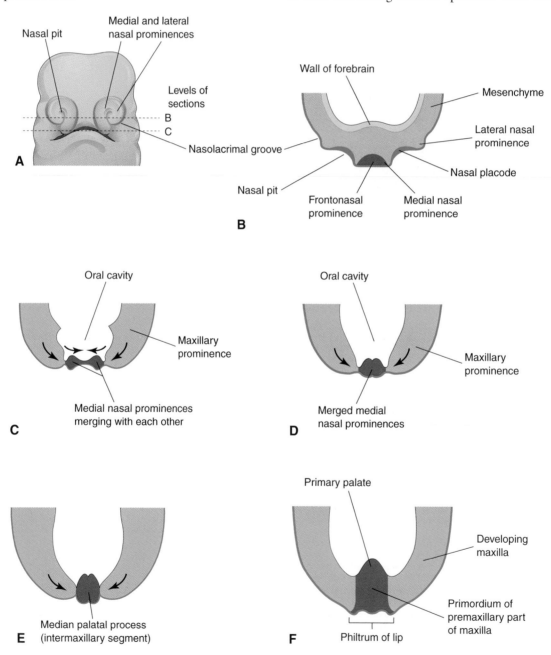

FIGURE 10-27. Illustrations of the early development of the maxilla, palate, and upper lip. **A,** Facial view of a 5-week embryo. **B** and **C,** Sketches of horizontal sections at the levels shown in **A.** The *arrows* indicate subsequent growth of the maxillary and medial nasal prominences toward the median plane and merging of the prominences with each other. **D** to **F,** Similar sections of older embryos showing merging of the medial nasal prominences with each other and with the maxillary prominences to form the upper lip.

mingling of the underlying mesenchyme. Merging of the medial nasal and maxillary prominences results in continuity of the upper jaw and lip and separation of the nasal pits from the stomodeum. As the medial nasal prominences merge, they form an intermaxillary segment (see Figs. 10-27C to F). The intermaxillary segment gives rise to the following:

● The deep middle part of the upper lip
● The premaxillary part of the maxilla and its associated gingiva (gum)
● The primary palate

The lateral parts of the upper lip, most of the maxilla, and the secondary palate form from the maxillary prominences (see Fig. 10-24D). These prominences merge laterally with the mandibular prominences. Recent studies show that the lower part of the medial nasal prominences becomes deeply positioned and are covered by medial extensions of the maxillary prominences to form the **philtrum**. The primordial lips and cheeks are invaded by myoblasts from the second pair of pharyngeal arches, which differentiate into the facial muscles (see Fig. 10-6 and Table 10-1). The myoblasts from the first pair of arches differentiate into the muscles of mastication.

◼ DEVELOPMENT OF THE NASAL CAVITIES

As the face develops, the **nasal placodes** become depressed, forming **nasal pits** (see Figs. 10-25 and 10-26). Proliferation of the surrounding mesenchyme forms the medial and lateral **nasal prominences** and results in deepening of the nasal pits and the formation of primordial **nasal sacs**. Each nasal sac grows dorsally, ventral to the developing forebrain (Fig. 10-28A). At first, the nasal sacs are separated from the oral cavity by the **oronasal membrane**. This membrane ruptures by the end of the sixth week of development, bringing the nasal and oral cavities into communication (see Fig. 10-28B and C). The regions of continuity between the nasal and oral cavities are the **primordial choanae**, which lie posterior to the primary palate. After the *secondary palate* develops, the choanae are located at the junction of the nasal cavity and pharynx (see Fig. 10-28D). While these changes are occurring, the superior, middle, and inferior **conchae** develop as elevations of the lateral walls of the nasal cavities (see Fig. 10-30D). Concurrently, the ectodermal epithelium in the roof of each nasal cavity becomes specialized to form the **olfactory epithelium**. Some epithelial cells differentiate into olfactory receptor cells. The axons of these cells constitute the **olfactory nerves**, which grow into the olfactory bulbs of the brain (see Fig. 10-28C and D).

Paranasal Sinuses

Some paranasal sinuses, in particular, the **maxillary sinuses**, begin to develop during late fetal life; the remainder of them develop after birth. They form from outgrowths, or diverticula, of the walls of the nasal cavities, becoming pneumatic (air-filled) extensions of the nasal cavities in the adjacent bones. The original

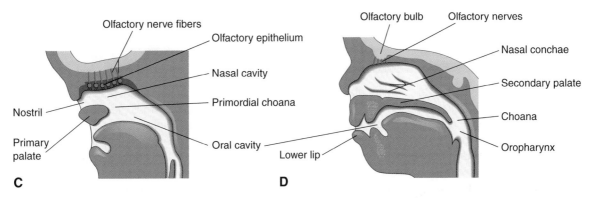

FIGURE 10-28. Sagittal sections of the head, showing development of the nasal cavities. The nasal septum has been removed. **A,** At 5 weeks. **B,** At 6 weeks, showing breakdown of the oronasal membrane. **C,** At 7 weeks, showing the nasal cavity communicating with the oral cavity and the development of the olfactory epithelium. **D,** At 12 weeks. The palate and the lateral wall of the nasal cavity are evident.

openings of the diverticula persist as the orifices of the adult sinuses.

■ DEVELOPMENT OF THE PALATE

The palate develops from two primordia: the primary palate and the secondary palate.

Palatogenesis begins in the sixth week, but is not completed until the 12th week. The critical period of development of the palate is from the end of the sixth week until the beginning of the ninth week.

Primary Palate

Early in the sixth week, the primary palate (**median palatine process**) begins to develop from the deep part of the intermaxillary segment of the maxilla (see Figs. 10-27F and 10-28). Initially, this segment is a wedge-shaped mass of mesenchyme between the internal surfaces of the maxillary prominences of the developing maxillae. The primary palate forms the **premaxillary part of the maxilla** (Fig. 10-29B). It represents only a small part of the adult hard palate (i.e., the part anterior to the incisive fossa).

Secondary Palate

The secondary palate is the primordium of the hard and soft parts of the palate (see Figs. 10-28D and 10-29A and B). The secondary palate begins to develop early in the sixth week from two mesenchymal projections that extend from the internal aspects of the maxillary prominences. Initially, these structures—called **lateral palatal processes** (palatal shelves)—project inferomedially on each side of the tongue (Figs. 10-30A to C). As the jaws develop, the tongue becomes relatively smaller and moves inferiorly. During the seventh and eighth weeks, the lateral palatine processes elongate and ascend to a horizontal position superior to the tongue. Gradually, the processes approach each other and fuse in the median plane (see Figs. 10-30E to H). They also fuse with the nasal septum and the posterior part of the primary palate. Elevation of the palatal processes, or shelves, to the horizontal position is believed to be caused by an intrinsic force that is generated by the hydration of hyaluronic acid in the mesenchymal cells within the palatal processes. The medial epithelial seam at the edges of the palatal shelves breaks down, which is a prerequisite for fusion of the palatal shelves.

The **nasal septum** develops in a downward growth pattern from internal parts of the merged medial nasal prominences (see Fig. 10-30C, E, and G). The fusion

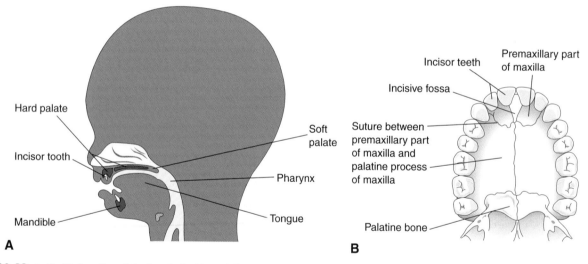

FIGURE 10-29. **A,** Sagittal section of the head of a 20-week fetus, showing the location of the palate. **B,** The bony palate and the alveolar arch of a young adult. The suture between the premaxillary part of the maxilla and the fused palatine processes of the maxillae is usually visible in the crania of young persons. It is not visible in the hard palates of most dried crania because they are usually from old adults.

PARANASAL SINUSES IN NEONATAL AND POSTNATAL DEVELOPMENT

Most of the paranasal sinuses are rudimentary or absent in newborns. The *maxillary sinuses* are small at birth. They grow slowly until puberty and are not fully developed until all of the permanent teeth have erupted in early adulthood. No frontal or sphenoid sinuses are present at birth. The ethmoid cells (sinuses) are small before 2 years, and they do not begin to grow rapidly until 6 to 8 years. At approximately 2 years, the two most anterior ethmoid cells grow into the frontal bone, forming a frontal sinus on each side. Usually, the frontal sinuses are visible on radiographs by 7 years. The two most posterior ethmoid cells grow into the sphenoid bone at approximately 2 years, forming two sphenoid sinuses. Growth of the paranasal sinuses is important in altering the size and shape of the face during infancy and childhood and in adding resonance to the voice during adolescence.

FIGURE 10-30. **A,** Sagittal section of the embryonic head at the end of the sixth week, showing the median palatine process, or primary palate. **B, D, F,** and **H,** The roof of the mouth from the sixth to 12th weeks, showing the development of the palate. The *broken lines* indicate the sites of fusion of the palatine processes. The *arrows* indicate medial and posterior growth of the lateral palatine processes. **C, E,** and **G,** Frontal sections of the head, showing fusion of the lateral palatine processes with each other and with the nasal septum, and separation of the nasal and oral cavities.

CLEFT LIP AND CLEFT PALATE

Clefts of the upper lip and palate are common. The defects are classified according to developmental criteria, with the incisive fossa and papilla used as reference landmarks (see Figs. 10-29*B* and 10-34*A*). Cleft lip ("harelip") and cleft palate are especially conspicuous because they result in an abnormal facial appearance and defective speech. Two major groups of cleft lip and cleft palate are recognized (see Figs. 10-32 to 10-34):

Anterior cleft anomalies include cleft lip, with or without cleft of the alveolar part of the maxilla. A complete cleft anomaly is one in which the cleft extends through the lip and the alveolar part of the maxilla to the incisive fossa, separating the anterior and posterior parts of the palate (see Fig. 10-34*E* and *F*). Anterior cleft anomalies result from a deficiency of mesenchyme in the maxillary prominences and the median palatal process (see Fig. 10-27*D* and *E*).

Posterior cleft anomalies include clefts of the secondary, or posterior, palate that extend through the soft and hard regions of the palate to the incisive fossa, separating the anterior and posterior parts of the palate (see Fig. 10-34*G* and *H*). Posterior cleft anomalies are caused by defective development of the secondary palate and result from growth distortions in the lateral palatine processes that, in turn, prevent the medial migration and fusion of these processes.

Clefts involving the upper lip, with or without cleft palate, occur in approximately 1 in 1000 births; however, their frequency varies widely, and 60% to 80% of those affected are boys. The clefts vary in severity from small notches in the vermilion border of the lip (see Fig. 10-33*G*) to larger clefts that extend into the floor of the nostril and through the alveolar part of the maxilla (see Figs. 10-32*A* and 10-34*E*). *Cleft lip can be unilateral or bilateral.*

Unilateral cleft lip (Figs. 10-31 and 10-32*A*) results from failure of the maxillary prominence on the affected side to unite with the merged medial nasal prominences (Fig. 10-33*A* to *H*), in turn, causing a persistent labial groove. The tissues in the floor of the persistent groove break down. As a result, the lip is divided into medial and lateral parts. Sometimes, a bridge of tissue, called a *Simonart band*, joins the parts of the incomplete cleft lip.

Bilateral cleft lip (Figs. 10-32*B* and 10-34*F*) results from failure of the mesenchymal masses in the maxillary prominences to meet and unite with the merged medial nasal prominences. When there is a complete bilateral cleft of the lip and the alveolar part of the maxilla, the intermaxillary segment hangs free and projects anteriorly. These defects are especially deforming because of the loss of continuity of the *orbicularis oris muscle*, which closes the mouth and purses the lips.

Median cleft lip is an extremely rare defect. It results from partial or complete failure of the medial nasal prominences to merge and form the intermaxillary segment. Median cleft of the lower lip is also very rare and is caused by failure of the mandibular prominences to merge completely.

The landmark for distinguishing anterior from posterior cleft anomalies is the incisive fossa. Anterior and posterior cleft anomalies are embryologically distinct.

Cleft palate, with or without cleft lip, occurs in approximately 1 in 2500 births and is more common in girls than in boys. The cleft may involve only the uvula, giving it a fishtail appearance (see Fig. 10-34*B*), or it may extend through the soft and hard regions of the palate (see Fig. 10-34*C* and *D*). In severe cases associated with cleft lip, the cleft in the palate extends through the alveolar part of the maxilla and the lips on both sides (see Fig. 10-34*G* and *H*).

Unilateral and bilateral clefts in the palate are classified into three groups:

* *Clefts of the anterior palate* result from failure of the lateral palatine processes to meet and fuse with the primary palate (see Fig. 10-34*F*).
* *Clefts of the posterior palate* result from failure of the lateral palatine processes to meet and fuse with each other and with the nasal septum (see Fig. 10-30*E*).
* *Clefts of the anterior and posterior parts of the palate* result from failure of the lateral palatine processes to meet and fuse with the primary palate, with each other, and with the nasal septum.

Most clefts of the lip and palate result from multiple factors (*multifactorial inheritance*; see Chapter 19). Some clefts of the lip, palate, or both appear as part of syndromes determined by single mutant genes. Other clefts are features of chromosomal syndromes, especially *trisomy 13*. A few cases of cleft lip or cleft palate appear to be caused by teratogenic agents (e.g., anticonvulsant drugs). A sibling of a child with a cleft palate has an elevated risk of having a cleft palate, but no increased risk of cleft lip. A cleft of the lip and the alveolar process of the maxilla that continues through the palate is usually transmitted through a male sex-linked gene.

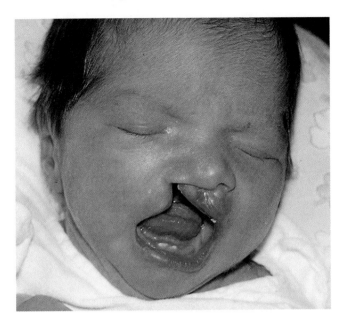

FIGURE 10-31. Infant with unilateral cleft lip and cleft palate. Clefts of the lip, with or without a cleft palate, occur in approximately 1 in 1000 births; most affected individuals are boys. (Courtesy of A.E. Chudley, MD, Professor of Pediatrics and Child Health, Children's Hospital and University of Manitoba, Winnipeg, Manitoba, Canada.)

FACIAL CLEFTS

Various types of facial cleft occur, but are all extremely rare. Severe clefts are usually associated with gross anomalies of the head. *Oblique facial clefts* (orbitofacial fissures) are often bilateral and extend from the upper lip to the medial margin of the orbit. When this occurs, the nasolacrimal ducts are open grooves (persistent nasolacrimal grooves). Oblique facial clefts associated with cleft lip result from failure of the maxillary prominences to merge with the lateral and medial nasal prominences. Lateral, or transverse, facial clefts run from the mouth toward the ear. Bilateral clefts result in a very large mouth, a condition called *macrostomia.* In severe cases, the clefts in the cheeks extend almost to the ears.

OTHER FACIAL ANOMALIES

Congenital microstomia (small mouth) results from excessive merging of the maxillary and mandibular prominences of the first arch. In severe cases, the abnormality may be associated with underdevelopment (hypoplasia) of the mandible. *Absence of the nose* occurs when no nasal placodes form. A *single nostril* results when only one nasal placode forms. *Bifid nose* results when the medial nasal prominences do not merge completely; in such cases, the nostrils are widely separated and the nasal bridge is bifid.

A

B

FIGURE 10-32. Congenital anomalies of the lip and palate. **A,** Infant with a left unilateral cleft lip and a cleft palate. **B,** Infant with a bilateral cleft lip and a cleft palate. (Courtesy of Dr. Barry H. Grayson and Dr. Bruno L. Vendittelli, New York University Medical Center, Institute of Reconstructive Plastic Surgery, New York, NY.)

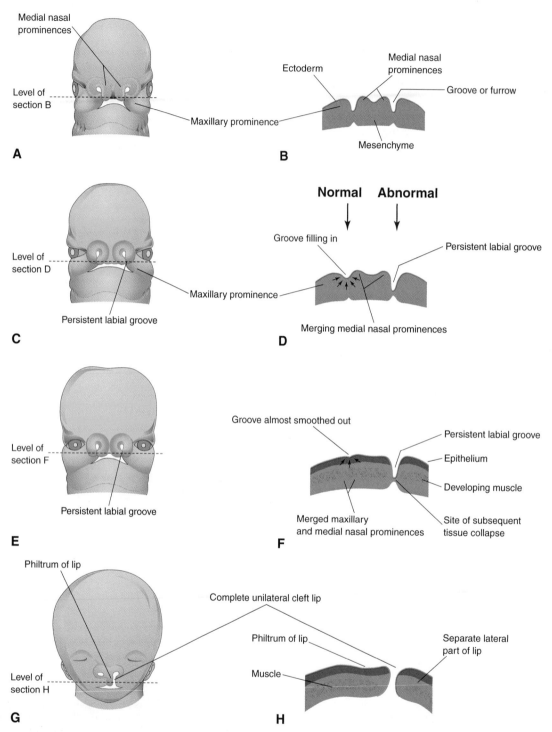

FIGURE 10-33. Illustrations of the embryologic basis for a complete unilateral cleft lip. **A,** A 5-week embryo. **B,** Horizontal section through the head, showing the grooves between the maxillary prominences and the merging medial nasal prominences. **C,** A 6-week embryo, showing a persistent labial groove on the left side. **D,** Horizontal section through the head, showing the groove gradually filling in on the right side after proliferation of the mesenchyme *(arrows).* **E,** A 7-week embryo. **F,** Horizontal section through the head, showing that the epithelium on the right has almost been pushed out of the groove between the maxillary and medial nasal prominences. **G,** A 10-week fetus with a complete unilateral cleft lip. **H,** Horizontal section through the head after stretching of the epithelium and breakdown of the tissues in the floor of the persistent labial groove on the left side, resulting in the formation of a complete unilateral cleft lip.

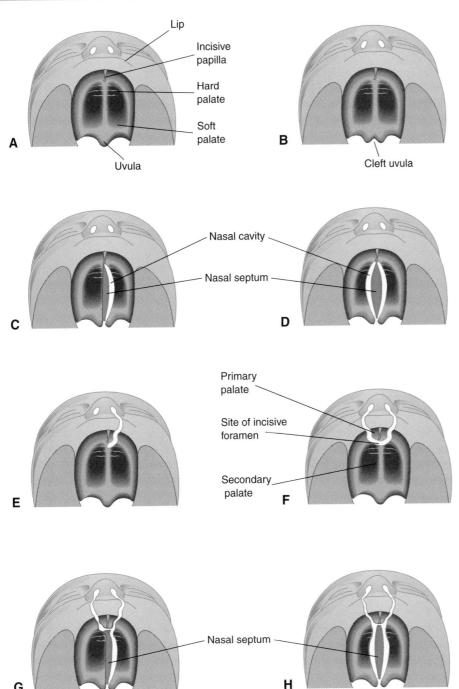

FIGURE 10-34. Various types of cleft lip and cleft palate. **A,** Normal lip and palate. **B,** Cleft uvula. **C,** Unilateral cleft of the posterior, or secondary, palate. **D,** Bilateral cleft of the posterior palate. **E,** Complete unilateral cleft of the lip and the alveolar process of the maxilla, with a unilateral cleft of the anterior, or primary, palate. **F,** Complete bilateral cleft of the lip and the alveolar processes of the maxillae, with bilateral cleft of the anterior palate. **G,** Complete bilateral cleft of the lip and the alveolar processes of the maxillae, with bilateral cleft of the anterior palate and unilateral cleft of the posterior palate. **H,** Complete bilateral cleft of the lip and the alveolar processes of the maxillae, with complete bilateral cleft of the anterior and posterior palate.

between the nasal septum and the palatal processes begins anteriorly during the ninth week and is completed posteriorly by the 12th week, superior to the primordium of the hard palate (see Fig. 10-30D and F). Bone gradually develops by intramembranous ossification (see Chapter 15) in the primary palate, forming the premaxillary part of the maxilla, which lodges the incisor teeth (see Fig. 10-29B). Concurrently, bone extends from the maxillae and the palatine bones into the lateral palatal processes to form the **hard palate** (see Fig. 10-30E and G). The posterior parts of these processes do not become ossified. They extend posteriorly beyond the nasal septum and

fuse to form the **soft palate**, including its soft, conical projection, the **uvula** (see Fig. 10-30D, F, and H). The **median palatal raphe** indicates the line of fusion of the lateral palatal processes. A small nasopalatine canal persists in the median plane of the palate, between the premaxillary part of the maxilla and the palatal processes of the maxillae. This canal is represented in the adult hard palate by the **incisive fossa** (see Fig. 10-29B). An irregular suture runs from the incisive fossa to the alveolar process of the maxilla, between the lateral incisor and the canine teeth on each side, indicating where the embryonic primary and secondary palates fused.

CLINICALLY ORIENTED QUESTIONS

1. What kind of lip defect is a "harelip"? What is the clinical name for this birth defect?

2. Some say that embryos have cleft lips and that this common facial anomaly represents a persistence of this embryonic condition. Are these statements accurate?

3. Neither Clare nor her husband has a cleft lip or a cleft palate, and no one in either one of their families is known to have or to have had these anomalies. What are their chances of having a child with a cleft lip, with or without a cleft palate?

4. Mary's son has a cleft lip and a cleft palate. Her brother has a similar defect involving his lip and palate. Although Mary does not plan to have any more children, her husband says that Mary is entirely to blame for their son's birth defects. Was the defect likely inherited only from Mary's side of the family?

5. A patient's son has minor anomalies involving his external ears, but he does not have hearing problems or a facial malformation. Would his ear abnormalities be considered branchial defects?

The answers to these questions are at the back of the book.

11

THE RESPIRATORY SYSTEM

The **lower respiratory organs** (larynx, trachea, bronchi, and lungs) begin to form during the fourth week. The primordium of the lower respiratory system—the **laryngotracheal groove** (Figs. 11-1*A* to *C*; see Fig. 11-3*A*) develops caudal to the fourth pair of pharyngeal pouches. The endoderm lining gives rise to the epithelium and the glands of the larynx, trachea, bronchi, and pulmonary epithelium. The connective tissue, cartilage, and smooth muscle in these structures develop from the splanchnic mesoderm surrounding the foregut (see Fig. 11-4*A*). By the end of the fourth week, a pouchlike **laryngotracheal diverticulum** (lung bud) forms (Fig. 11-2*A*) and is located ventral to the caudal part of the foregut. As this diverticulum elongates, its distal end enlarges to form a globular **respiratory bud**. The laryngotracheal diverticulum soon separates from the **primordial pharynx**. A partition known as the **tracheoesophageal septum** forms (see Fig. 11-2*D* and *E*), dividing the cranial part of the foregut into a *ventral part*, the **laryngotracheal tube** (primordium of the larynx, trachea, bronchi, and lungs),

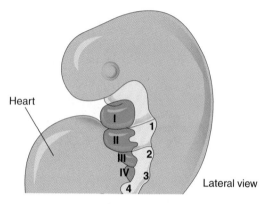

Heart

I
II
III
IV

1
2
3
4

Lateral view

Roman numerals indicate pharyngeal arches and numbers indicate pharyngeal pouches

A

FIGURE 11-1. **A,** Lateral view of a 4-week-old embryo, showing the relationship of the pharyngeal apparatus to the developing respiratory system. **B,** Sagittal section of the cranial half of the embryo. **C,** Horizontal section of the embryo, showing the floor of the primordial pharynx and the location of the laryngotracheal groove.

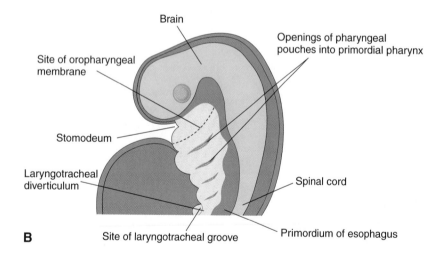

Brain

Site of oropharyngeal membrane

Openings of pharyngeal pouches into primordial pharynx

Stomodeum

Laryngotracheal diverticulum

Spinal cord

Site of laryngotracheal groove

Primordium of esophagus

B

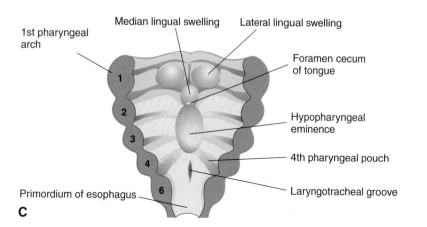

1st pharyngeal arch

Median lingual swelling

Lateral lingual swelling

Foramen cecum of tongue

1
2
3
4
6

Hypopharyngeal eminence

4th pharyngeal pouch

Primordium of esophagus

Laryngotracheal groove

C

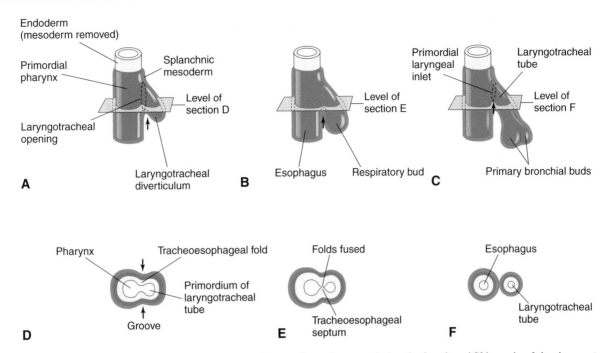

FIGURE 11-2. Successive stages in the development of the tracheoesophageal septum during the fourth and fifth weeks of development. **A to C,** Lateral views of the caudal part of the primordial pharynx, showing the laryngotracheal diverticulum and partitioning of the foregut into the esophagus and the laryngotracheal tube. **D to F,** Transverse sections, showing the formation of the tracheoesophageal septum and how it separates the foregut into the laryngotracheal tube and the esophagus. The *arrows* represent cellular changes resulting from growth.

and a *dorsal part* (primordium of the oropharynx and esophagus) (see Fig. 11-2*F*).

■ DEVELOPMENT OF THE LARYNX

The epithelial lining of the larynx develops from the endoderm of the cranial end of the laryngotracheal tube. The cartilages of the larynx develop from the cartilages in the fourth and sixth pairs of pharyngeal arches (see Chapter 10). The **laryngeal cartilages** develop from mesenchyme that is derived from *neural crest cells*. The mesenchyme at the cranial end of the laryngotracheal tube proliferates rapidly, producing paired **arytenoid swellings** (Fig. 11-3*B*). The laryngeal epithelium proliferates rapidly, resulting in *temporary occlusion of the laryngeal lumen*. Recanalization of the larynx occurs by the 10th week. The laryngeal ventricles form during this recanalization process. These recesses are bound by the folds of mucous membrane that become the *vocal folds* (cords) and the *vestibular folds*. The **epiglottis** develops from the caudal part of the *hypopharyngeal eminence* (see Fig.10-22), a prominence produced by the proliferation of the mesenchyme in the ventral ends of the third and fourth pharyngeal arches (see Fig. 11-3*B* to *D*). The rostral part of this eminence forms the posterior third or pharyngeal part of the tongue (see Chapter 10). Because the **laryngeal muscles** develop from myoblasts in the fourth and sixth pairs of pharyngeal arches, they are innervated by the laryngeal branches of the vagus nerves (cranial nerve X) that supply these arches (see Table 10-1). Growth of the larynx and the epiglottis is rapid during the first 3 years after birth. By 3 years of age, the epiglottis has reached its adult form. There is gradual descent of both structures during early childhood.

LARYNGEAL ATRESIA

Laryngeal atresia (obstruction) is a rare anomaly that results in obstruction of the upper fetal airway; it is also known as **congenital high airway obstruction syndrome**. Distal to the atresia or stenosis (narrowing), the airways become dilated, the lungs are enlarged and echogenic (capable of producing echoes during ultrasonography because they are filled with liquid), the diaphragm is either flattened or inverted, and fetal ascites, hydrops, or both (accumulation of serous fluid) is present. Prenatal ultrasonography permits diagnosis of these anomalies.

■ DEVELOPMENT OF THE TRACHEA

The endodermal lining of the laryngotracheal tube distal to the larynx differentiates into the epithelium and the glands of the trachea and the pulmonary epithelium. The cartilage, connective tissue, and muscles of the trachea are derived from the splanchnic mesoderm surrounding the laryngotracheal tube (Fig. 11-4*A* to *D*).

■ DEVELOPMENT OF THE BRONCHI AND LUNGS

The respiratory bud (lung bud) that develops at the caudal end of the laryngotracheal diverticulum during the fourth week (Fig. 11-2*B*) soon divides into two outpouchings called **primary bronchial buds** (see Figs. 11-2*C* and 11-7*A*).

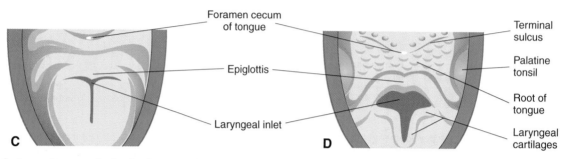

FIGURE 11-3. Successive stages in the development of the larynx. **A,** At 4 weeks. **B,** At 5 weeks. **C,** At 6 weeks. **D,** At 10 weeks. The epithelium lining the larynx is of endodermal origin. The cartilages and muscles of the larynx arise from the mesenchyme in the fourth and sixth pairs of pharyngeal arches. Note that the laryngeal inlet changes in shape from a slitlike opening to a T-shaped inlet as the mesenchyme surrounding the developing larynx proliferates.

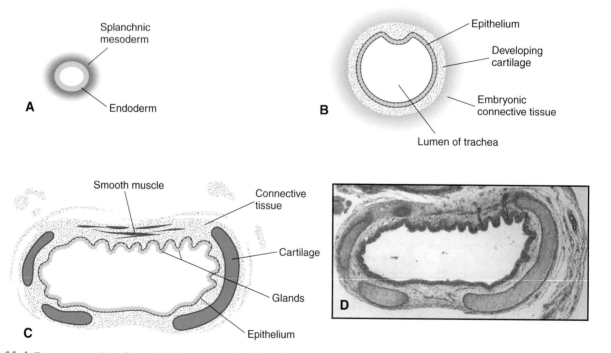

FIGURE 11-4. Transverse sections through the laryngotracheal tube, showing progressive stages in the development of the trachea. **A,** At 4 weeks. **B,** At 10 weeks. **C,** At 11 weeks. Note that the endoderm of the tube gives rise to the epithelium and the glands of the trachea and that the mesenchyme surrounding the tube forms the connective tissue, muscle, and cartilage (drawing of the micrograph shown in **D**). **D,** Photomicrograph of a transverse section of the developing trachea at 12 weeks. (From Moore KL, Persaud TVN, Shiota K: Color Atlas of Clinical Embryology, 2nd ed. Philadelphia, WB Saunders, 2000.)

TRACHEOESOPHAGEAL FISTULA

A **tracheoesophageal fistula (TEF)** is an abnormal passage between the trachea and the esophagus (Fig. 11-5). It occurs at a rate of approximately 1 in 3000 to 1 in 4500 live births, and it predominantly affects boys. In most cases, the fistula is associated with **esophageal atresia**. TEF results from incomplete division of the cranial part of the foregut into respiratory and esophageal parts during the fourth week. Incomplete fusion of the tracheoesophageal folds results in a **defective tracheoesophageal septum** and communication between the trachea and esophagus.

TEF is the most common anomaly of the lower respiratory tract. Four main varieties of TEF may develop. The usual anomaly is a blind ending of the superior part of the esophagus (*esophageal atresia*) and a joining of the inferior part to the trachea near its bifurcation (Figs. 11-5*A* and 11-6). Infants with this type of TEF and esophageal atresia cough and choke when swallowing because of the accumulation of excessive amounts of liquid in the mouth and upper respiratory tract. When the infant attempts to swallow milk, it rapidly fills the esophageal pouch and is regurgitated. Gastric contents may also reflux from the stomach through the fistula into the trachea and lungs and may result in pneumonia or pneumonitis (inflammation of the lungs). Other varieties of TEF are shown in Figure 11-5*B* to *D*. **Polyhydramnios** (see Chapter 8) is often associated with esophageal atresia and TEF. Excess amniotic fluid accumulates because fluid cannot pass to the stomach and intestines for absorption and subsequent transfer through the placenta to the mother's blood for disposal.

TRACHEAL STENOSIS AND ATRESIA

Narrowing (stenosis) and obstruction (atresia) of the trachea are uncommon anomalies that are usually associated with one of the varieties of TEF. Stenoses and atresias probably result from unequal partitioning of the foregut into the esophagus and the trachea. In some cases, a web of tissue obstructs airflow (*incomplete tracheal atresia*).

Later, **secondary bronchial buds** form and grow laterally into the *pericardioperitoneal canals* (see Fig. 11-7*A*). Together with the surrounding splanchnic mesoderm, the bronchial buds differentiate into the bronchi and their ramifications in the lungs (Fig. 11-7*B*). Early in the fifth week, the connection of each bronchial bud with the trachea enlarges to form the primordium of a main bronchus (Fig. 11-8). The embryonic right main bronchus is slightly larger than the left one and is oriented more vertically. The main bronchi subdivide into **secondary bronchi** (see Fig. 11-8). On the right, the superior secondary bronchus supplies the superior (upper) lobe of the lung, whereas the inferior secondary bronchus subdivides into two bronchi, one connecting to the middle lobe of the right lung and the other connecting to the inferior (lower) lobe. On the left, the two secondary bronchi supply the superior and inferior lobes of the lung. Each secondary bronchus undergoes progressive branching. The **segmental bronchi**—10 in the right lung and 8 or 9 in the left lung—begin to form by the seventh week. As this development occurs, the surrounding mesenchyme also divides. Each segmental bronchus, with its surrounding mass of mesenchyme, is the primordium of a **bronchopulmonary segment**. By 24 weeks, approximately 17 orders of branches have formed and **respiratory bronchioles** have developed (Fig. 11-9*B*). An additional seven orders of airways develop after birth.

As the bronchi develop, cartilaginous plates are formed from the surrounding splanchnic mesoderm. The bronchial smooth muscle and connective tissue and the pulmonary connective tissue and capillaries are also derived from this mesoderm. As the lungs develop, they acquire a layer of **visceral pleura** from the splanchnic mesoderm (Fig. 11-7*B*). With expansion, the lungs and pleural cavities grow caudally into the mesenchyme of the body wall and soon lie close to the heart. The thoracic body wall becomes lined by a layer of **parietal pleura**, derived from the somatic mesoderm.

Maturation of the Lungs

Maturation of the lungs is divided into four stages: pseudoglandular, canalicular, terminal saccular, and alveolar.

Pseudoglandular Period (6–16 Weeks)

The developing lungs somewhat histologically resemble an exocrine gland during the early part of this period (see Fig. 11-9*A*). By 16 weeks, all of the major elements of the lung have formed, except those involved with gas exchange. Respiration is not possible; hence, *fetuses born during this period are unable to survive.*

Canalicular Period (16–26 Weeks)

The canalicular period overlaps the pseudoglandular period because cranial segments of the lungs mature faster than caudal segments. During the canalicular period, the lumina of the bronchi and the terminal bronchioles become larger and the lung tissue becomes highly vascular (see Fig. 11-9*B*). By 24 weeks, each terminal bronchiole has given rise to two or more **respiratory bronchioles**, each of which then divides into three to six tubular passages called the primordial **alveolar ducts**. Respiration is possible toward the end of the canalicular stage because

FIGURE 11-5. The main varieties of tracheoesophageal fistula, shown in order of frequency. Possible directions of the flow of the contents are indicated by *arrows*. **A,** Esophageal atresia is associated with tracheoesophageal fistula in more than 85% of cases. **B,** Fistula between the trachea and the esophagus; this type of anomaly accounts for approximately 4% of cases. **C,** Air cannot enter the distal esophagus and the stomach. **D,** Atresia of the proximal segment of the esophagus, with fistulas between the trachea and both the proximal and the distal segments of the esophagus. All infants born with tracheoesophageal fistula have esophageal dysmotility, and most have reflux.

FIGURE 11-6. Tracheoesophageal fistula in a 17-week male fetus. The upper esophageal segment ends blindly (pointer). (From Kalousek DK, Fitch N, Paradice BA: Pathology of the Human Embryo and Previable Fetus. New York, Springer Verlag, 1990.)

some thin-walled **terminal sacs** (primordial alveoli) have developed at the ends of the respiratory bronchioles and the lung tissue is well vascularized. Although a fetus born at 24 to 26 weeks may survive if given intensive care, a fetus born at this time often has respiratory distress because of pulmonary surfactant deficiency.

Terminal Sac Stage (26 Weeks to Birth)

During this period, many more terminal sacs develop (see Fig. 11-9C), and their epithelium becomes very thin. Capillaries begin to bulge into these developing alveoli. The intimate contact between epithelial and endothelial cells establishes the **blood-air barrier**, which permits adequate gas exchange for survival of the fetus if it is born prematurely. By 26 weeks, the terminal sacs are lined mainly by squamous epithelial cells of endodermal origin—**type I alveolar cells**, or pneumocytes—across which gas exchange occurs. The capillary network proliferates rapidly in the mesenchyme around the developing alveoli, and there is concurrent active development of lymphatic capillaries. Scattered among the squamous epithelial cells are rounded secretory epithelial cells—**type II alveolar cells**, or pneumocytes—*which secrete pulmonary surfactant*, a complex mixture of phospholipids and proteins.

The maturation of alveolar type II cells and the production of surfactant vary widely in fetuses of different ages. The production of **surfactant** increases during the terminal stages of pregnancy, particularly during the last 2 weeks before birth. Surfactant counteracts the forces of pulmonary surface tension and facilitates expansion of the terminal sacs (primordial alveoli) by preventing atelectasis (collapse of terminal sacs during exhalation).

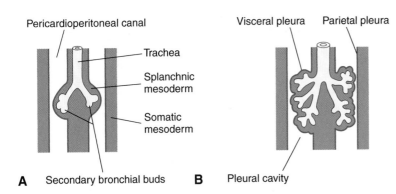

FIGURE 11-7. Illustrations of the growth of the developing lungs into the splanchnic mesoderm adjacent to the medial walls of the pericardioperitoneal canals (primordial pleural cavities). Development of the layers of the pleura is also shown. **A,** At 5 weeks. **B,** At 6 weeks.

Surfactant production begins by 20 weeks, but surfactant is present in only small amounts in premature infants. It does not reach adequate levels until the late fetal period. Both increased surfactant production induced by antenatal corticosteroids and surfactant replacement therapy have increased the rates of survival of these infants.

Alveolar Period (32 Weeks to 8 Years)

Exactly when the terminal saccular period ends and the alveolar period begins depends on the definition of the term **alveolus** (see Fig. 11-9D). At the beginning of the alveolar period, each respiratory bronchiole terminates in a cluster of thin-walled terminal sacs that are separated from one another by loose connective tissue. These terminal sacs represent future alveolar ducts. The **alveolocapillary membrane** (pulmonary diffusion barrier, or respiratory membrane) is sufficiently thin to allow gas exchange. The transition

from dependence on the placenta for gas exchange to autonomous gas exchange requires the following adaptive changes in the lungs:

● Production of surfactant in the alveolar sacs
● Transformation of the lungs from secretory organs into gas-exchanging organs
● Establishment of parallel pulmonary and systemic circulations

Approximately 95% of characteristic **mature alveoli** develop postnatally. Before birth, the primordial alveoli appear as small bulges on the walls of the respiratory bronchioles and terminal sacs (future alveolar ducts). After birth, the primordial alveoli enlarge as the lungs expand; however, most of the increase in the size of the lungs results from an increase in the number of respiratory bronchioles and primordial alveoli rather than from an increase in the size of the alveoli. Alveolar development is largely complete by 3 years of age, but new alveoli may be added until approximately 8 years of age. Unlike mature

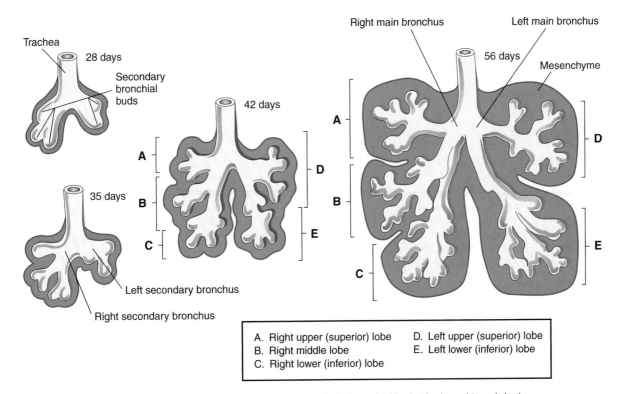

A. Right upper (superior) lobe	D. Left upper (superior) lobe
B. Right middle lobe	E. Left lower (inferior) lobe
C. Right lower (inferior) lobe	

FIGURE 11-8. Successive stages in the development of the bronchial buds, the bronchi, and the lungs.

A Pseudoglandular period (6–16 weeks)

B Canalicular period (16–26 weeks)

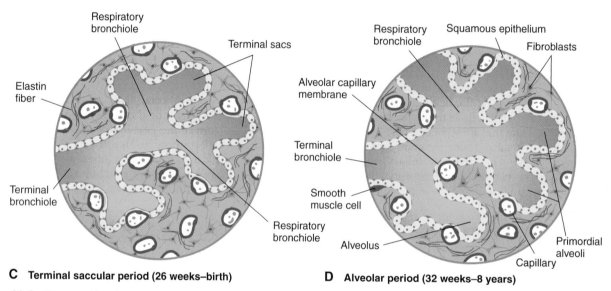

C Terminal saccular period (26 weeks–birth)

D Alveolar period (32 weeks–8 years)

FIGURE 11-9. Diagram of histologic sections, showing progressive stages of lung development. **A** and **B**, Early stages of lung development. In **C** and **D**, note that the alveolocapillary membrane is thin and that some capillaries bulge into the terminal saccules.

alveoli, immature alveoli have the potential for forming additional primordial alveoli. As these alveoli increase in size, they become mature alveoli.

Approximately 150 million primordial alveoli, one half the number in adults, are present in the lungs of a full-term newborn infant. On chest radiographs, therefore, the lungs of newborn infants appear denser than adult lungs. Between the third and the eighth year, the adult complement of 300 million alveoli is achieved.

Three factors are important for normal lung development:
● Adequate thoracic space for lung growth
● Fetal breathing movements
● Adequate amniotic fluid volume

Fetal breathing movements occur before birth, exerting sufficient force to cause aspiration of some amniotic fluid into the lungs. These fetal breathing movements occur approximately 50% of the time and only during rapid eye movement sleep; they are essential for normal lung development. These movements stimulate lung development, possibly by creating a pressure gradient between the lungs and the amniotic fluid. By birth, the fetus has had the advantage of several months of breathing exercise. Fetal breathing movements increase as the time of delivery approaches.

At birth, the lungs are approximately half-filled with fluid derived from the amniotic cavity, the lungs, and the tracheal glands. Aeration of the lungs at birth occurs not so much by the inflation of empty collapsed organs as by the rapid replacement of intra-alveolar fluid by air. The fluid in the lungs is cleared at birth by three routes:
● Through the mouth and nose by pressure on the thorax during vaginal delivery
● Into the pulmonary capillaries and pulmonary arteries and veins
● Into the lymphatics

OLIGOHYDRAMNIOS AND LUNG DEVELOPMENT

When oligohydramnios (an insufficient amount of amniotic fluid) is severe and chronic (e.g., because of amniotic fluid leakage), lung development is retarded because restriction of the fetal thorax impedes lung growth. Pulmonary hypoplasia occurs as a result and may be severe.

RESPIRATORY DISTRESS SYNDROME

Respiratory distress syndrome (RDS) affects approximately 2% of live newborn infants, and those born prematurely are the most susceptible. RDS is also known as *hyaline membrane disease*. These affected infants have rapid, labored breathing shortly after birth. An estimated 30% of all neonatal disease results from RDS or its complications. *Surfactant deficiency is a major cause of RDS.* The lungs are underinflated, and the alveoli contain fluid with high protein content that appears glassy—*hyaline membrane*. This membrane is believed to be derived from a combination of substances in the circulation and from the injured pulmonary epithelium. Prolonged intrauterine asphyxia may produce irreversible changes in type II alveolar cells, making them incapable of producing surfactant. Not all of the growth factors and hormones that control surfactant production have been identified, but *corticosteroids* and *thyroxine* are potent stimulators of surfactant production.

Glucocorticoid treatment during pregnancy accelerates fetal lung development and surfactant production. This finding has led to the routine clinical use of corticosteroids (betamethasone) for the prevention of RDS in preterm labor. In addition, the intratracheal administration of *exogenous* surfactant (**surfactant replacement therapy**) reduces both the severity of RDS and the neonatal mortality rate.

LUNGS OF NEWBORN INFANTS

Fresh, healthy neonatal lungs always contain some air; consequently, pulmonary tissue samples float in water. By contrast, a diseased lung that is partially filled with fluid may not float. Of medicolegal significance is the fact that the lungs of a stillborn infant are firm and sink when placed in water because they contain fluid, not air.

LUNG HYPOPLASIA

In infants with a congenital diaphragmatic hernia (see Chapter 9), the lung is unable to develop normally because it is compressed by the abnormally positioned abdominal viscera. Lung hypoplasia is characterized by markedly reduced lung volume. Most infants with a congenital diaphragmatic hernia die of pulmonary insufficiency, despite optimal postnatal care, because their lungs are too hypoplastic to support extrauterine life.

CLINICALLY ORIENTED QUESTIONS

1. What stimulates the infant to start breathing at birth? Is "slapping the buttocks" necessary?
2. An infant reportedly died approximately 72 hours after birth from the effects of respiratory distress syndrome. What is respiratory distress syndrome? By what other name is this condition known? Is its cause genetic or environmental?
3. Can an infant born 22 weeks after fertilization survive?

The answers to these questions are at the back of the book.

THE ALIMENTARY OR DIGESTIVE SYSTEM

A the beginning of the fourth week of development, the **primordial gut** is closed at its cranial end by the **oropharyngeal membrane** (see Fig. 11-1*B*) and at its caudal end by the **cloacal membrane** (Fig. 12-1). The primordial gut forms during the fourth week as the head, tail, and lateral folds incorporate the dorsal part of the umbilical vesicle into the embryo (see Chapter 6). The endoderm of the primordial gut gives rise to most of the epithelium and glands of the alimentary tract. The epithelium at the cranial and caudal extremities of the tract is derived from the ectoderm of the **stomodeum** and the **proctodeum** (anal pit), respectively (see Fig. 12-1). The muscular tissue, connective tissue, and other layers of the wall of the digestive tract are derived from the splanchnic mesenchyme surrounding the primordial gut. The primordial gut is divided into three parts: foregut, midgut, and hindgut. The regional differentiation of the primordial gut is established by *homeobox genes* that are expressed in the endoderm and the surrounding mesoderm. The endoderm provides temporal and positional information for the development of the gut.

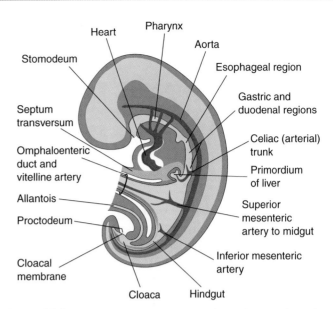

FIGURE 12-1. Median section of a 4-week embryo, showing the early alimentary, or digestive, system and its blood supply. The primordial gut is a long tube extending the length of the embryo. Its blood vessels are derived from the vessels that supplied the umbilical vesicle.

■ THE FOREGUT

The derivatives of the foregut are as follows:
● The *primordial pharynx* and its derivatives
● The *lower respiratory system*
● The *esophagus* and *stomach*
● The *duodenum*, just distal to the opening of the bile duct
● The *liver, biliary apparatus* (hepatic ducts, gallbladder, and bile duct), and pancreas

All of these foregut derivatives except the pharynx, the respiratory tract, and most of the esophagus are supplied by the celiac trunk, the artery of the foregut (Figs. 12-1 and 12-2*A*).

Development of the Esophagus

The separation of the esophagus from the laryngotracheal tube by the **tracheoesophageal septum** is described in Chapter 11. Initially, the esophagus is short, but it elongates rapidly and reaches its final relative length by the seventh week. Its epithelium and glands are derived from the endoderm. The epithelium proliferates and partly or completely obliterates the lumen; however, recanalization of the esophagus normally occurs by the end of the eighth week. The striated muscle of the esophagus is derived from the mesenchyme in the caudal pharyngeal arches. The smooth muscle, mainly in the inferior third of the esophagus, develops from the surrounding splanchnic mesenchyme.

Development of the Stomach

Approximately in the middle of the fourth week, a slight dilation of the tubelike foregut indicates the site of the primordial stomach. It first appears as a fusiform enlargement that is oriented in the median plane (see

---

ESOPHAGEAL ATRESIA

Blockage of the esophagus occurs in approximately 1 in 3000 to 1 in 4500 live births. Approximately one third of affected infants are born prematurely. Esophageal atresia is frequently associated with **tracheoesophageal fistula** (see Fig. 11-5). Esophageal atresia results from deviation of the *tracheoesophageal septum* in a posterior direction (see Figs. 11-2 and 11-6); as a result, separation of the esophagus from the laryngotracheal tube is incomplete. In some cases, the atresia results from *failure of esophageal recanalization* during the eighth week of development. A fetus with esophageal atresia is unable to swallow amniotic fluid, resulting in polyhydramnios, the accumulation of an excessive amount of amniotic fluid.

ESOPHAGEAL STENOSIS

Narrowing of the lumen of the esophagus (stenosis) can occur anywhere along the esophagus, but it usually occurs in the distal one third, either as a web or as a long segment of esophagus with a threadlike lumen. The stenosis usually results from incomplete recanalization of the esophagus during the eighth week, but it may result from a failure of esophageal blood vessels to develop in the affected area.

Fig. 12-2*B*). The primordial stomach enlarges and broadens ventrodorsally. Its dorsal border grows more quickly than its ventral border. This site of rapid growth demarcates the **greater curvature of the stomach** (see Fig. 12-2*D*).

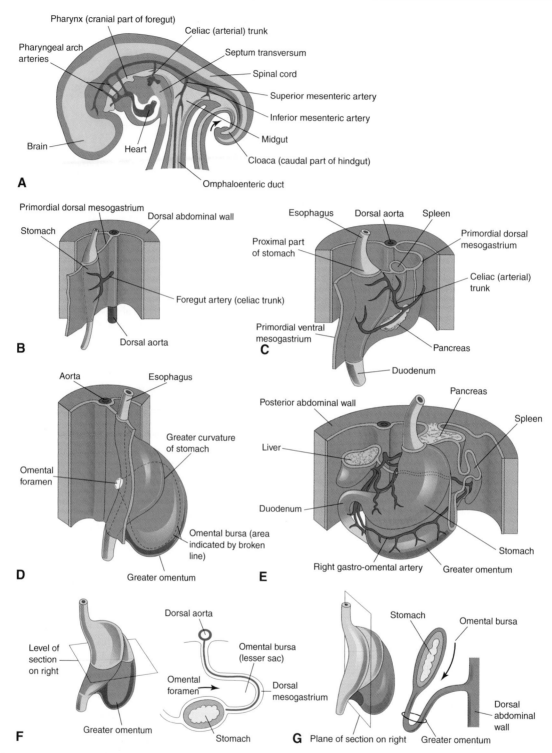

FIGURE 12-2. Illustrations of the development and rotation of the stomach and the formation of the omental bursa (lesser sac) and the greater omentum. **A,** Median section of a 28-day embryo. **B,** Anterolateral view of a 28-day embryo. **C,** Embryo at approximately 35 days. **D,** Embryo at approximately 40 days. **E,** Embryo at approximately 48 days. **F,** Lateral view of the stomach and greater omentum of an embryo at approximately 52 days. The transverse section shows the omental foramen and omental bursa. **G,** Sagittal section, showing the omental bursa and greater omentum. The *arrow* in **F** and **G** indicates the site of the omental foramen.

Rotation of the Stomach

As the stomach enlarges, it rotates 90 degrees in a clockwise direction around its longitudinal axis. The effects of rotation on the stomach are as follows (Figs. 12-2 and 12-3):

- The ventral border (lesser curvature) moves to the right, and the dorsal border (greater curvature) moves to the left (see Fig. 12-2C to F).
- Before rotation, the cranial and caudal ends of the stomach are in the median plane (see Fig. 12-2B).

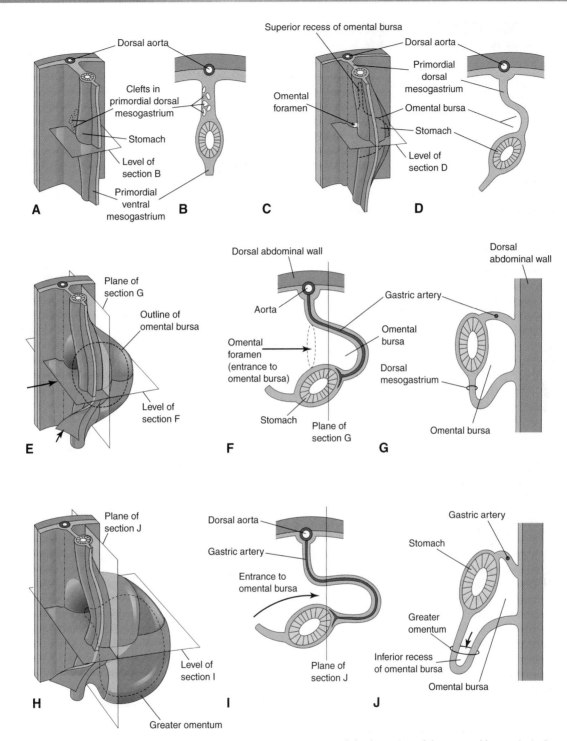

FIGURE 12-3. Illustrations of the development of the stomach and its mesenteries and the formation of the omental bursa. **A,** At 5 weeks. **B,** Transverse section, showing clefts in the dorsal mesogastrium. **C,** Later stage, after coalescence of the clefts to form the omental bursa. **D,** Transverse section, showing the initial appearance of the omental bursa. **E,** The dorsal mesentery has elongated and the omental bursa has enlarged. **F** and **G,** Transverse and sagittal sections, respectively, showing elongation of the dorsal mesogastrium and expansion of the omental bursa. **H,** At 6 weeks, showing the greater omentum and expansion of the omental bursa. **I** and **J,** Transverse and sagittal sections, respectively, showing the inferior recess of the omental bursa and the omental foramen. The *arrows* in **E, F,** and **I,** indicate the site of the omental foramen. In **J,** the *arrow* indicates the recess of the omental bursa.

● During rotation and growth of the stomach, its cranial region moves to the left and slightly inferiorly, and its caudal region moves to the right and superiorly (see Fig 12-2C to E).

● After rotation, the stomach assumes its final position, with its long axis almost transverse to the long axis of the body (see Fig. 12-2E). The rotation and growth of the stomach explain why the left vagus nerve supplies the anterior wall of the adult stomach and the right vagus nerve innervates its posterior wall.

Mesenteries of the Stomach

The stomach is suspended from the dorsal wall of the abdominal cavity by a dorsal mesentery—the primordial **dorsal mesogastrium** (see Figs. 12-2*B* and *C* and 12-3*A* to *D*). This mesentery, originally located in the median plane, is carried to the left during rotation of the stomach. The primordial **ventral mesogastrium**—attaches the stomach and duodenum to the liver and the ventral abdominal wall (see Figs. 12-2*C* and 12-3*A* and *B*).

The Omental Bursa

Isolated clefts develop in the mesenchyme that forms the thick dorsal mesogastrium (see Fig. 12-3*A* and *B*). The clefts soon coalesce to form a single cavity—the **omental bursa** *(lesser sac)*, a large recess of the peritoneal cavity (see Figs. 12-2*F* and *G* and 12-3*C* and *D*). Rotation of the stomach pulls the dorsal mesogastrium to the left, thereby enlarging the bursa. The omental bursa lies between the stomach and the posterior abdominal wall. As the stomach enlarges, the omental bursa expands and hangs over the developing intestines. This part of the omental bursa is called the **greater omentum** (see Figs. 12-3*G* to *J* and 12-14*A*). The two layers of the greater omentum eventually fuse (see Fig. 12-14*F*). The omental bursa communicates with the main part of the peritoneal cavity through a small opening known as the **omental foramen** (see Figs. 12-2*D* and *F* and 12-3*C* and *F*).

Development of the Duodenum

Early in the fourth week, the duodenum develops just distal to the origin of the bile duct from the caudal part of the foregut and the cranial part of the midgut (Fig. 12-4*A*). The developing duodenum elongates, forming a C-shaped loop that projects ventrally (see Fig. 12-4*B* to *D*). As the stomach rotates, the duodenal loop rotates to the right and comes to lie retroperitoneally (external to the peritoneum). Because of its derivation from the foregut and the midgut, the duodenum is supplied by branches of both the celiac and the superior mesenteric arteries (see Fig. 12-1). The lumen of the duodenum is temporarily obliterated because of the proliferation of its epithelial cells. Normally, the duodenum becomes recanalized by the end of the embryonic period.

Development of the Liver and the Biliary Apparatus

The liver, gallbladder, and biliary duct system arise as a ventral outgrowth (hepatic diverticulum) from the caudal part of the foregut early in the fourth week (Figs. 12-4*A* and 12-7*A*). The **hepatic diverticulum** extends into the septum transversum (see Fig. 12-7*B*), a mass of splanchnic mesoderm between the developing heart and the midgut. The hepatic diverticulum enlarges and divides into two parts as it grows between the layers of the **ventral mesogastrium** (see Fig. 12-4*A*). The larger, cranial part of the hepatic diverticulum is the **primordium of the liver**. The proliferating endodermal cells give rise to interlacing cords of hepatocytes and to the epithelial lining of the intrahepatic part of the biliary apparatus. The **hepatic cords** anastomose around endothelium-lined spaces, the primordia of the hepatic sinusoids. The fibrous and

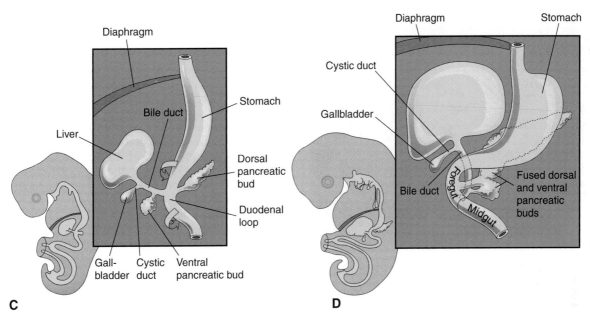

FIGURE 12-4. Illustrations of progressive stages in the development of the duodenum, liver, pancreas, and extrahepatic biliary apparatus. **A,** At 4 weeks. **B** and **C,** At 5 weeks. **D,** At 6 weeks.

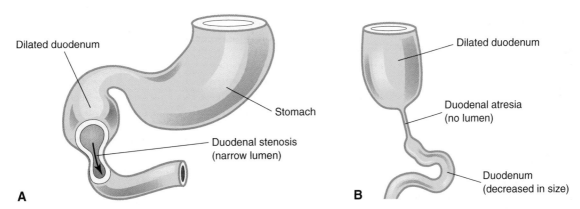

FIGURE 12-5. Illustrations of the embryologic basis of the two common types of congenital intestinal obstruction. **A,** Duodenal stenosis. The *arrow* is in the stenotic lumen of the duodenum. **B,** Duodenal atresia. Most duodenal atresias occur in the descending and horizontal parts of the duodenum.

FIGURE 12-6. Ultrasound scans of a fetus at 33 weeks' gestation (31 weeks after fertilization), showing duodenal atresia. **A,** An oblique scan shows the dilated, fluid-filled stomach (St) entering the proximal duodenum (D), which is also enlarged because of the atresia (blockage) distal to it. **B,** Transverse ultrasound scan, showing the characteristic "double-bubble" appearance of the stomach and duodenum when there is duodenal atresia. (Courtesy of Dr. Lyndon M. Hill, Magee-Women's Hospital, Pittsburgh, PA.)

hematopoietic tissue and Kupffer cells of the liver are derived from the mesenchyme in the septum transversum.

The liver grows rapidly and soon fills a large part of the abdominal cavity (see Figs. 12-7C and D and 12-13). **Hematopoiesis** (formation of various types of blood cells and other formed elements) begins during the sixth week. By the ninth week, the liver accounts for approximately 10% of the total weight of the fetus. **Bile formation** by the hepatic cells begins during the 12th week.

The small, caudal part of the hepatic diverticulum becomes the **gallbladder**, and the stalk of the diverticulum forms the **cystic duct** (see Fig. 12-4B and C). Initially, the *extrahepatic biliary apparatus* is occluded with epithelial cells. The stalk connecting the hepatic and cystic ducts to the duodenum becomes the **bile duct** (common bile duct). Initially, this duct attaches to the ventral aspect of the duodenal loop; however, as the duodenum grows and

---

ANOMALIES OF THE LIVER AND THE BILIARY DUCTS

Minor variations of liver lobulation are common, but congenital anomalies of the liver are rare. Variations of the hepatic ducts, bile duct, and cystic duct are common. For example, **accessory hepatic ducts** may be present, and an awareness of their possible presence is important from a surgical perspective.

EXTRAHEPATIC BILIARY ATRESIA

Extrahepatic biliary atresia, the most serious anomaly involving the extrahepatic biliary system, is uncommon. Failure of the bile ducts to canalize often results from persistence of the solid stage of duct development. Jaundice occurs soon after birth.

rotates, the entrance of the bile duct is carried to the dorsal aspect of the duodenum (see Fig. 12-4C and D).

The Ventral Mesentery

The thin, *double-layered ventral mesentery* (Figs. 12-7C and D and 12-8) gives rise to two structures:
- The **lesser omentum**, which passes from the liver to the lesser curvature of the stomach (hepatogastric ligament) and from the liver to the duodenum *(hepatoduodenal ligament)*
- The **falciform ligament**, which extends from the liver to the ventral abdominal wall

The **umbilical vein** passes in the free border of the falciform ligament on its way from the umbilical cord to the liver. The ventral mesentery, derived from the mesogastrium, also forms the visceral peritoneum of the liver.

Development of the Pancreas

The pancreas develops from the dorsal and ventral **pancreatic buds**, which arise from the caudal part of the foregut (Fig. 12-9A). Most of the pancreas is derived from the **dorsal pancreatic bud**, which appears first. It grows rapidly between the layers of the dorsal mesentery. The **ventral pancreatic bud** develops near the entry of the bile duct into the duodenum and grows between the layers of the ventral mesentery (see Fig. 12-9A and B). As the duodenum rotates to the right and becomes C-shaped, the ventral pancreatic bud is carried dorsally with the bile duct (see Fig. 12-9C to F). It soon lies posterior to the dorsal pancreatic bud and later fuses with it (see Fig. 12-9G).

Formation of the dorsal pancreatic bud depends on signals from the notochord (activin and fibroblast growth factor 2) that block the expression of Sonic hedgehog (Shh) in the endoderm.

The ventral pancreatic bud forms the *uncinate process* and part of the *head of the pancreas*. As the stomach, duodenum, and ventral mesentery rotate, the pancreas comes to lie along the dorsal abdominal wall (see Fig. 12-11D and E). As the pancreatic buds fuse, their ducts anastomose. The

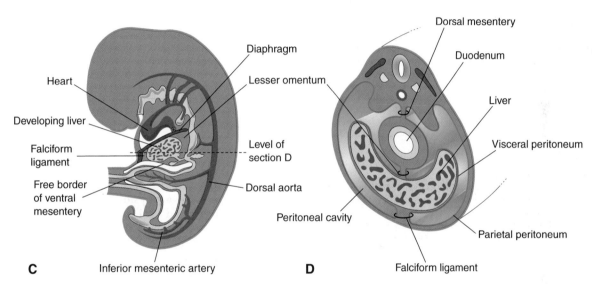

FIGURE 12-7. Illustrations of how the caudal part of the septum transversum becomes stretched and membranous as it forms the ventral mesentery. **A,** Median section of a 4-week embryo. **B,** Transverse section of the embryo, showing expansion of the peritoneal cavity *(arrows)*. **C,** Sagittal section of a 5-week embryo. **D,** Transverse section of the embryo after formation of the dorsal and ventral mesenteries.

pancreatic duct forms from the duct of the ventral bud and the distal part of the duct of the dorsal bud (see Fig. 12-9*G*). In approximately 9% of people, the proximal part of the duct of the dorsal bud often persists as an **accessory pancreatic duct** that opens into the *minor duodenal papilla*. The connective tissue sheath and the interlobular septa of the pancreas develop from the surrounding splanchnic mesenchyme. **Insulin secretion** begins at approximately 10 weeks. The glucagon- and somatostatin-containing cells develop before differentiation of the insulin-secreting cells occurs. With increasing fetal age, total pancreatic insulin and glucagon content also increases.

■ DEVELOPMENT OF THE SPLEEN

The spleen is derived from a mass of mesenchymal cells located between the layers of the dorsal mesogastrium (Fig. 12-11*A* and *B*). The spleen begins to develop during the fifth week, but does not acquire its characteristic shape

ANULAR PANCREAS

Anular pancreas is an uncommon anomaly, but it warrants description because it may cause duodenal obstruction (Fig. 12-10C). The ringlike, anular part of the pancreas consists of a thin, flat band of pancreatic tissue surrounding the descending, or second, part of the duodenum. An anular pancreas may cause obstruction of the duodenum shortly after birth, but many cases are not diagnosed until adulthood. Boys are affected much more frequently than girls. Anular pancreas probably results from the growth of a bifid ventral pancreatic bud around the duodenum (see Fig. 12-10A to C). The parts of the bifid ventral bud then fuse with the dorsal bud, forming a pancreatic ring.

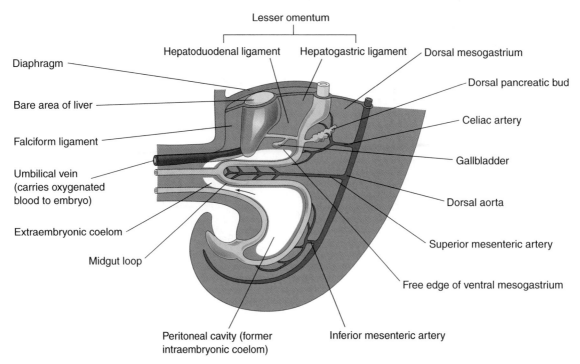

FIGURE 12-8. Median section of the caudal half of an embryo at the end of the fifth week, showing the liver and its associated ligaments. The *arrow* indicates the communication of the peritoneal cavity with the extraembryonic coelom. Because of the rapid growth of the liver and the midgut loop, the abdominal cavity temporarily becomes too small to contain the developing intestines; consequently, they enter the extraembryonic coelom in the proximal part of the umbilical cord.

ACCESSORY SPLEENS

One or more small splenic masses (polysplenia) may develop, commonly near the hilum of the spleen or adjacent to the tail of the pancreas. An accessory spleen (approximately 1 cm in diameter) occurs in approximately 10% of people.

---

until early in the fetal period. The spleen is lobulated in the fetus, but the lobules normally disappear before birth. The notches in the superior border of the adult spleen are remnants of the grooves that separated the fetal lobules.

■ THE MIDGUT

The derivatives of the midgut are as follows:
● The small intestine, including the duodenum distal to the opening of the bile duct
● The cecum, appendix, ascending colon, and right one half to two thirds of the transverse colon

All of these derivatives are supplied by the **superior mesenteric artery** (see Fig. 12-1). The midgut loop is suspended from the dorsal abdominal wall by an elongated mesentery (see Fig. 12-8). The midgut elongates and forms a ventral, U-shaped **midgut loop of the intestine** that projects into the proximal part of the umbilical cord. At this stage, the intraembryonic coelom communicates with the extraembryonic coelom at the umbilicus (see Fig. 12-8). This

projection of the intestine, occurring at the beginning of the sixth week, is called a **physiologic umbilical herniation** (Figs. 12-12*A* to *C* and 12-13). Umbilical herniation occurs because there is not enough room in the abdomen for the rapidly growing midgut.

The midgut loop communicates with the umbilical vesicle through the narrow **omphaloenteric duct** (yolk stalk) until the 10th week (see Fig. 12-12*A*). This loop has both cranial and caudal limbs. The cranial limb grows rapidly and forms small intestinal loops. The caudal limb undergoes very little change, except for the development of the **cecal diverticulum**, which is the primordium of the cecum and the appendix (see Fig. 12-12*C* to *E*).

Rotation of the Midgut Loop

While in the umbilical cord, the midgut loop rotates 90 degrees counterclockwise around the axis of the **superior mesenteric artery** (see Fig. 12-12*B*). This rotation brings the cranial limb (small intestine) of the midgut loop to the right and the caudal limb (large intestine) to the left. During rotation, the cranial limb elongates and forms loops of small intestine.

Return of the Midgut to the Abdomen

During the 10th week, with enlargement of the abdominal cavity, the intestines return to the abdomen (*reduction of the physiologic midgut hernia*) (see Fig. 12-12*C* and *D*). The small intestine returns first, passing posterior to the superior mesenteric artery, and occupies the central part of

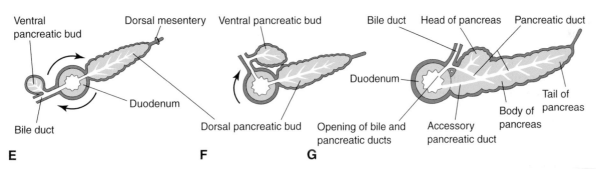

FIGURE 12-9. **A** to **D**, Illustrations of successive stages in the development of the pancreas from the fifth to the eighth weeks. **E** to **G**, Transverse sections through the duodenum and the developing pancreas. Growth and rotation *(arrows)* of the duodenum bring the ventral pancreatic bud toward the dorsal bud; these two structures subsequently fuse. Note that the bile duct initially attaches to the ventral aspect of the duodenum and is carried around to the dorsal aspect as the duodenum rotates. The pancreatic duct is formed by the union of the distal part of the dorsal pancreatic duct and the entire ventral pancreatic duct. The proximal part of the dorsal pancreatic duct usually obliterates, but it may persist as an accessory pancreatic duct.

the abdomen. As the large intestine returns, it undergoes a further 180-degree counterclockwise rotation (see Fig. 12-12C_1 and D_1). Later, it comes to occupy the right side of the abdomen. The ascending colon becomes recognizable as the posterior abdominal wall progressively elongates (see Figs. 12-12E and 12-14A).

Fixation of the Intestines

Rotation of the stomach and the duodenum causes the duodenum and the pancreas to fall to the right, where they are pressed against the posterior abdominal wall by the colon. The adjacent layers of peritoneum fuse

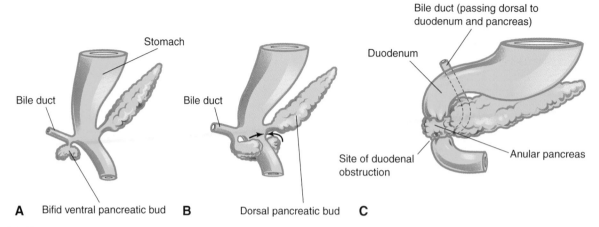

A Bifid ventral pancreatic bud **B** Dorsal pancreatic bud **C**

Figure 12-10. **A** and **B**, Illustrations of the probable embryologic basis of an anular pancreas. **C**, An anular pancreas encircling the duodenum. This anomaly sometimes produces complete obstruction (atresia) or partial obstruction (stenosis) of the duodenum.

and subsequently disappear (see Fig. 12-14C and F); consequently, most of the duodenum and the head of the pancreas become retroperitoneal (posterior to the peritoneum). The mesentery of the ascending colon fuses with the parietal peritoneum on this wall and also becomes retroperitoneal (see Fig. 12-14B and E). Other derivatives of the midgut loop (e.g., the jejunum and ileum) retain their mesenteries.

The Cecum and the Appendix

The *primordium of the cecum and the appendix* appears in the sixth week as a swelling on the antimesenteric border of the caudal limb of the midgut loop (Figs. 12-12C to E and 12-15A). Initially, the appendix is a small diverticulum of the cecum. It subsequently increases rapidly in length so that, at birth, it is a relatively long tube arising from the distal end of the cecum (see Fig. 12-15B to D). After birth, the wall of the cecum grows unequally, and as a result, the appendix comes to enter its medial side (see Fig. 12-15E). *The appendix is subject to considerable variation in position.* As the ascending colon elongates, the appendix may pass posterior to the cecum (*retrocecal* appendix—64% of people) or the colon (*retrocolic appendix*). It may also descend over the brim of the pelvis (*pelvic appendix*).

■ THE HINDGUT

The derivatives of the hindgut are as follows:
● The left one third to one half of the transverse colon, the descending colon and sigmoid colon, the rectum and the superior part of the anal canal
● The epithelium of the urinary bladder and most of the urethra

All of these derivatives are supplied by the **inferior mesenteric artery** (see Fig. 12-1). The junction between the segment of transverse colon derived from the midgut and that originating from the hindgut is indicated by the change in blood supply from a branch of the superior mesenteric artery to a branch of the inferior mesenteric artery. The descending colon becomes retroperitoneal as its

---

CONGENITAL OMPHALOCELE

Congenital omphalocele is a persistence of the herniation of the abdominal contents into the proximal part of the umbilical cord (Figs. 12-16 and 12-17). Herniation of the intestines occurs in approximately 1 in 5000 births, whereas herniation of the liver and intestines occurs in approximately 1 in 10,000 births. The size of the hernia depends on its contents. The abdominal cavity is proportionately small when an omphalocele is present because the impetus for it to grow is absent.

UMBILICAL HERNIA

When the intestines herniate through an imperfectly closed umbilicus, an umbilical hernia forms. This common type of hernia differs from an omphalocele. In umbilical hernias, the protruding mass (usually consisting of part of the greater omentum and small intestine) is covered by subcutaneous tissue and skin. The hernia protrudes during crying, straining, or coughing and can easily be reduced through the fibrous ring at the umbilicus. Surgery is not usually performed unless the hernia persists to the age of 3 to 5 years.

---

mesentery fuses with the peritoneum on the left posterior abdominal wall (see Fig. 12-14B and E). The mesentery of the sigmoid colon is retained.

The Cloaca

The expanded terminal part of the hindgut, the cloaca, is an endoderm-lined chamber that is in contact with the

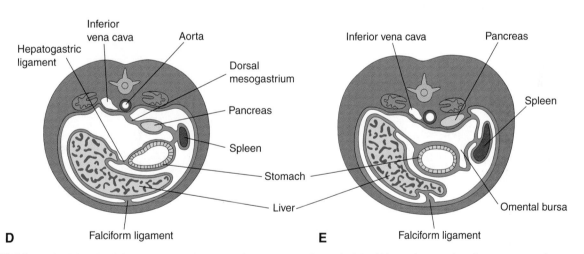

FIGURE 12-11. **A,** The left side of the stomach and associated structures at the end of the fifth week. Note that the pancreas, spleen, and celiac trunk are located between the layers of the dorsal mesogastrium. **B,** Transverse section of the liver, stomach, and spleen at the level shown in **A,** showing their relationship to the dorsal and ventral mesenteries. **C,** Transverse section of a fetus, showing fusion of the dorsal mesogastrium with the peritoneum on the posterior abdominal wall. **D** and **E,** Similar sections, showing movement of the liver to the right and rotation of the stomach. Observe the fusion of the dorsal mesogastrium to the dorsal abdominal wall, which results in the pancreas becoming retroperitoneal.

surface ectoderm at the cloacal membrane (see Fig. 12-22A and B). This membrane is composed of the endoderm of the cloaca and the ectoderm of the proctodeum (see Fig. 12-22C and D). The cloaca receives the allantois ventrally (see Fig. 12-22A).

Partitioning of the Cloaca

The cloaca is divided into dorsal and ventral parts by the mesenchyme—the **urorectal septum**—that develops in the angle between the allantois and the hindgut (see

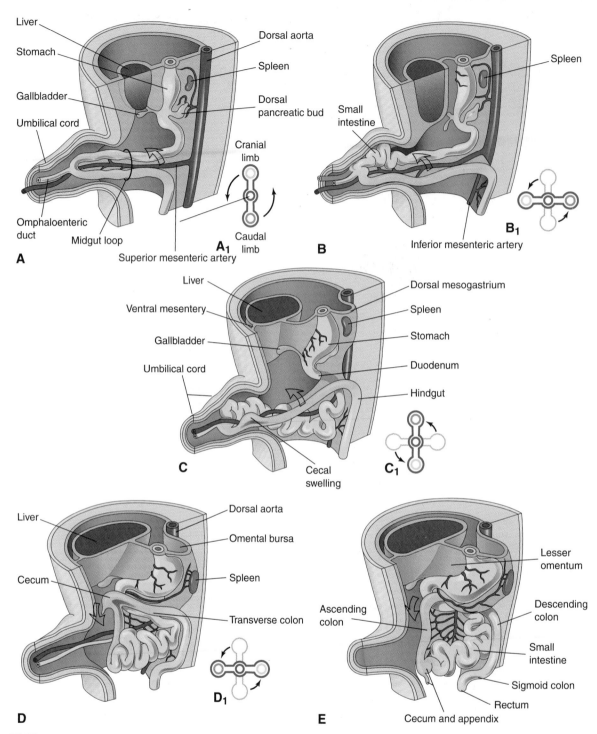

FIGURE 12-12. Illustrations of the rotation of the midgut, as seen from the left. **A,** During the sixth week, the midgut loop is situated in the proximal part of the umbilical cord. **A₁,** Transverse section through the midgut loop, showing the initial relationship of the limbs of the midgut loop to the superior mesenteric artery. **B,** A later stage, showing the beginning of midgut rotation. **B₁,** Illustration of the 90-degree counterclockwise rotation that carries the cranial limb of the midgut to the right. **C,** At approximately 10 weeks, the intestines return to the abdomen. **C₁,** Illustration of a further rotation of 90 degrees. **D,** By approximately 11 weeks, all of the intestines return to the abdomen. **D₁,** A further 90-degree rotation of the gut, for a total of 270 degrees. **E,** The later fetal period, showing the cecum rotating to its normal position in the lower right quadrant of the abdomen.

Fig. 12-22C and D). As the septum grows toward the cloacal membrane, it develops forklike extensions that produce infoldings of the lateral walls of the cloaca (see Fig. 12-22B₁). These folds grow toward each other and fuse, forming a partition that divides the cloaca into two parts

(see Fig. 12-22D to F₁): the rectum and the cranial part of the **anal canal** dorsally, and the **urogenital sinus** ventrally.

By the seventh week, the urorectal septum has fused with the cloacal membrane, dividing it into a smaller, dorsal **anal membrane** and a larger, ventral urogenital membrane (see

Figure 12-13. Physiologic hernia in a 58-day embryo attached to its chorionic sac. Note the herniated intestine derived from the midgut loop in the proximal part of the umbilical cord. (Courtesy of Dr. D.K. Kalousek, Department of Pathology, University of British Columbia, Children's Hospital, Vancouver, British Columbia, Canada.)

Gastroschisis and Congenital Epigastric Hernia

Gastroschisis results from a defect near the median plane of the abdominal wall (Fig. 12-18). The viscera protrude into the amniotic cavity and are bathed by amniotic fluid. The term *gastroschisis*, which literally means "split stomach," is a misnomer because the anterior abdominal wall, not the stomach, is split. The defect usually occurs on the right side, lateral to the median plane, and is more common in boys than in girls. The anomaly results from incomplete closure of the lateral folds during the fourth week of development (see Chapter 6).

Nonrotation of the Midgut

Nonrotation of the midgut (*left-sided colon*) is a relatively common condition (Fig. 12-19A and B). As a result of nonrotation, the caudal limb of the loop returns to the abdomen first, the small intestine lies on the right side of the abdomen, and the entire large intestine lies on the left. Although patients are generally asymptomatic, if volvulus (twisting) occurs, the superior mesenteric artery may be obstructed, resulting in infarction and gangrene of the intestine supplied by it.

Fig. 12-22E and F). The area of fusion of the urorectal septum with the cloacal membrane is represented in the adult by the **perineal body**, the tendinous center of the perineum. Mesenchymal proliferations produce elevations of the surface ectoderm around the **anal membrane**. As a result, this membrane is soon located at the bottom of

Mixed Rotation and Volvulus

With mixed rotation and volvulus, the cecum lies just inferior to the pylorus of the stomach and is fixed to the posterior abdominal wall by peritoneal bands that pass over the duodenum (see Fig. 12-19B). These bands and the volvulus usually cause **duodenal obstruction**. This type of malrotation results from failure of the midgut loop to complete the final 90 degrees of rotation (see Fig. 12-12D); consequently, the terminal part of the ileum returns to the abdomen first.

Reversed Rotation

In very unusual cases, the midgut loop rotates in a clockwise rather than a counterclockwise direction (see Fig. 12-19C). As a result, the duodenum lies anterior to the superior mesenteric artery rather than posterior to it, and the transverse colon lies posterior to the superior mesenteric artery instead of anterior to it. In these infants, the transverse colon may be obstructed by pressure from the superior mesenteric artery.

Subhepatic Cecum and Appendix

If the cecum adheres to the inferior surface of the liver when it returns to the abdomen (see Fig. 12-12D), it is drawn superiorly as the liver decreases in size. As a result, the cecum remains in its fetal position (see Fig. 12-19D). Subhepatic cecum and appendix is more common in boys than in girls. This anomaly may not be detected until adulthood. Subhepatic cecum is not common in adults; however, when it occurs, it may create problems in the diagnosis of appendicitis and during surgical removal of the appendix.

Internal Hernia

In the case of an internal hernia, the small intestine passes into the mesentery of the midgut loop during the return of the intestines to the abdomen (see Fig. 12-19E). As a result, a hernia-like sac forms. This very uncommon condition usually does not produce symptoms and is often detected at autopsy or during anatomic dissection.

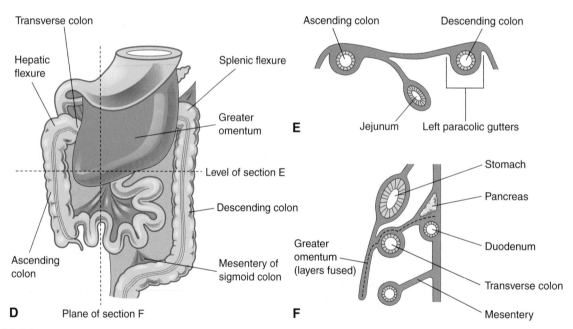

Figure 12-14. Fixation of the intestines. **A,** Ventral view of the intestines before their fixation. **B,** Transverse section at the level shown in **A**. The *arrows* indicate areas of subsequent fusion. **C,** Sagittal section at the plane shown in **A**, illustrating the greater omentum overhanging the transverse colon. The *arrows* indicate areas of subsequent fusion. **D,** Ventral view of the intestines after their fixation. **E,** Transverse section at the level shown in **D** after disappearance of the mesentery of the ascending and descending colon. **F,** Sagittal section at the plane shown in **D**, illustrating fusion of the greater omentum with the mesentery of the transverse colon and fusion of the layers of the greater omentum.

an ectodermal depression—the *proctodeum*, or anal pit (see Fig. 12-22F). The anal membrane usually ruptures at the end of the eighth week of development, bringing the anal canal into communication with the amniotic cavity.

The Anal Canal

The superior two thirds of the adult anal canal are derived from the **hindgut**; the inferior one third develops from the

proctodeum (Fig. 12-23). The junction of the epithelium derived from the ectoderm of the proctodeum and that derived from the endoderm of the hindgut is roughly indicated by an irregular **pectinate line** located at the inferior limit of the anal valves. This line also indicates the approximate former site of the anal membrane. At the anus, the epithelium is keratinized and continuous with the skin around it. The other layers of the wall of the anal canal are derived from the splanchnic mesenchyme.

FIGURE 12-15. Successive stages in the development of the cecum and the appendix. **A,** At 6 weeks. **B,** At 8 weeks. **C,** At 12 weeks. **D,** At birth. Note that the appendix is relatively long and is continuous with the apex of the cecum. **E,** Adult. Note that the appendix is now relatively short and lies on the medial side of the cecum.

MIDGUT VOLVULUS

Midgut volvulus is an anomaly in which the small intestine does not enter the abdominal cavity normally and the mesenteries do not undergo normal fixation. As a result, twisting of the intestines occurs (see Fig. 12-19F). Only two parts of the intestine—the duodenum and the proximal colon—are attached to the posterior abdominal wall. The small intestine hangs by a narrow stalk that contains the superior mesenteric artery and vein. These vessels are usually twisted in this stalk and become obstructed at or near the duodenojejunal junction. The circulation to the twisted intestine is often restricted; if the vessels are completely obstructed, gangrene develops.

STENOSIS AND ATRESIA OF THE INTESTINE

Partial occlusion (stenosis) and complete occlusion (atresia) of the intestinal lumen (see Fig. 12-5) account for approximately one third of cases of intestinal obstruction. The obstructive lesion occurs most often in the ileum (50%) and the duodenum (25%). *These anomalies result from failure of recanalization of the intestine.* Most atresias of the ileum are probably *caused by infarction of the fetal bowel as a result of impairment of its blood supply* secondary to volvulus. This impairment most likely occurs during the 10th week as the intestines return to the abdomen.

FIGURE 12-17. Sonogram of the abdomen of a fetus (28 weeks' gestation), showing a large omphalocele, with much of the liver protruding from the abdomen. The mass also contains a small, membrane-covered sac *(arrows).* The umbilical cord was integrally involved in the anomaly. (Courtesy of Dr. C.R. Harman, Department of Obstetrics, Gynecology and Reproductive Sciences, Women's Hospital and University of Maryland, Baltimore, MD.)

FIGURE 12-16. An infant with an omphalocele. The defect resulted in herniation of intra-abdominal structures (liver and intestine) into the proximal end of the umbilical cord. The omphalocele is covered by a membrane composed of peritoneum and amnion. (Courtesy of Dr. N.E. Wiseman, Pediatric Surgeon, Children's Hospital, Winnipeg, Manitoba, Canada.)

ILEAL DIVERTICULUM AND OTHER OMPHALOENTERIC DUCT REMNANTS

A congenital ileal diverticulum (Meckel diverticulum) (Fig. 12-20) occurs in 2% to 4% of infants and is three to five times more prevalent in boys than in girls. *An ileal diverticulum is of clinical significance because it sometimes becomes inflamed and causes symptoms that mimic appendicitis.* The wall of the diverticulum contains all layers of the ileum and may contain small patches of gastric and pancreatic tissues. The gastric mucosa often secretes acid, producing ulceration and bleeding (Fig. 12-21A). An ileal diverticulum represents a remnant of the proximal portion of the omphaloenteric duct. It typically appears as a fingerlike pouch approximately 3 to 6 cm long that arises from the *antimesenteric border of the ileum,* 40 to 50 cm from the ileocecal junction. An ileal diverticulum may be connected to the umbilicus by a fibrous cord or an **omphaloenteric (umbilicoileal) fistula** (see Fig. 12-21B and C); other possible remnants of the omphaloenteric duct are shown in Figure 12-21D to F.

CONGENITAL MEGACOLON

In infants with congenital megacolon, or **Hirschsprung disease** (Fig. 12-24), a part of the colon is dilated because of the *absence of autonomic ganglion cells* in the myenteric plexus distal to the dilated segment of colon. The enlarged colon—**megacolon**—has the normal number of ganglion cells. The dilation results from failure of peristalsis in the aganglionic segment, which prevents movement of the intestinal contents. Boys are affected more often than girls (4 to 1). Congenital megacolon results from failure of neural crest cells to migrate into the wall of the colon during the fifth to seventh weeks of development. Of the genes involved in the pathogenesis of Hirschsprung disease, the RET proto-oncogene accounts for most cases.

FIGURE 12-18. **A,** A newborn infant with an anterior abdominal wall defect—gastroschisis. The defect was relatively small (2–4 cm long) and involved all layers of the abdominal wall. It was located to the right of the umbilicus. **B,** The same infant after the viscera were returned to the abdomen and the defect was surgically closed. **C,** Sonogram of a fetus (20 weeks' gestation) with gastroschisis. Loops of small bowel can be seen floating freely in the amniotic fluid *(arrow)* anterior to the fetal abdomen *(left).* (**A** and **B,** Courtesy of A.E. Chudley, MD, Section of Genetics and Metabolism, Department of Pediatrics and Child Health, Children's Hospital, Winnipeg, Manitoba, Canada. **C,** Courtesy of Dr. C.R. Harman, Department of Obstetrics, Gynecology and Reproductive Services, Women's Hospital and University of Maryland, Baltimore, MD.)

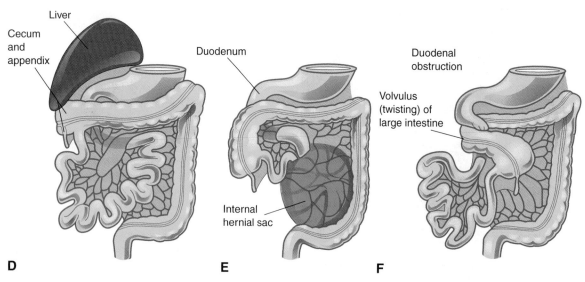

FIGURE 12-19. Various abnormalities of midgut rotation. **A,** Nonrotation. **B,** Mixed rotation and volvulus. The *arrow* indicates the twisting of the intestine. **C,** Reversed rotation. **D,** Subhepatic cecum and appendix. **E,** Internal hernia. **F,** Midgut volvulus.

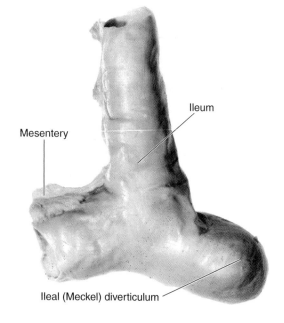

FIGURE 12-20. A typical ileal diverticulum (cadaveric specimen), commonly referred to clinically as *Meckel diverticulum.* (From Moore KL, Persaud TVN, Shiota K: Color Atlas of Clinical Embryology, 2nd ed. Philadelphia, WB Saunders, 2000.)

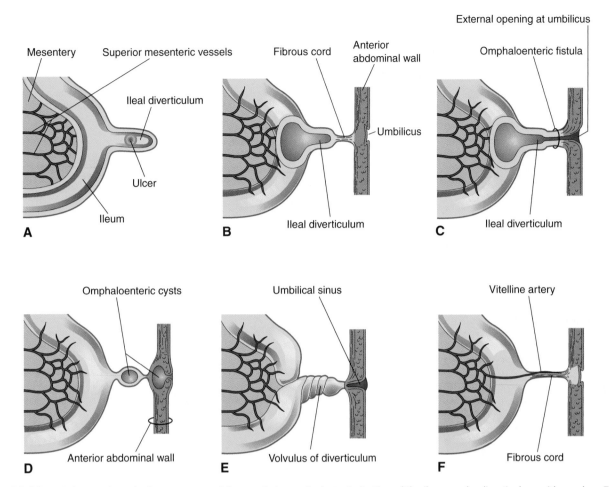

Figure 12-21. Ileal diverticula and other remnants of the omphaloenteric duct. **A,** Section of the ileum and a diverticulum with an ulcer. **B,** A diverticulum connected to the umbilicus by a fibrous cord. **C,** Omphaloenteric fistula resulting from persistence of the entire intra-abdominal portion of the omphaloenteric duct. **D,** Omphaloenteric cysts at the umbilicus and in a fibrous remnant of the omphaloenteric duct. **E,** Umbilical sinus resulting from the persistence of the omphaloenteric duct near the umbilicus. **F,** The omphaloenteric duct has persisted as a fibrous cord connecting the ileum with the umbilicus. A persistent vitelline artery extends along the fibrous cord to the umbilicus. This artery carried blood from the embryo to the omphaloenteric duct.

Because of its hindgut origin, the superior two thirds of the anal canal are supplied mainly by the *superior rectal artery*, the continuation of the *inferior mesenteric artery*. Its nerves are derived from the autonomic nervous system. Because of its origin from the proctodeum, the inferior one third of the anal canal is supplied mainly by the *inferior rectal arteries*, branches of the internal pudendal artery. Its nerve supply is from the inferior rectal nerve, and it is sensitive to pain, temperature, touch, and pressure.

The differences in blood supply, nerve supply, and venous and lymphatic drainage of the two parts of the anal canal are important clinically because the characteristics of carcinomas involving the two parts differ. Tumors in the superior part are painless and arise from the columnar epithelium, whereas those in the inferior part are painful and arise from the squamous epithelium.

IMPERFORATE ANUS AND ANORECTAL ANOMALIES

Imperforate anus occurs in approximately 1 in 5000 newborn infants, and it is more common in boys (Figs. 12-25 and 12-26C). *Most anorectal anomalies result from abnormal development of the urorectal septum,* resulting in incomplete separation of the cloaca into urogenital and anorectal parts (Fig. 12-26A). Lesions are classified as low or high, depending on whether the rectum ends superior or inferior to the puborectalis muscle.

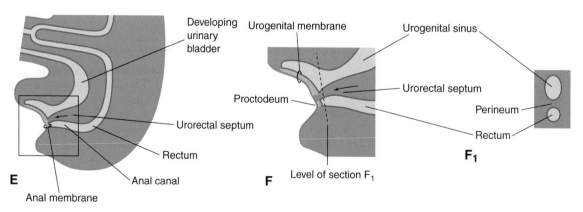

FIGURE 12-22. Illustrations of successive stages in the partitioning of the cloaca into the rectum and the urogenital sinus by the urorectal septum. **A, C,** and **E,** Views from the left side at 4, 6, and 7 weeks, respectively. **B, D,** and **F,** Enlargements of the cloacal region. **B₁, D₁,** and **F₁,** Transverse sections of the cloaca at the levels shown in **B, D,** and **F,** respectively. Note that the postanal gut, or tailgut (shown in **B**), degenerates and disappears as the rectum forms from the dorsal part of the cloaca (shown in **C**). The *arrows* indicate the growth of the urorectal septum.

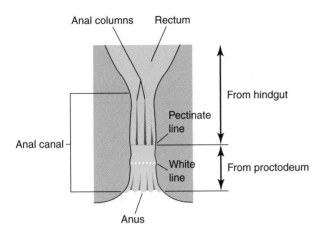

FIGURE 12-23. The rectum and the anal canal, showing their developmental origins. Note that the superior two thirds of the anal canal are derived from the hindgut and are endodermal in origin, whereas the inferior one third of the anal canal is derived from the proctodeum and is ectodermal in origin. Because of their different embryologic origins, the superior and inferior parts of the anal canal are supplied by different arteries and nerves and have different venous and lymphatic drainages.

FIGURE 12-25. Female neonate with membranous anal atresia (imperforate anus). In most cases of anal atresia, a thin layer of tissue separates the anal canal from the exterior. (Courtesy of A.E. Chudley, MD, Section of Genetics and Metabolism, Department of Pediatrics and Child Health, Children's Hospital, Winnipeg, Manitoba, Canada.)

FIGURE 12-24. Radiograph of the colon after a barium enema in a 1-month-old infant with megacolon (Hirschsprung disease). The distal, aganglionic segment is narrow, with a dilated proximal colon full of fecal material above it. Note the transition zone *(arrow)*. (Courtesy of Dr. Martin H. Reed, Department of Radiology, University of Manitoba and Children's Hospital, Winnipeg, Manitoba, Canada.)

LOW RECTAL ANOMALIES

Anal Agenesis, With or Without a Fistula

The anal canal may end blindly, or there may be an **ectopic anus** or an **anoperineal fistula** that opens into the perineum (see Fig. 12-26D and E). The abnormal canal may, however, open into the vagina in girls or the urethra in boys (see Fig. 12-26F and G). Most low anorectal anomalies are associated with an external fistula. **Anal agenesis with a fistula** results from incomplete separation of the cloaca by the urorectal septum.

Anal Stenosis

In anal stenosis, the anus is in a normal position, but the anus and the anal canal are narrow (see Fig. 12-26B). This anomaly is probably caused by a slight dorsal deviation of the urorectal septum as it grows caudally to fuse with the cloacal membrane. As a result, the anal canal is small.

Membranous Atresia of the Anus

In membranous anal atresia, the anus is in the normal position, but a thin layer of tissue separates the anal canal from the exterior (Figs. 12-25 and 12-26C). The anal membrane is thin enough to bulge on straining. This anomaly results from failure of the anal membrane to perforate at the end of the eighth week.

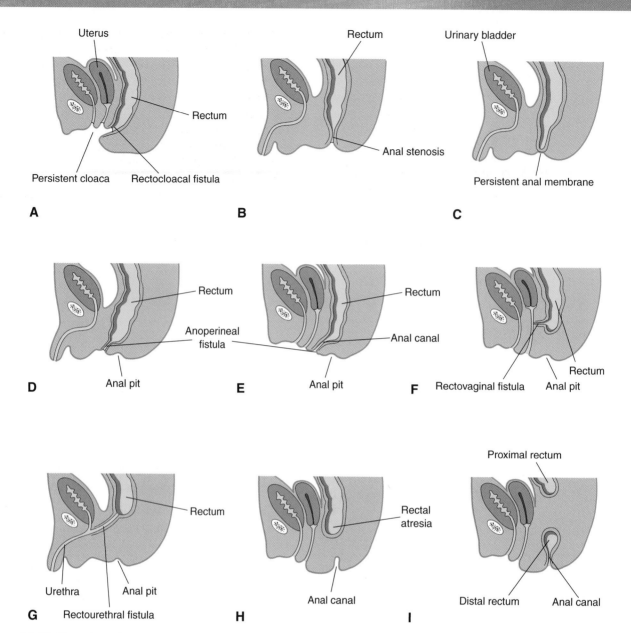

FIGURE 12-26. Illustrations of various types of anorectal anomalies. **A,** Persistent cloaca. Note the common outlet of the intestinal, urinary, and reproductive tracts. **B,** Anal stenosis. **C,** Membranous anal atresia. **D** and **E,** Anal agenesis with a perineal fistula. **F,** Anorectal agenesis with a rectovaginal fistula. **G,** Anorectal agenesis with a rectourethral fistula. **H** and **I,** Rectal atresia.

HIGH ANORECTAL ANOMALIES

Anorectal Agenesis, With or Without a Fistula

In anorectal agenesis, the rectum ends superior to the puborectalis muscle. This is the most common type of anorectal anomaly, and it accounts for approximately two thirds of anorectal defects. Although the rectum ends blindly, there is usually a fistula to the bladder (rectovesical fistula) or the urethra (rectourethral fistula) in boys, or to the vagina (rectovaginal fistula) or the vestibule of the vagina (rectovestibular fistula) in girls (see Fig. 12-26F and G). Anorectal agenesis with a fistula is the result of incomplete separation of the cloaca by the urorectal septum.

Rectal Atresia

With rectal atresia, the anal canal and the rectum are present, but are separated (see Fig. 12-26H and I). Sometimes the two segments of bowel are connected by a fibrous cord, the remnant of the atretic portion of the rectum. The cause of rectal atresia may be abnormal recanalization of the colon or, more likely, a defective blood supply, as discussed for atresia of the small intestine.

CLINICALLY ORIENTED QUESTIONS

1. Approximately 2 weeks after birth, an infant began to vomit shortly after feeding. Each time, the vomitus was propelled approximately 2 feet. The physician told the mother that the infant had a benign stomach tumor resulting in a narrow outlet from the stomach. Is there an embryologic basis for this anomaly? Is the tumor malignant?

2. Some say that infants with Down syndrome have an increased incidence of duodenal atresia. Is this true? Can the condition be corrected?

3. A man claimed that his appendix was on his left side. Is this possible and, if so, how could this happen?

4. A nurse reported that a patient supposedly had two appendices and had had separate operations to remove them. Do people ever have two appendices?

5. What is Hirschsprung disease? Some sources state that it is a congenital condition resulting from large bowel obstruction. Is this correct? If so, what is its embryologic basis?

6. A nurse once stated that feces can sometimes be expelled from a baby's umbilicus. Can this really happen? If so, what conditions would likely be present?

The answers to these questions are at the back of the book.

13

THE UROGENITAL SYSTEM

Embryologically, the urinary (excretory) system and the genital (reproductive) system are closely associated. During folding of the embryo (see Chapter 6), the intermediate mesoderm is carried ventrally and loses its connection with the somites. A longitudinal elevation of the mesoderm—the **urogenital ridge**—forms on each side of the dorsal aorta. It gives rise to parts of the urinary and genital systems. The part of the urogenital ridge that gives rise to the urinary system is the **nephrogenic cord** (Fig. 13-1D and F); the part that gives rise to the genital system is the **gonadal ridge** (see Fig. 13-18C).

FIGURE 13-1. **A,** Dorsal view of an embryo during the third week (approximately 18 days). **B,** Transverse section of the embryo, showing the position of the intermediate mesenchyme before lateral folding occurs. **C,** Lateral view of an embryo during the fourth week (approximately 24 days). **D,** Transverse section of the embryo after the commencement of folding. **E,** Lateral view of an embryo later in the fourth week (approximately 26 days). **F,** Transverse section of the embryo, showing the lateral folds meeting each other ventrally.

■ DEVELOPMENT OF THE URINARY SYSTEM

The urinary system consists of the kidneys, the ureters, the urinary bladder, and the urethra.

Development of the Kidneys and Ureters

Three sets of excretory organs, or kidneys, develop in human embryos: the *pronephros, mesonephros,* and *metanephros.*

Pronephroi

The transitory, rudimentary pronephroi appear early in the fourth week of development. They are represented by a few cell clusters in the neck region (Fig. 13-2*A*). The pronephric ducts run caudally and open into the *cloaca* (see Fig. 13-2*B*). The pronephroi soon degenerate; however, most of the pronephric ducts persist and are used by the next set of excretory organs.

Mesonephroi

The mesonephroi appear late in the fourth week caudal to the pronephroi (see Fig. 13-2). The mesonephroi function until the permanent kidneys develop (Fig. 13-3). The mesonephroi consist of glomeruli and **mesonephric tubules** (see Fig. 13-3 *C* to *F*). The tubules open into the **mesonephric ducts,** originally the pronephric ducts. The mesonephric ducts open into the cloaca. The mesonephroi degenerate toward the end of the first trimester; however, their tubules become the efferent ductules of the testes, and the mesonephric ducts have several adult derivatives in the male (Table 13-1).

Metanephroi

The metanephroi—the **primordia of the permanent kidneys**—begin to develop early in the fifth week and start to function approximately 4 weeks later. Urine is excreted into the amniotic cavity and mixes with the amniotic fluid. The definitive kidneys develop from two sources (Fig. 13-4*A*):

● The metanephric diverticulum (ureteric bud)
● The metanephric mass of the intermediate mesoderm (metanephric blastema)

Both primordia of the metanephroi are of mesodermal origin. The **metanephric diverticulum** is an outgrowth from the mesonephric duct, near its entrance into the cloaca, and is the primordium of the ureter, the renal pelvis, the calices, and the collecting tubules (see Fig. 13-4*B* to *E*). The elongating diverticulum penetrates the **metanephrogenic blastema**—a mass of cells that forms the nephrons (see Fig. 13-4*B*). The stalk of the metanephric diverticulum becomes the **ureter,** and its cranial end forms the renal pelvis. Branching of the mesonephric buds results in formation of the collecting tubules.

The **straight collecting tubules** undergo repeated branching, forming successive generations of collecting tubules. The first four generations of tubules enlarge and become confluent to form the **major calices** (see Fig. 13-4*C* to *E*); the second four generations coalesce to form the **minor calices.** The remaining generations of tubules form the collecting tubules. The end of each **arched collecting tubule** induces clusters of mesenchymal cells in the metanephric mass of the mesoderm to form small **metanephric vesicles** (Fig. 13-5*A*). These vesicles elongate and become the **renal tubules** (see Fig. 13-5*B* and *C*). The proximal ends of these tubules are invaginated by glomeruli. The renal corpuscle (glomerulus and glomerular capsule) and its proximal convoluted tubule, **nephron loop** (of Henle), and distal convoluted tubule constitute a **nephron** (see Fig. 13-5*D*). Each distal convoluted tubule contacts an arched collecting tubule, and the tubules become confluent, forming a **uriniferous tubule.**

Branching of the metanephric diverticulum depends on an inductive signal from the metanephric mesoderm,

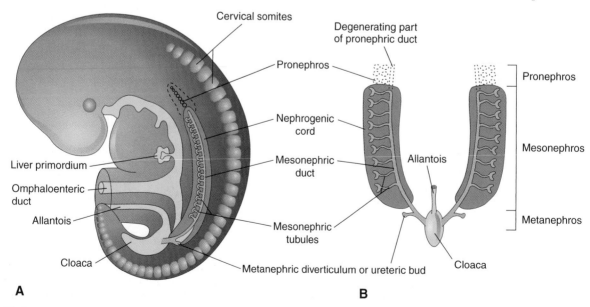

FIGURE 13-2. The three sets of excretory organs in an embryo during the fifth week. **A,** Lateral view. **B,** Ventral view. In this diagram, the mesonephric tubules have been pulled laterally; their normal position is shown in **A.**

A, Lateral view of a 5-week embryo, showing the extent of the mesonephros and the primordium of the metanephros, or permanent kidney. **B,** Transverse section of the embryo, showing the nephrogenic cords from which the mesonephric tubules develop. **C** to **F,** Transverse sections, showing successive stages in the development of a mesonephric tubule between the 5th and 11th weeks. Note that the mesenchymal cell cluster in the nephrogenic cord develops a lumen, thereby forming a mesonephric vesicle. The vesicle soon becomes an S-shaped mesonephric tubule and extends laterally to join the mesonephric duct. The expanded medial end of the mesonephric tubule is invaginated by blood vessels to form a glomerular capsule (Bowman capsule). The cluster of capillaries projecting into this capsule is the glomerulus.

and differentiation of the nephrons depends on induction by the collecting tubules. The **molecular aspects** of the reciprocal interactions between the metanephric mesenchyme and the collecting tubules are shown in Figure 13-6.

The **fetal kidneys** are subdivided into lobes. The lobulation usually disappears during infancy as the nephrons increase and grow. At term, nephron formation is complete—each kidney containing approximately 2 million nephrons. Functional maturation of the kidneys occurs after birth.

TABLE 13-1. Adult Derivatives and Vestigial Remains of Embryonic Urogenital Structures*

MALE	EMBRYONIC STRUCTURE	FEMALE
Testis	**Indifferent gonad**	*Ovary*
Seminiferous tubules	**Cortex**	*Ovarian follicles*
Rete testis	**Medulla**	Rete ovarii
Gubernaculum	**Gubernaculum**	*Ovarian ligament*
		Round ligament of uterus
Efferent ductules of testis	**Mesonephric tubules**	Epoophoron
Paradidymis		Paroophoron
Appendix of epididymis	**Mesonephric duct**	Appendix vesiculosa
Duct of epididymis		Duct of epoophoron
Ductus deferens		Longitudinal duct; Gartner duct
Ureter, pelvis, calices, and collecting tubules		*Ureter, pelvis, calices, and collecting tubules*
Ejaculatory duct and seminal gland		
Appendix of testis	**Paramesonephric Duct**	Hydatid (of Morgagni)
		Uterine tube
		Uterus
Urinary bladder	**Urogenital sinus**	*Urinary bladder*
Urethra (except navicular fossa)		*Urethra*
Prostatic utricle		*Vagina*
Prostate		*Urethral and paraurethral glands*
Bulbourethral glands		*Greater vestibular glands*
Seminal colliculus	**Sinus tubercle**	Hymen
Penis	**Phallus**	*Clitoris*
Glans of penis		*Glans of clitoris*
Corpora cavernosa of penis		*Corpora cavernosa of clitoris*
Corpus spongiosum of penis		*Bulb of vestibule*
Ventral aspect of penis	**Urogenital folds**	*Labia minora*
Scrotum	**Labioscrotal swellings**	*Labia majora*

*Functional derivatives are shown in italics.

FIGURE 13-4. Development of the metanephros, the primordium of the permanent kidney. **A,** Lateral view of a 5-week embryo, showing the primordium of the metanephros. **B** to **E,** Successive stages in the development of the metanephric diverticulum (fifth to eighth weeks). Observe the development of the ureter, the renal pelvis, the calices, and the collecting tubules.

A

- Capsule of kidney
- Metanephrogenic blastema
- Cell cluster
- Arched collecting tubule
- Metanephric vesicle
- Straight collecting tubule

B

- Metanephric vesicle
- Arched collecting tubule
- Site of contact of tubules
- Metanephric tubule
- Mesenchyme

C

- Site of contact
- S-shaped metanephric tubule
- Site of continuity of tubules
- Branch of renal artery
- Nephron loop

D

- Straight collecting tubule
- Distal convoluted tubule
- Proximal convoluted tubule
- Glomerulus
- Glomerular capsule
- Descending and ascending limbs of nephron loop

FIGURE 13-5. Illustrations of stages in nephrogenesis—the development of nephrons. **A,** Nephrogenesis commences approximately at the beginning of the eighth week. **B** and **C,** Note that the metanephric tubules, the primordia of the nephrons, become continuous with the collecting tubules to form uriniferous tubules. **D,** The number of nephrons more than doubles from 20 weeks to 38 weeks. Observe that nephrons are derived from the metanephric mass of the mesoderm and that the collecting tubules are derived from the metanephric diverticulum.

Positional Changes of the Kidneys

The metanephric kidneys lie close to each other in the pelvis (Fig. 13-7A). As the abdomen grows, the kidneys gradually come to lie in the abdomen and move farther apart (Fig. 13-7B and C). The caudal part of the embryo grows away from the kidneys so that the kidneys occupy progressively higher cranial levels. As the kidney "ascends," it rotates medially almost 90 degrees. By the ninth week, the kidneys come in contact with the suprarenal glands as they attain their adult position (Fig. 13-7C and D).

Changes in the Blood Supply of the Kidneys

Initially, the renal arteries are branches of the common iliac arteries (see Fig. 13-7A and B). Later, the kidneys receive their blood supply from the distal end of the aorta (see Fig. 13-7C). The kidneys receive their most cranial arterial branches from the abdominal aorta. The primordial

ACCESSORY RENAL ARTERIES

The common variations in the blood supply to the kidneys reflect the manner in which the blood supply continually changes during embryonic and early fetal life (see Fig. 13-7). Approximately 25% of adult kidneys have accessory (supernumerary) renal arteries, usually arising from the aorta, superior or inferior to the main renal artery (Fig. 13-8A and B). An accessory artery to the inferior pole (polar renal artery) may cross anterior to the ureter and obstruct it, causing **hydronephrosis**, or distention of the pelvis and calices with urine (see Fig. 13-8B). Renal arteries are end arteries; consequently, if an accessory artery is damaged or ligated, the part of the kidney supplied by it will become ischemic. Accessory arteries are approximately twice as common as accessory veins.

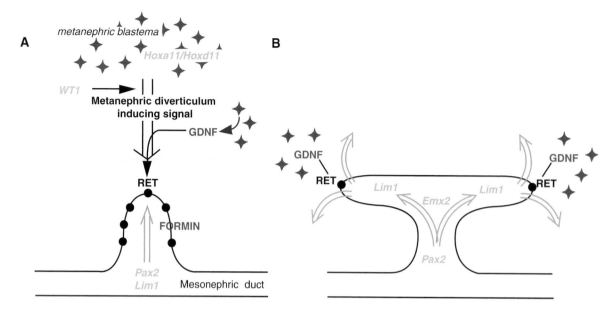

FIGURE 13-6. Molecular control of kidney development. **A,** Formation of the metanephric diverticulum requires inductive signals derived from the metanephrogenic blastema under the control of transcription factors *(yellow text),* such as WT1, and signaling molecules *(red text),* including GDNF and its epithelial receptor, RET. Normal metanephric diverticulum (ureteric bud) response to these inductive signals is under the control of transcription factors, such as Pax2, Lim1, and the FORMIN gene. **B,** Branching of the metanephric diverticulum is initiated and maintained by interaction with the mesenchyme under the regulation of genes such as Emx2 and specified expression of GDNF and RET at the tips of the invading metanephric diverticulum. (From Piscione TD, Rosenblum ND: The malformed kidney: disruption of the glomerular and tubular development. Clin Genet 56: 342–356, 1999.)

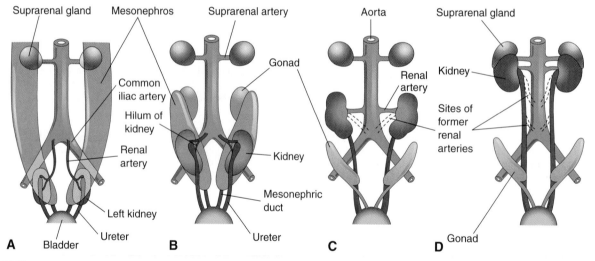

FIGURE 13-7. Ventral views of the abdominopelvic region of embryos and fetuses (sixth to ninth weeks), showing medial rotation and "ascent" of the kidneys from the pelvis to the abdomen. **A** and **B,** Observe also the size regression of the mesonephroi. **C** and **D,** Note that, as the kidneys "ascend," they are supplied by arteries at successively higher levels, and that the hilum of the kidney (where the vessels and nerves enter) is eventually directed anteromedially.

arteries become the renal arteries. Normally, the caudal branches undergo involution and disappear.

Development of the Urinary Bladder

Division of the cloaca by the **urorectal septum** (see Fig. 13-11*A*) into a dorsal rectum and a ventral **urogenital sinus** is described in Chapter 12. For descriptive purposes, the urogenital sinus is divided into three parts (see Fig. 13-11*A* and *C*):

● A cranial *vesical part* that forms most of the bladder and is continuous with the allantois

● A middle *pelvic part* that becomes the urethra in the neck of the bladder, the prostatic part of the urethra in males, and the entire urethra in females
● A caudal *phallic part* that grows toward the genital tubercle—the primordium of the penis or the clitoris

Initially, the bladder is continuous with the **allantois** (see Fig. 13-11*C*). The allantois soon constricts and becomes a thick, fibrous cord, the **urachus** (see Fig. 13-11*G*). In adults, the urachus is represented by the **median umbilical ligament**. As the bladder enlarges, distal parts of the mesonephric ducts are incorporated into its dorsal wall (see Fig. 13-11*B* to *H*) and contribute to the formation of the

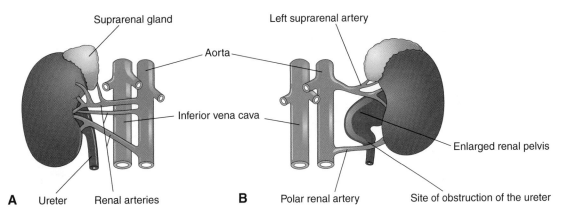

FIGURE 13-8. Common variations of the renal vessels. **A** and **B**, Multiple renal arteries. The polar renal artery shown in **B** has obstructed the ureter and produced an enlarged renal pelvis.

CONGENITAL ANOMALIES OF THE KIDNEYS AND URETERS

Unilateral renal agenesis occurs in approximately 1 in 1000 newborn infants (Fig. 13-9A). Boys are affected more often than girls, and the left kidney is usually the one that is absent. The other kidney usually undergoes compensatory hypertrophy and performs the function of the missing kidney. **Bilateral renal agenesis** *is associated with oligohydramnios* (small amount of amniotic fluid) because little or no urine is excreted into the amniotic cavity. This condition occurs in approximately 1 in 3000 births, is three times more common in boys, and is incompatible with postnatal life. These infants also have pulmonary hypoplasia. Failure of the metanephric diverticulum to penetrate the metanephrogenic blastema results in an absence of renal development because no nephrons are induced by the collecting tubules to develop from the metanephrogenic blastema. Renal agenesis probably has a multifactorial cause.

MALROTATION OF THE KIDNEYS

If the kidney does not rotate, the hilum faces anteriorly (embryonic position) [see Figs. 13-7 and 13-9C]. If the hilum faces posteriorly, then rotation has progressed too far; if it faces laterally, then medial rotation has occurred. Abnormal rotation of the kidneys is often associated with ectopic kidneys.

Ectopic Kidneys

One or both kidneys may be in an abnormal position (Fig. 13-9B and E). Most ectopic kidneys are located in the pelvis, but some lie in the inferior part of the abdomen. Pelvic kidneys and other forms of ectopia result from failure of the kidneys to "ascend."

FUSION ANOMALIES

Crossed Fused Ectopia

Sometimes, a kidney crosses to the other side, resulting in crossed renal ectopia, with or without fusion. An unusual kidney abnormality is unilateral fused kidney (see Fig. 13-9D). In such cases, the developing kidneys fuse while they are in the pelvis, and one kidney "ascends" to its normal position, carrying the other one with it.

Horseshoe Kidney

In approximately 1 in 500 persons, the poles of the kidneys are fused (usually the inferior poles) (Fig. 13-10). Normal ascent of the fused kidneys is prevented because they are caught by the root of the inferior mesenteric artery.

DUPLICATIONS OF THE URINARY TRACT

Duplications of the abdominal part of the ureter and the renal pelvis are common, but a **supernumerary kidney** is rare (see Fig. 13-9C and F). These anomalies result from division of the metanephric diverticulum. Incomplete division of the ureteric primordium results in a divided kidney with a bifid ureter (see Fig. 13-9B). Complete division results in a double kidney with a bifid ureter or with separate ureters (Fig. 13-11). A supernumerary kidney with its own ureter probably results from the formation of two metanephric diverticula.

FIGURE 13-9. Various anomalies of the urinary system. The small sketch at the *lower right* of each illustration shows the probable embryologic basis of the anomaly. **A,** Unilateral renal agenesis. **B,** On the right side of the fetus, a pelvic kidney; on the left side of the fetus, a divided kidney with a bifid ureter. **C,** On the right side of the fetus, malrotation of the kidney; on the left side of fetus, a bifid ureter and a supernumerary kidney. **D,** Crossed fused renal ectopia. The left kidney has crossed over and fused with the right kidney. **E,** Discoid kidney resulting from fusion of the kidneys while they were in the pelvis. **F,** Supernumerary left kidney resulting from the development of two metanephric diverticula.

connective tissue in the *trigone of the bladder*. The epithelium of the entire bladder is derived from the endoderm of the urogenital sinus. The other layers of the bladder wall develop from the adjacent splanchnic mesenchyme. As the mesonephric ducts are absorbed, the ureters come to open separately into the urinary bladder (see Fig. 13-11*C* to *H*). The orifices of the mesonephric ducts move close together and enter the prostatic part of the urethra as the caudal

ends of these ducts become the *ejaculatory ducts*. In females, the distal ends of the mesonephric ducts degenerate.

Development of the Urethra

The epithelium of most of the male urethra and the entire female urethra is derived from the endoderm

FIGURE 13-10. Horseshoe kidney in a female fetus (13 weeks). This anomaly resulted from fusion of the inferior poles of the kidneys while they were in the pelvis. (Courtesy of Dr. D.K. Kalousek, Department of Pathology, University of British Columbia, Children's Hospital, Vancouver, British Columbia, Canada.)

CYSTIC KIDNEY DISEASE

In *autosomal recessive polycystic kidney disease*, both kidneys contain many hundreds of small cysts, resulting in **renal insufficiency**. This disease is diagnosed at birth or in utero by ultrasonography. Death of the infant often occurs shortly after birth; however, an increasing number of these infants are surviving because of postnatal dialysis and kidney transplantation. The outcome for children with **multicystic dysplastic kidney** disease is generally good because in 75% of cases the disease is unilateral. In multicystic dysplastic kidney, fewer cysts are seen than in autosomal recessive polycystic kidney disease. For many years, it was believed that the cysts were the result of failure of the metanephric vesicles to join the tubules derived from the metanephrogenic blastema (see Fig. 13-5B). It is now believed that the cysts are wide dilations of parts of the otherwise continuous nephrons.

ECTOPIC URETER

In males, an ectopic ureter may open into the neck of the bladder, the prostatic part of the urethra, the ductus deferens, the prostatic utricle, or the seminal gland. In females, an ectopic ureter may enter the neck of the bladder, the urethra, the vagina, or the vestibule of the vagina. An ectopic ureter results when the ureter is carried caudally with the mesonephric duct and is incorporated into the caudal portion of the vesical part of the urogenital sinus.

URACHAL ANOMALIES

A remnant of the lumen usually persists in the inferior part of the urachus in infants, and in approximately 50% of cases, the lumen is continuous with the cavity of the bladder. Remnants of the epithelial lining of the urachus may give rise to **urachal cysts** (Fig. 13-12A). The patent inferior end of the urachus may dilate to form a **urachal sinus** that opens into the bladder. The lumen in the superior part of the urachus may also remain patent and form a urachal sinus that opens at the umbilicus (see Fig. 13-12B). Very rarely, the entire urachus remains patent and forms a **urachal fistula** that allows urine to escape from its umbilical orifice (see Fig. 13-12C).

EXSTROPHY OF THE BLADDER

Exstrophy of the bladder is a severe anomaly that occurs in approximately 1 in 10,000 to 1 in 40,000 births, predominantly affecting boys (Fig. 13-13). *Exposure and protrusion of the mucosal surface of the posterior wall of the bladder* characterize this congenital anomaly. The trigone of the bladder and the ureteric orifices are exposed, and urine dribbles intermittently from the everted bladder. **Epispadias**, in which the urethra opens on the dorsum of the penis, and wide separation of the pubic bones are associated with complete exstrophy of the bladder. In some cases, the penis is divided into two parts, and the scrotum is bifid (split). Exstrophy of the bladder is believed to be caused by failure of the mesenchymal cells to migrate between the ectoderm and the endoderm of the infra-abdominal wall (cloacal membrane) during the fourth week (Fig. 13-14B and C). As a result, no muscle and connective tissue form in the abdominal wall over the urinary bladder. Rupture of the fragile cloacal membrane results in wide communication between the exterior and the mucous membrane of the bladder. Rupture of the membrane before division of the cloaca by the urorectal septum leads to exstrophy of the cloaca, resulting in exposure of both the bladder and the hindgut.

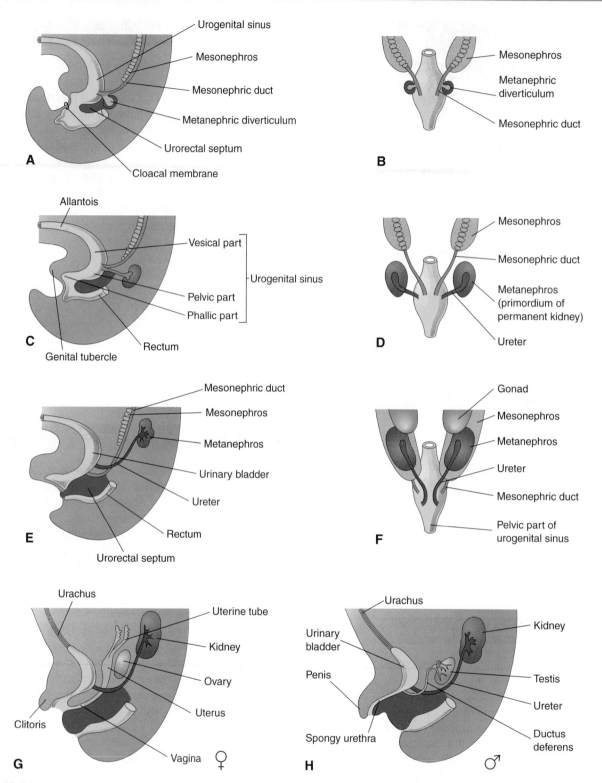

FIGURE 13-11. Division of the cloaca into the urogenital sinus and the rectum; absorption of the mesonephric ducts; development of the urinary bladder, urethra, and urachus; and changes in the location of the ureters. **A,** Lateral view of the caudal half of a 5-week embryo. **B, D,** and **F,** Dorsal views. **C, E, G,** and **H,** Lateral views. The stages shown in **G** and **H** are reached by the 12th week of development.

of the urogenital sinus (see Figs. 13-11 and 13-15). The distal part of the urethra in the glans of the penis is derived from a solid cord of ectodermal cells that grows from the tip of the glans penis to meet the part of the spongy urethra derived from the phallic part of the urogenital sinus (see Fig.

13-15*A* to *C*). The ectodermal cord canalizes and joins the rest of the spongy urethra; consequently, *the epithelium of the terminal part of the urethra is derived from the surface ectoderm.* The connective tissue and the smooth muscle of the urethra in both sexes are derived from the splanchnic mesenchyme.

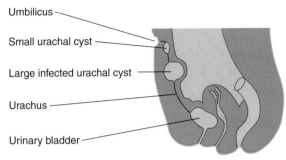

Umbilicus

Small urachal cyst

Large infected urachal cyst

Urachus

Urinary bladder

A

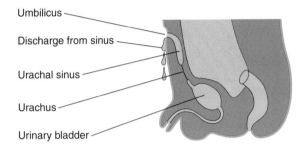

Umbilicus

Discharge from sinus

Urachal sinus

Urachus

Urinary bladder

B

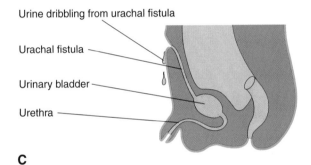

Urine dribbling from urachal fistula

Urachal fistula

Urinary bladder

Urethra

C

FIGURE 13-12. Urachal anomalies. **A,** Urachal cysts. The most common site for these cysts is in the superior end of the urachus, just inferior to the umbilicus. **B,** Two types of urachal sinuses are shown: one that opens into the bladder and one that opens at the umbilicus. **C,** Patent urachus or urachal fistula connecting the bladder and the umbilicus.

FIGURE 13-13. A male infant with exstrophy of the bladder. Because of defective closure of the inferior part of the anterior abdominal wall and the anterior wall of the bladder, the urinary bladder appears as an everted, bulging mass inferior to the umbilicus. (Courtesy of A.E. Chudley, MD, Department of Pediatrics and Child Health, University of Manitoba, Children's Hospital, Winnipeg, Manitoba, Canada.)

CONGENITAL ADRENAL HYPERPLASIA: ADRENOGENITAL SYNDROME

Congenital adrenal hyperplasia represents a group of *autosomal recessive disorders* in which an abnormal increase in the cells of the suprarenal cortex results in excessive androgen production during the fetal period. In girls, this usually causes masculinization of the external genitalia and enlargement of the clitoris (Fig. 13-17). Affected boys have normal external genitalia and may remain undiagnosed in early infancy. Later in childhood, in both sexes, excess androgen leads to rapid growth and accelerated skeletal maturation. Congenital adrenal hyperplasia (CAH) is usually caused by a genetically determined mutation in the cytochrome-P450c 21-steroid, 21-hydroxylase gene, which causes a deficiency of suprarenal cortical enzymes that are necessary for the biosynthesis of various steroid hormones. The reduced hormone output results in increased release of adrenocorticotrophic hormone, which causes CAH and overproduction of androgens by the hyperplastic suprarenal glands.

■ DEVELOPMENT OF THE SUPRARENAL GLANDS

The **cortex** of the suprarenal (adrenal) gland develops from the mesenchyme lining the posterior abdominal wall, whereas the **medulla** differentiates from the adjacent sympathetic ganglion derived from the **neural crest cells** (Fig. 13-16*A* and *B*). These cells differentiate into the secretory cells of the suprarenal medulla. The cortex is evident during the sixth week as an aggregation of mesenchymal cells seen bilaterally between the root of the dorsal mesentery and the developing gonad (see Fig. 13-18*C*). Differentiation of the characteristic suprarenal cortical zones begins during the late fetal period (see Fig. 13-16*C* to *E*). The *zona glomerulosa* and the *zona fasciculata* are present at birth, but the *zona reticularis* is not recognizable until the end of the third year (see Fig. 13-16*H*). Relative to body weight, the fetal suprarenal glands are 10 to 20 times larger than the adult glands due to the extensive size of the fetal cortex. The suprarenal medulla remains small until after birth (see Fig. 13-16*F*). The suprarenal glands rapidly become smaller as the cortex regresses during the first year of infancy (see Fig. 13-16*G*).

■ DEVELOPMENT OF THE GENITAL SYSTEM

The early genital systems in the two sexes are similar; therefore, the initial period of genital development is referred to as the *indifferent state of sexual development*.

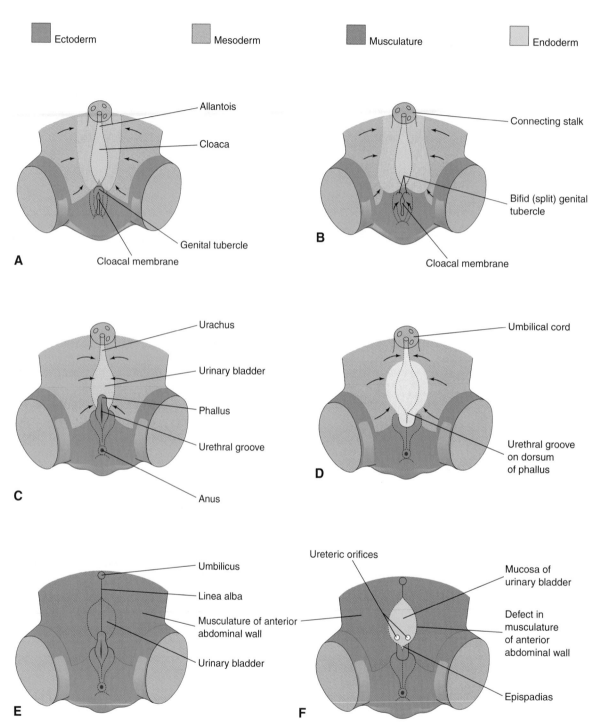

Ectoderm   Mesoderm   Musculature   Endoderm

A
Allantois
Cloaca
Genital tubercle
Cloacal membrane

B
Connecting stalk
Bifid (split) genital tubercle
Cloacal membrane

C
Urachus
Urinary bladder
Phallus
Urethral groove
Anus

D
Umbilical cord
Urethral groove on dorsum of phallus

E
Umbilicus
Linea alba
Musculature of anterior abdominal wall
Urinary bladder

F
Ureteric orifices
Mucosa of urinary bladder
Defect in musculature of anterior abdominal wall
Epispadias

FIGURE 13-14. **A, C,** and **E,** Normal stages in the development of the infraumbilical abdominal wall and the penis during the fourth to eighth weeks. Note that mesoderm and (later) muscle reinforce the ectoderm of the developing anterior abdominal wall. **B, D,** and **F,** Probable stages in the development of exstrophy of the bladder and epispadias. In **B** and **D,** note that the mesenchyme (embryonic connective tissue) does not extend into the anterior abdominal wall anterior to the urinary bladder. Also note that the genital tubercle is located in a more caudal position than usual, and that the urethral groove has formed on the dorsal surface of the penis. In **F,** the surface ectoderm and the anterior wall of the bladder have ruptured, resulting in exposure of the posterior wall of the bladder. Note that the musculature of the anterior abdominal wall is present on each side of the defect. (Based on Patten BM, Barry A: The genesis of exstrophy of the bladder and epispadias. Am J Anat 90:35, 1952.)

FIGURE 13-15. Schematic longitudinal sections of the distal part of the developing penis, showing the development of the prepuce and the distal part of the spongy urethra. **A,** At 11 weeks. **B,** At 12 weeks. **C,** At 14 weeks.

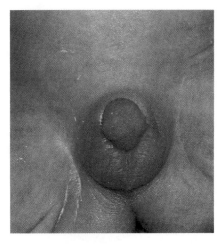

FIGURE 13-17. External genitalia of a newborn female infant with congenital adrenal hyperplasia. The virilization was caused by excessive androgens produced by the suprarenal glands during the fetal period. Note the enlarged clitoris and fusion of the labia majora. (Courtesy of Dr. Heather Dean, Department of Pediatrics and Child Health, University of Manitoba, Winnipeg, Manitoba, Canada.)

Development of the Gonads

The gonads (testes and ovaries) are derived from three sources:
- The mesodermal epithelium lining the posterior abdominal wall
- The underlying mesenchyme (embryonic connective tissue)
- The primordial germ cells

Indifferent Gonads

Gonadal development begins during the fifth week, when a thickened area of mesothelium develops on the medial side of the mesonephros (Fig. 13-18*A* to *C*). Proliferation of this epithelium and the underlying mesenchyme produces a bulge on the medial side of the mesonephros, called the **gonadal ridge** (see Fig. 13-18*A* and *C*). Finger-like epithelial cords—**gonadal cords**—soon grow into the underlying

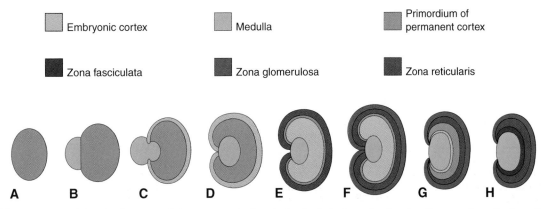

FIGURE 13-16. Illustrations of the development of the suprarenal adrenal glands. **A,** At 6 weeks, showing the mesodermal primordium of the fetal cortex. **B,** At 7 weeks, showing the addition of neural crest cells. **C,** At 8 weeks, showing the fetal cortex and the early permanent cortex beginning to encapsulate the medulla. **D** and **E,** Later stages of encapsulation of the medulla by the cortex. **F,** Neonatal period, showing the fetal cortex and two zones of the permanent cortex. **G,** At 1 year of age. Note that the fetal cortex has almost disappeared. **H,** At 4 years of age. Note the adult pattern of cortical zones. Observe that the fetal cortex has disappeared and that the gland is smaller than it was at birth (**F**).

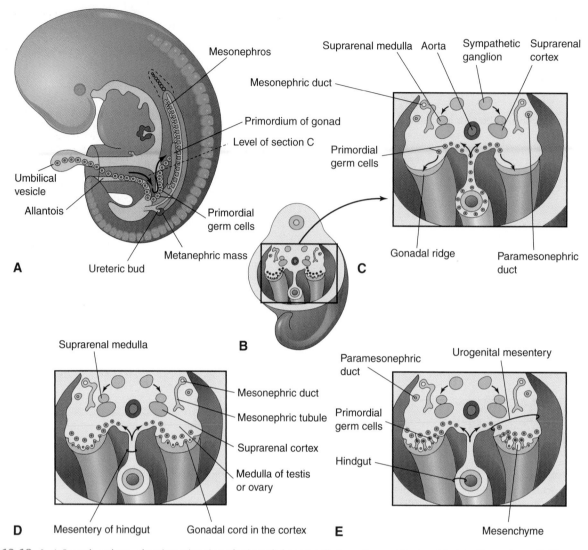

FIGURE 13-18. **A,** A 5-week embryo, showing migration of primordial germ cells from the umbilical vesicle into the embryo. **B,** Three-dimensional sketch of the caudal region of the 5-week embryo, showing the location and extent of the gonadal ridges. **C,** Transverse section, showing the primordium of the suprarenal glands, the gonadal ridges, and the migration of primordial germ cells into the developing gonads. **D,** Transverse section of a 6-week embryo, showing the gonadal cords. **E,** Similar section at a later stage, showing the indifferent gonads and the paramesonephric ducts.

mesenchyme (see Fig. 13-18D). The **indifferent gonads** now consist of an external cortex and an internal medulla. In embryos with an XX sex chromosome complex, the cortex of the gonad differentiates into an ovary and the medulla regresses. In embryos with an XY sex chromosome complex, the medulla differentiates into a testis and the cortex regresses, except for vestigial remnants (see Table 13-1).

Primordial Germ Cells

The **primordial germ cells** originate in the wall of the umbilical vesicle and migrate along the dorsal mesentery of the gut to the gonadal ridges (see Fig. 13-18A). During the sixth week, the primordial germ cells enter the underlying mesenchyme and are incorporated into the **gonadal cords** (see Fig. 13-18E). They eventually differentiate into oocytes or sperms.

Sex Determination

Chromosomal sex, established at fertilization, depends on whether an X-bearing sperm or a Y-bearing sperm fertilizes the X-bearing oocyte. The type of gonads that develop is determined by the sex chromosome complex of the embryo (XX or XY). Before the seventh week, the gonads of the two sexes are identical in appearance and are called **indifferent gonads** (Fig. 13-19). Development of the male phenotype requires a Y chromosome, but only the short arm of this chromosome is critical for sex determination. Two X chromosomes are required for the development of the female phenotype.

Development of the Testes

Testes usually develop in embryos with a normal Y chromosome in their sex chromosome complement. A

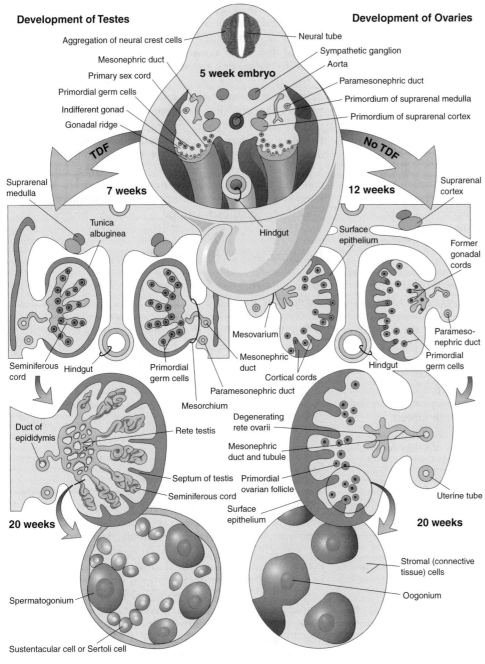

Development of Testes

Aggregation of neural crest cells
Mesonephric duct
Primary sex cord
Primordial germ cells
Indifferent gonad
Gonadal ridge

5 week embryo

Neural tube
Sympathetic ganglion
Aorta
Paramesonephric duct
Primordium of suprarenal medulla
Primordium of suprarenal cortex

Development of Ovaries

TDF

No TDF

7 weeks

12 weeks

Suprarenal medulla

Tunica albuginea

Hindgut

Surface epithelium

Suprarenal cortex

Former gonadal cords

Seminiferous cord

Hindgut

Primordial germ cells

Mesovarium

Mesonephric duct

Cortical cords

Paramesonephric duct

Mesorchium

Hindgut

Paramesonephric duct

Primordial germ cells

Duct of epididymis

Rete testis

Degenerating rete ovarii

Mesonephric duct and tubule

Septum of testis

Seminiferous cord

Primordial ovarian follicle

Surface epithelium

Uterine tube

20 weeks

20 weeks

Spermatogonium

Stromal (connective tissue) cells

Oogonium

Sustentacular cell or Sertoli cell

Section of seminiferous tubule

Section of ovarian cortex

FIGURE 13-19. Differentiation of the indifferent gonads of a 5-week embryo *(top)* into ovaries or testes. The *left side* of the drawing shows the development of testes resulting from the effects of the testis-determining factor (TDF) located on the Y chromosome. Note that the gonadal cords become seminiferous cords, the primordia of the seminiferous tubules. The parts of the gonadal cords that enter the medulla of the testis form the rete testis. In the section of the testis at the *bottom left*, observe that there are two kinds of cells: spermatogonia, derived from the primordial germ cells; and sustentacular or Sertoli, cells, derived from the mesenchyme. The *right side* shows the development of ovaries in the absence of TDF. Cortical cords have extended from the surface epithelium of the gonad, and primordial germ cells have entered them. They are the primordia of the oogonia. Follicular cells are derived from the surface epithelium of the ovary. The *arrows* indicate the changes that occur as the gonads (testes and ovaries) develop.

ABNORMAL SEX CHROMOSOME COMPLEXES

In embryos with abnormal sex chromosome complexes, such as XXX or XXY, the number of X chromosomes appears to be unimportant in sex determination. If a normal Y chromosome is present, the embryo develops as a male. If no Y chromosome is present or if the testis-determining region of the Y chromosome has been lost, female development occurs. The loss of an X chromosome does not appear to interfere with the migration of primordial germ cells to the gonadal ridges because some germ cells have been observed in the fetal gonads of 45, X females with Turner syndrome. Two X chromosomes are needed, however, to bring about complete ovarian development.

coordinated sequence of genes induces the development of testes. The *SRY gene for the testis-determining factor* (TDF) on the short arm of the Y chromosome acts as the switch that directs the development of the indifferent gonad into a testis. Expression of the transcription factor SOX9 is also essential for testicular determination. The testis-determining factor induces the gonadal cords to condense and extend into the medulla of the indifferent gonad, where they branch and anastomose to form the **rete testis**. The connection of the prominent gonadal cords—the seminiferous cords—with the surface epithelium is lost when the **tunica albuginea** develops (see Fig. 13-19). The dense tunica albuginea, a thick, fibrous capsule, is a characteristic feature of testicular development in the fetus. Gradually, the testis separates from the degenerating mesonephros and becomes suspended by its own mesentery, the **mesorchium**. The seminiferous cords develop into the seminiferous tubules, the straight tubules (tubuli recti), and the rete testis.

The **seminiferous tubules** are separated by the mesenchyme, giving rise to the **interstitial cells** (of Leydig). By the eighth week, these cells secrete **androgenic hormones**—*testosterone* and *androstenedione*—that induce masculine differentiation of the mesonephric ducts and the external genitalia. Testosterone production is stimulated by **human chorionic gonadotropin**, which reaches peak amounts during the 8- to 12-week period of embryonic and fetal development. The fetal testes also produce a glycoprotein known as antimüllerian hormone, or **müllerian-inhibiting substance (MIS)**. MIS is produced by the sustentacular (Sertoli) cells, which are present until puberty, at which time the levels of MIS decrease. MIS suppresses the development of the paramesonephric (Müllerian) ducts, which form the uterus and uterine tubes. The seminiferous tubules remain solid (i.e., without lumina) until puberty, when lumina begin to develop. The walls of the seminiferous tubules are composed of two kinds of cells (see Fig. 13-19):

- Sertoli cells, supporting cells derived from the surface epithelium of the testis
- Spermatogonia, primordial sperm cells derived from the primordial germ cells

Sertoli cells constitute most of the seminiferous epithelium in the fetal testis (see Fig. 13-19). The **rete testis** becomes continuous with 15 to 20 mesonephric tubules that become **efferent ductules**. These ductules are connected with the mesonephric duct, which becomes the **ductus epididymis** (see Figs. 13-19 and 13-20*A*).

Development of the Ovaries

Gonadal development occurs slowly in female embryos. The X chromosomes bear genes for ovarian development, and an autosomal gene also appears to play a role in ovarian organogenesis. The ovary is not identifiable by histologic examination until approximately the 10th week of development. **Gonadal cords** extend into the medulla and form a rudimentary *rete ovarii*. This structure normally degenerate and disappear (see Fig. 13-19). **Cortical cords** extend from the surface epithelium of the developing ovary into the underlying mesenchyme during the early fetal period. As the cortical cords increase in size, **primordial germ cells** are incorporated into them. At approximately 16 weeks, these cortical cords begin to break up into

isolated cell clusters—called **primordial follicles**—each of which consists of an **oogonium** (derived from a primordial germ cell), surrounded by a single layer of follicular cells derived from the cortical cord (see Fig. 13-19). Active mitosis produces thousands of oogonia during fetal life.

No oogonia form postnatally. Although many oogonia degenerate before birth, 2 million or so enlarge to become primary oocytes before birth. After birth, the surface epithelium of the ovary flattens to a single layer of cells that is continuous with the mesothelium of the peritoneum at the hilum of the ovary. The surface epithelium becomes separated from the follicles in the cortex by a thin, fibrous capsule, the **tunica albuginea**. As the ovary separates from the regressing mesonephros, it is suspended by its mesentery, the **mesovarium**.

Development of the Genital Ducts

Both male and female embryos have two pairs of genital ducts: the mesonephric ducts (Wolffian ducts) and the paramesonephric ducts (Müllerian ducts) (Fig. 13-21*A*).

The **mesonephric ducts** play an essential role in the development of the **male reproductive system** (see Fig. 13-20*A*). In female fetuses, the mesonephric ducts almost completely disappear, leaving only a few nonfunctional remnants (see Fig. 13-20*B* and *C* and Table 13-1). The **paramesonephric ducts** play an essential role in the development of the **female reproductive system** (see Fig. 13-20*B* and *C*).

Development of the Male Genital Ducts and Glands

The fetal testes produce testosterone and MIS. **Testosterone** stimulates the mesonephric ducts to form male genital ducts; MIS causes the paramesonephric ducts to disappear by epithelial-mesenchymal transformation. As the mesonephros degenerates, some mesonephric tubules persist and are transformed into efferent ductules (see Fig. 13-20*A*). These ductules open into the mesonephric duct, which has been transformed into the **duct of the epididymis** in this region. Distal to the epididymis, the mesonephric duct acquires a thick investment of smooth muscle and becomes the **ductus deferens**. A lateral outgrowth from the caudal end of each mesonephric duct gives rise to the **seminal gland** (vesicle). The secretions of this pair of glands nourish the sperms. The part of the mesonephric duct between the duct of this gland and the urethra becomes the **ejaculatory duct**.

PROSTATE

Multiple endodermal outgrowths arise from the prostatic part of the urethra and grow into the surrounding mesenchyme (Fig. 13-22). The glandular epithelium of the prostate differentiates from these endodermal cells, and the associated mesenchyme differentiates into the dense stroma and the smooth muscle of the prostate. Secretions from the prostate make up a portion of the fluid in ejaculate.

BULBOURETHRAL GLANDS

The bulbourethral glands are pea-sized structures that develop from paired outgrowths from the spongy part of the

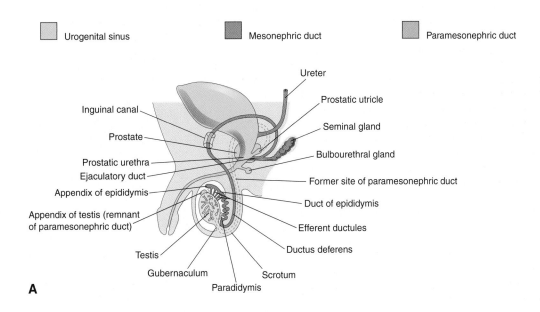

Urogenital sinus Mesonephric duct Paramesonephric duct

A, Reproductive system in a newborn male infant.

Inguinal canal
Prostate
Prostatic urethra
Ejaculatory duct
Appendix of epididymis
Appendix of testis (remnant of paramesonephric duct)
Testis
Gubernaculum
Paradidymis
Scrotum

Ureter
Prostatic utricle
Seminal gland
Bulbourethral gland
Former site of paramesonephric duct
Duct of epididymis
Efferent ductules
Ductus deferens

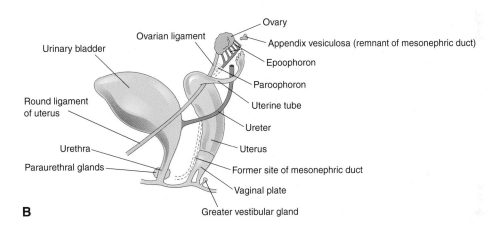

B

Urinary bladder
Round ligament of uterus
Urethra
Paraurethral glands

Ovarian ligament
Ovary
Appendix vesiculosa (remnant of mesonephric duct)
Epoophoron
Paroophoron
Uterine tube
Ureter
Uterus
Former site of mesonephric duct
Vaginal plate
Greater vestibular gland

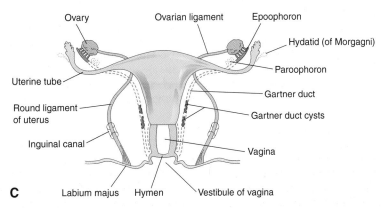

C

Ovary
Ovarian ligament
Epoophoron
Hydatid (of Morgagni)
Paroophoron
Gartner duct
Gartner duct cysts
Vagina
Vestibule of vagina
Uterine tube
Round ligament of uterus
Inguinal canal
Labium majus
Hymen

FIGURE 13-20. Development of the male and female reproductive systems from the genital ducts and the urogenital sinus. Vestigial structures are also shown. **A,** Reproductive system in a newborn male infant. **B,** Female reproductive system in a 12-week fetus. **C,** Reproductive system in a newborn female infant.

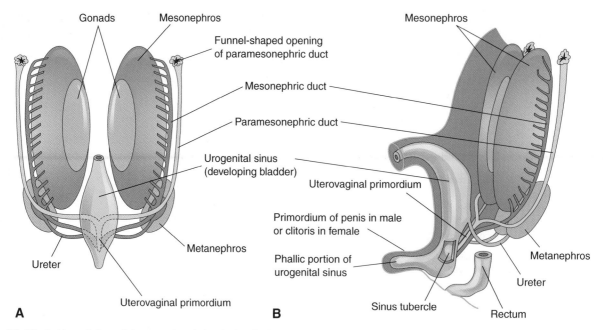

FIGURE 13-21. **A,** Ventral view of the posterior abdominal wall of a 7-week embryo, showing the two pairs of genital ducts that are present during the indifferent state of sexual development. **B,** Lateral view of a 9-week fetus, showing the sinus tubercle (Müller tubercle) on the posterior wall of the urogenital sinus. It becomes the hymen in females and the seminal colliculus in males.

urethra (see Fig. 13-20*A*). The smooth muscle fibers and the stroma differentiate from the adjacent mesenchyme. The secretions of these glands contribute to semen.

Development of the Female Genital Ducts and Glands

In female embryos, the mesonephric ducts regress because of lack of testosterone, and the paramesonephric ducts develop because of the absence of MIS. Female sexual development does not depend on the presence of ovaries or hormones. The **paramesonephric ducts** form most of the female genital tract. The **uterine tubes** develop from the unfused cranial parts of the paramesonephric ducts (see Fig. 13-20*B* and *C*). The caudal, fused portions of these ducts form the **uterovaginal primordium**, which gives rise to the uterus and the superior portion of the vagina. The endometrial stroma and the myometrium are derived from the splanchnic mesenchyme. Fusion of the paramesonephric ducts also brings together two peritoneal folds that form the right and left **broad ligament** and two peritoneal compartments, the **rectouterine pouch** and the **vesicouterine pouch** (Fig. 13-23*B* to *D*).

DEVELOPMENT OF THE VAGINA
The vaginal epithelium is derived from the endoderm of the urogenital sinus, and the fibromuscular wall of the vagina develops from the surrounding mesenchyme. Contact of the *uterovaginal primordium* with the urogenital sinus, forming the **sinus tubercle** (see Fig. 13-21*B*), induces the formation of paired endodermal outgrowths called **sinovaginal bulbs** (see Fig. 13-23*A*). They extend from the urogenital sinus to the caudal end of the uterovaginal primordium. The sinovaginal bulbs fuse to form a vaginal plate (Fig. 13-20*B*). The central cells of this plate break

down, forming the lumen of the vagina. The peripheral cells of the plate form the vaginal epithelium, or lining (see Fig. 13-20*C*). Until late in fetal life, the lumen of the vagina is separated from the cavity of the urogenital sinus by a membrane called the **hymen** (Fig. 13-24*H*; see also Fig. 13-20*C*). The hymen is formed by invagination of the posterior wall of the urogenital sinus.

FEMALE AUXILIARY GENITAL GLANDS
Buds grow from the urethra into the surrounding mesenchyme, forming the mucus-secreting **urethral and paraurethral glands**. Outgrowths from the urogenital sinus form bilateral greater vestibular glands (of Bartholin) in the lower one third of the labia majora. These tubuloalveolar glands also secrete mucus (see Table 13-1).

VESTIGIAL STRUCTURES DERIVED FROM THE EMBRYONIC GENITAL DUCTS
During conversion of the mesonephric and paramesonephric ducts into adult structures, parts of the ducts remain as vestigial structures (see Table 13-1 and Fig. 13-20*A* to *C*). These vestiges are rarely seen unless pathologic changes develop in them.

Development of the External Genitalia

From the fourth week to the early part of the seventh week, the external genitalia are sexually undifferentiated (see Fig. 13-24*A* and *B*). Distinguishing sexual characteristics begin to appear during the 9th week, but the external genitalia are not fully differentiated until the 12th week. Early in the fourth week, the proliferating mesenchyme produces a **genital tubercle** in both sexes at the cranial end of the cloacal membrane. **Labioscrotal swellings** and **urogenital folds** soon develop on each side of the

FIGURE 13-22. **A,** Dorsal view of the developing prostate in an 11-week fetus. **B,** Median section of the developing urethra and prostate. Note the numerous endodermal outgrowths from the prostatic urethra. The vestigial prostatic utricle is also shown. **C,** Section of the prostate (at 16 weeks) at the level shown in **B**.

cloacal membrane. The genital tubercle soon elongates to form a **primordial phallus**. When the urorectal septum fuses with the cloacal membrane at the end of the sixth week, it divides the cloacal membrane into a dorsal anal membrane and a ventral urogenital membrane (see Fig. 13-24B). The **urethral membrane** lies in the floor of a median cleft, the **urethral groove**, which is bound by the urogenital folds. The anal and urogenital membranes rupture approximately 1 week later, forming the **anus** and the **urogenital orifice**, respectively. In the female fetus, the urethra and the vagina open into a common cavity, the **vestibule**.

Development of the Male External Genitalia

Masculinization of the indifferent external genitalia is induced by **testosterone** (see Fig. 13-24C, E, and G). As the phallus enlarges and elongates to become the penis,

the urogenital folds form the lateral walls of the **urethral groove** on the ventral surface of the penis. This groove is lined by a proliferation of endodermal cells, the **urethral plate** (see Fig. 13-24C), which extends from the phallic portion of the urogenital sinus. The **urethral folds** fuse with each other along the ventral surface of the penis to form the **spongy urethra** (see Fig. 13-24E_1 to E_3). The surface ectoderm fuses in the median plane of the penis, forming the **penile raphe** and enclosing the spongy urethra within the penis. At the tip of the **glans penis**, an ectodermal ingrowth forms a cellular ectodermal cord, which grows toward the root of the penis to meet the spongy urethra (see Fig. 13-15A). This cord canalizes and joins the previously formed spongy urethra (see Fig. 13-16B). This juncture completes the terminal part of the urethra and moves the external urethral orifice to the tip of the glans penis (see Fig. 13-15C). During the 12th week, a circular ingrowth of ectoderm occurs at the periphery of the glans (see Fig. 13-15B). When this ingrowth breaks down, it forms the **prepuce** (foreskin) (see Fig. 13-15C). The **corpora cavernosa** penis and the **corpus spongiosum** penis develop from mesenchyme in the phallus. The **labioscrotal swellings** grow toward each other and fuse to form the **scrotum** (see Fig. 13-24E and G). The line of fusion of these folds is clearly visible as the **scrotal raphe** (see Fig. 13-24G).

Development of the Female External Genitalia

Growth of the phallus in the female fetus gradually decreases, with the structure becoming the **clitoris**. The clitoris develops in the same way as the penis, but the urogenital folds do not fuse, except posteriorly, where they join to form the **frenulum of the labia minora**. The unfused parts of the urogenital folds form the **labia minora**. The labioscrotal folds fuse posteriorly to form the **posterior labial commissure** and anteriorly to form the **anterior labial commissure** and the **mons pubis** (see Fig. 13-24D, F, and H). Most

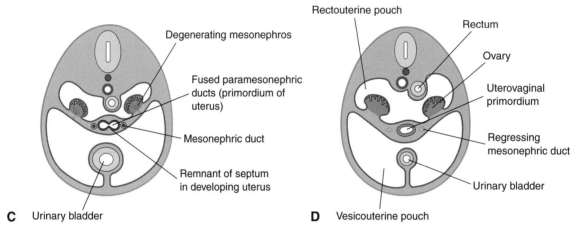

FIGURE 13-23. Early development of the ovaries and the uterus. **A,** Sagittal section of the caudal region of an 8-week female embryo. **B,** Transverse section, showing the paramesonephric ducts approaching each other. **C,** Similar section at a more caudal level, showing fusion of the paramesonephric ducts. A remnant of the septum that initially separated them is shown. **D,** Similar section, showing the uterovaginal primordium, broad ligament, and pouches in the pelvic cavity.

TRUE HERMAPHRODITISM

Persons with the extremely rare intersexual condition of true hermaphroditism usually have a 46, XX sex chromosome constitution. True hermaphroditism results from an error in sex determination. The phenotype may be male or female, but the external genitalia are always ambiguous.

FEMALE PSEUDOHERMAPHRODITISM

Female pseudohermaphroditism results from exposure of a female fetus to excessive androgens, the principal effect of which is virilization of the external genitalia (Fig. 13-25). Persons with this intersexual condition have *chromatin-positive nuclei* and a 46, XX chromosome constitution. The common cause of

female pseudohermaphroditism is **congenital adrenal hyperplasia**. There is no ovarian abnormality, but the excessive production of androgens by the fetal suprarenal glands causes masculinization of the external genitalia, varying from enlargement of the clitoris to almost masculine genitalia. Commonly, **clitoral hypertrophy**, partial fusion of the labia majora, and a persistent urogenital sinus are noted.

MALE PSEUDOHERMAPHRODITISM

Persons with the uncommon intersexual condition of male pseudohermaphroditism have sex *chromatin-negative nuclei* and a 46, XY chromosome constitution. The external and internal genitalia are variable, owing to varying degrees of development. These anomalies are caused by inadequate production of testosterone and MIS by the fetal testes. Testicular development ranges from rudimentary to normal.

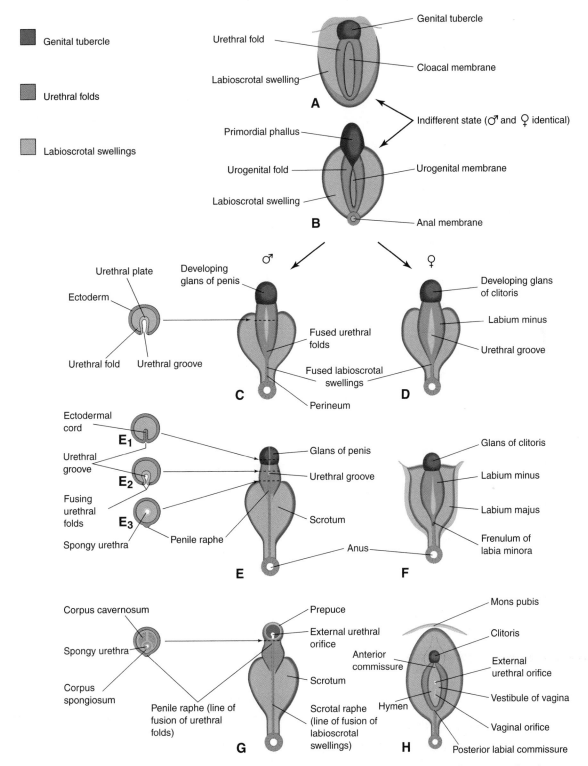

FIGURE 13-24. Development of the external genitalia. **A** and **B,** Appearance of the genitalia during the indifferent state (fourth to seventh weeks). **C, E,** and **G,** Stages in the development of the male external genitalia at 9, 11, and 12 weeks, respectively. On the *left* are schematic transverse sections of the developing penis, showing the formation of the spongy urethra. **D, F,** and **H,** Stages in the development of the female external genitalia at 9, 11, and 12 weeks, respectively.

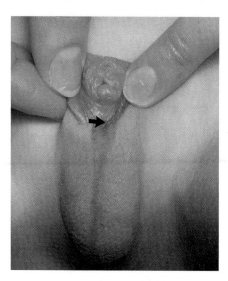

FIGURE 13-25. External genitalia of a 6-year-old girl, showing an enlarged clitoris and a scrotum-like structure formed by fusion of the labia majora. The *arrow* indicates the opening into the urogenital sinus. This extreme masculinization is the result of congenital adrenal hyperplasia. (Courtesy of Dr. Heather Dean, Department of Pediatrics and Child Health, University of Manitoba, Winnipeg, Manitoba, Canada.)

FIGURE 13-26. Glanular hypospadias in an infant. There is a shallow pit in the glans penis at the usual site of the urethral orifice. (Courtesy of A.E. Chudley, MD, Department of Pediatrics and Child Health, University of Manitoba, Children's Hospital, Winnipeg, Manitoba, Canada.)

ANDROGEN INSENSITIVITY SYNDROME

Androgen insensitivity syndrome (AIS)—also called **testicular feminization syndrome**—occurs in 1 in 20,000 live births. Individuals with this unusual condition are normal-appearing females, despite the presence of testes and a 46, XY chromosome constitution. The external genitalia are female, but the vagina usually ends in a blind pouch and the uterus and the uterine tubes are absent or rudimentary. At puberty, there is normal development of breasts and female characteristics, but menstruation does not occur and pubic hair is scanty or absent. The failure of masculinization to occur in these individuals results from a resistance to the action of testosterone at the cellular level in the genital tubercle and the labioscrotal and urogenital folds.

HYPOSPADIAS

There are four types of hypospadias: glanular hypospadias (the most common type), penile hypospadias, penoscrotal hypospadias, and perineal hypospadias. Hypospadias is the most common anomaly involving the penis and is found in 1 in 300 male infants. In **glanular hypospadias,** the external urethral orifice is on the ventral surface of the glans penis. In **penile hypospadias** the external urethral orifice is on the ventral surface of the body of the penis. The glans and penile types of hypospadias constitute most cases (Fig. 13-26). In **penoscrotal hypospadias,** the urethral orifice is at the junction of the penis and the scrotum. In **perineal hypospadias**, the external urethral orifice is located between the unfused halves of the scrotum. Hypospadias results from inadequate production of androgens by the fetal testes, inadequate receptor sites for these hormones, or both.

EPISPADIAS

In a rare condition known as **epispadias**, the urethra opens on the dorsal surface of the penis. It is *often associated with exstrophy of the bladder* (see Fig. 13-13). Epispadias may result from inadequate ectodermal-mesenchymal interactions during development of the genital tubercle. As a consequence, the genital tubercle develops more dorsally than in normal embryos. Consequently, when the urogenital membrane ruptures, the urogenital sinus opens on the dorsal surface of the penis. Urine is expelled at the root of the malformed penis.

ANOMALIES OF THE FEMALE GENITAL TRACT

Various types of uterine duplication and vaginal anomalies result from developmental arrest of the uterovaginal primordium during the eighth week of development (Fig. 13-27*B* to *G*). These developmental anomalies may include:

- Incomplete fusion of the paramesonephric ducts
- Incomplete development of one or both paramesonephric ducts

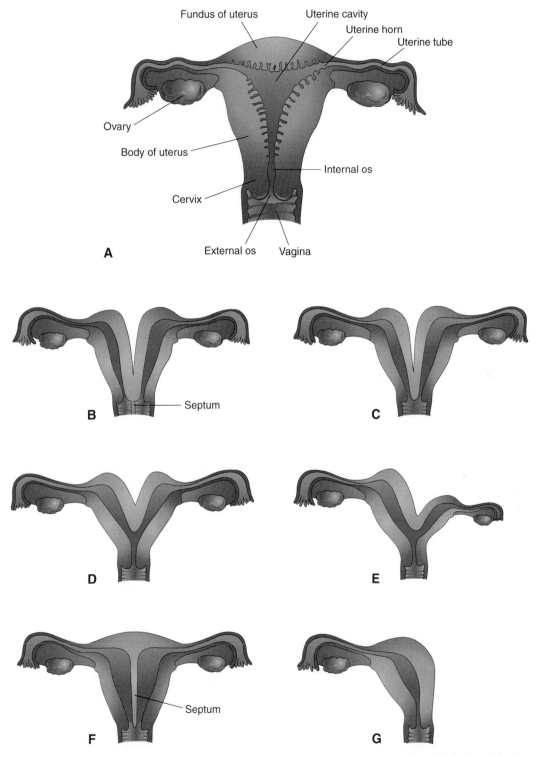

FIGURE 13-27. Various types of uterine anomalies. **A,** Normal uterus and vagina. **B,** Double uterus (uterus didelphys) and double vagina. **C,** Double uterus with a single vagina. **D,** Bicornuate uterus (two uterine horns). **E,** Bicornuate uterus with a rudimentary left horn. **F,** Septate uterus. **G,** Unicornuate uterus.

- Failure of parts of one or both paramesonephric ducts to develop
- Incomplete canalization of the vaginal plate that forms the vagina

A **double uterus** (uterus didelphys) results from failure of fusion of the inferior parts of the paramesonephric ducts. It may be associated with a double or a single vagina (see Fig. 13-27B and C). In some cases, the uterus is divided internally by a thin septum (see Fig. 13-27F). If the duplication involves only the superior part of the body of the uterus, the condition is called **bicornuate uterus** (see Fig. 13-27D and E). If growth of one paramesonephric duct is retarded and the duct does not fuse with the other one, a **bicornuate uterus with a rudimentary horn** develops (see Fig. 13-27E). The rudimentary horn may not communicate with the cavity of the uterus. A **unicornuate uterus** develops when one paramesonephric duct does not develop; this results in a uterus with one uterine tube (see Fig. 13-27G). In many of these cases, the individuals are fertile, but may have an increased incidence of premature delivery.

Agenesis of the vagina results from failure of the sinovaginal bulbs to develop and form the vaginal plate (see Fig. 13-20B). When the vagina is absent, the uterus is usually absent also, because the developing uterus (uterovaginal primordium) induces the formation of sinovaginal bulbs, which fuse to form the vaginal plate. Failure of canalization of the vaginal plate results in blockage of the vagina. Failure of the inferior end of the vaginal plate to perforate results in an **imperforate hymen**.

parts of the **labioscrotal folds** remain unfused and form two large folds of skin, the **labia majora**.

■ DEVELOPMENT OF THE INGUINAL CANALS

The inguinal canals form pathways for the testes to descend from their intra-abdominal position through the anterior abdominal wall and into the scrotum. *Inguinal canals develop in both sexes* because of the morphologically indifferent state of sexual development. As the mesonephros degenerates, a ligament called the **gubernaculum** develops on each side of the abdomen from the inferior pole of the gonad (Fig. 13-28A). The gubernaculum passes obliquely through the developing anterior abdominal wall at the site of the future inguinal canal. The gubernaculum attaches caudally to the internal surface of the *labioscrotal swellings*. The **processus vaginalis** is an evagination of peritoneum. The processus vaginalis develops ventral to the gubernaculum and herniates through the abdominal wall, along the path formed by the gubernaculum (see Fig. 13-28B to E). The vaginal process carries along extensions of the layers of the abdominal wall, which form the walls of the inguinal

canal. In males, these layers also form the coverings of the spermatic cord and the testis (see Fig. 13-28E and F). The opening in the transversalis fascia produced by the vaginal process becomes the **deep inguinal ring**, and the opening created in the external oblique aponeurosis forms the **superficial inguinal ring**.

Descent of the Testes

By 26 weeks, the testes have descended retroperitoneally from the posterior abdominal wall to the deep inguinal rings (see Fig. 13-28B and C). This change in position occurs as the fetal pelvis enlarges and the trunk of the embryo elongates. Transabdominal movement of the testes is largely a relative movement that results from growth of the cranial part of the abdomen away from the future pelvic region.

Testicular descent through the inguinal canals and into the scrotum is controlled by androgens (e.g., testosterone) produced by the fetal testes. The gubernaculum appears to guide the testes during their descent. Descent of the testes through the inguinal canals and into the scrotum usually begins during the 26th week and takes 2 to 3 days. In more than 97% of full-term newborn boys, both testes are in the scrotum. During the first 3 months after birth, most undescended testes descend into the scrotum. When the testis descends, it carries its ductus deferens and vessels with it. As the testis and the ductus deferens descend, they are ensheathed by the fascial extensions of the abdominal wall (see Fig. 13-28F):

- The extension of the transversalis fascia becomes the **internal spermatic fascia**.
- The extensions of the internal oblique muscle and the fascia become the **cremasteric muscle** and **fascia**.
- The extension of the external oblique aponeurosis becomes the **external spermatic fascia**.

Within the scrotum, the testis projects into the distal end of the processus vaginalis. During the perinatal period, the connecting stalk of the process is usually obliterated, isolating the **tunica vaginalis** as a peritoneal sac related to the testis (see Fig. 13-28F).

CRYPTORCHIDISM

Cryptorchidism (undescended testes) occurs in up to 30% of premature male infants and in approximately 3% to 4% of full-term male infants. Cryptorchidism may be unilateral or bilateral. In most cases, the testes descend into the scrotum by the end of the first year. If both testes remain within or just outside the abdominal cavity, they do not mature and sterility is common. If uncorrected, these patients have a significantly higher risk of germ cell tumors, especially in cases of abdominal cryptorchidism. **Cryptorchid testes** may be in the abdominal cavity or anywhere along the usual path of descent of the testis, but they are usually in the inguinal canal (Fig. 13-29A). The cause of most cases of cryptorchidism is unknown, but a deficiency of androgen production by the fetal testes is an important factor.

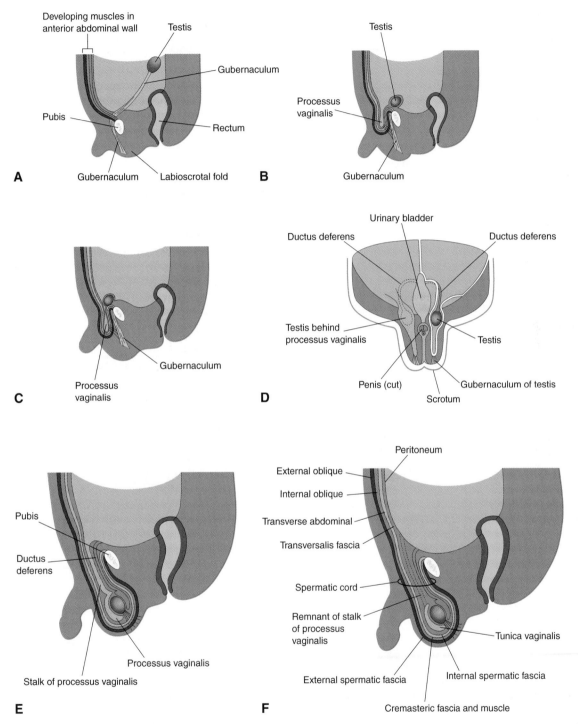

FIGURE 13-28. Formation of the inguinal canals and descent of the testes. **A,** Sagittal section of a 7-week embryo, showing the testis adjacent to the dorsal abdominal wall. **B** and **C,** Similar sections at approximately 28 weeks, showing the processus vaginalis and the testis beginning to pass through the inguinal canal. Note that the processus vaginalis carries fascial layers of the abdominal wall before it. **D,** Frontal section of a fetus approximately 3 days later, showing descent of the testis posterior to the processus vaginalis. The processus vaginalis has been cut away on the *left side* to show the testis and the ductus deferens. **E,** Sagittal section of a newborn male infant, showing the processus vaginalis communicating with the peritoneal cavity by a narrow stalk. **F,** Similar section of a 1-month-old male infant after obliteration of the stalk of the processus vaginalis. Note that the extended fascial layers of the abdominal wall now form the coverings of the spermatic cord.

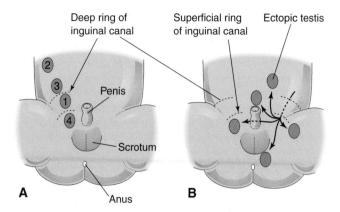

A, Deep ring of inguinal canal, Penis, Scrotum, Anus

B, Superficial ring of inguinal canal, Ectopic testis

FIGURE 13-29. Possible sites of cryptorchid and ectopic testes. **A**, Positions of cryptorchid testes, numbered 1 to 4 in order of frequency. **B**, Usual locations of ectopic testes.

- Interstitial (external to the aponeurosis of the external oblique muscle)
- In the proximal part of the medial thigh
- Dorsal to the penis
- On the opposite side (crossed ectopia)

All types of ectopic testis are rare, but **interstitial ectopia** occurs most frequently. Ectopic testis occurs when a part of the gubernaculum passes to an abnormal location and the testis follows it.

ECTOPIC TESTES

After traversing the inguinal canal, the testis may deviate from its usual path of descent and lodge in various abnormal locations (see Fig. 13-29B):

CONGENITAL INGUINAL HERNIA

If the communication between the tunica vaginalis and the peritoneal cavity does not close, a **persistent processus vaginalis** occurs. A loop of intestine may herniate through it into the scrotum or the labium majus (Fig. 13-30A and B). Embryonic remnants resembling the ductus deferens or the epididymis are often found in inguinal hernial sacs. Congenital inguinal hernia is much more common in males than in females, and it is often associated with cryptorchidism and, in females, with androgen insensitivity syndrome.

FIGURE 13-30. Sagittal sections, showing conditions resulting from failure of closure of the processus vaginalis. **A**, Incomplete congenital inguinal hernia resulting from persistence of the proximal part of the processus vaginalis. **B**, Complete congenital inguinal hernia into the scrotum resulting from persistence of the processus vaginalis. Cryptorchidism, a commonly associated condition, is also shown. **C**, Large cyst or hydrocele that arose from an unobliterated portion of the processus vaginalis. **D**, Hydrocele of the testis and the spermatic cord resulting from peritoneal fluid passing into a patent processus vaginalis.

HYDROCELE

Occasionally, the abdominal end of the processus vaginalis remains open, but is too small to permit herniation of the intestine (see Fig. 13-30D). In such cases, peritoneal fluid passes into the patent processus vaginalis and forms a **hydrocele of the testis.** If the middle part of the processus vaginalis remains open, fluid may accumulate and give rise to a **hydrocele of the spermatic cord** (see Fig. 13-30C).

Descent of the Ovaries

The ovaries also descend from the posterior abdominal wall to the pelvis, just inferior to the pelvic brim. The gubernaculum is attached to the uterus near the attachment of the uterine tube. The cranial part of the gubernaculum becomes the **ovarian ligament**, and the caudal part forms the **round ligament** of the uterus (see Fig. 13-20C). The round ligaments pass through the inguinal canals and terminate in the labia majora. The relatively small processus vaginalis in the female is usually obliterated, and it disappears long before birth.

CLINICALLY ORIENTED QUESTIONS

1. Does a horseshoe kidney usually function normally? What sort of problems may occur with this anomaly, and how can they be corrected?
2. A patient was told that he has two kidneys on one side and none on the other. How did this abnormality probably happen? Are there likely to be any problems associated with this condition?
3. Are true hermaphrodites ever fertile?
4. When a baby is born with ambiguous external genitalia, how long does it take to assign the appropriate sex? What does the physician tell the parents? How is the appropriate sex determined?
5. What is the most common type of disorder that produces ambiguous external genitalia? Will masculinizing, or androgenic, hormones given during the fetal period of development cause ambiguity of the external genitalia in female fetuses?

The answers to these questions are at the back of the book.

THE CARDIOVASCULAR SYSTEM

*T*he cardiovascular system is the first major system to function in the embryo. The primordial heart and vascular system appear in the middle of the third week of embryonic development (Fig. 14-1). The heart begins to beat at 22 to 23 days (Fig. 14-2). This precocious development is necessary because the rapidly growing embryo can no longer satisfy its nutritional and oxygen requirements by diffusion alone.

■ EARLY DEVELOPMENT OF THE HEART AND BLOOD VESSELS

Paired endothelial strands—**angioblastic cords**—appear in the cardiogenic mesoderm during the third week of development (see Fig. 14-1B and C). These cords canalize to form thin **heart tubes** that fuse to form the tubular heart late in the third week (see Fig. 14-5). An inductive influence from the anterior endoderm stimulates early formation of the heart. Cardiac morphogenesis is controlled by a cascade of *regulatory genes and transcription factors.*

Development and Fate of the Veins Associated with the Heart

Three paired veins drain into the tubular heart of a 4-week embryo (see Fig. 14-2):
- *Vitelline veins* return poorly oxygenated blood from the umbilical vesicle (yolk sac).
- *Umbilical veins* carry well-oxygenated blood from the chorion; only the left umbilical vein persists.
- *Common cardinal veins* return poorly oxygenated blood from the body of the embryo.

The **vitelline veins** enter the **sinus venosus** (see Figs. 14-2 and 14-4A and B). As the liver primordium grows into the septum transversum, the hepatic cords anastomose around pre-existing endothelium-lined spaces. These spaces, the primordia of the hepatic sinusoids, later become linked to the vitelline veins. The **hepatic veins** form from the remains of the right vitelline vein in the region of the developing liver. The **portal vein** develops from an anastomotic network of vitelline veins around the duodenum (see Fig. 14-4B). The fate of the umbilical veins may be summarized as follows (see Fig. 14-4B):
- The right umbilical vein and the caudal part of the left umbilical vein between the liver and the sinus venosus degenerate.
- The persistent caudal part of the left umbilical vein becomes the **umbilical vein**, which carries well-oxygenated blood from the placenta to the embryo.
- A large venous shunt—the **ductus venosus**—develops within the liver and connects the umbilical vein with the inferior vena cava (IVC). The ductus venosus forms a bypass through the liver, enabling most of the blood from the placenta to pass directly to the heart without passing through the capillary networks of the liver.

The **cardinal veins** (Figs. 14-2 and 14-3A) constitute the main venous drainage system of the embryo. The anterior and posterior cardinal veins drain the cranial and caudal parts of the embryo, respectively (see Fig. 14-3A). The anterior and posterior cardinal veins join the **common cardinal veins**, which enter the **sinus venosus** (Fig. 14-4A). During the eighth week, the **anterior cardinal veins** are connected by an oblique anastomosis (see Fig. 14-4B) that shunts blood from the left to the right anterior cardinal vein. This anastomotic shunt becomes the **left brachiocephalic vein** when the caudal part of the left anterior cardinal vein degenerates (see Figs.

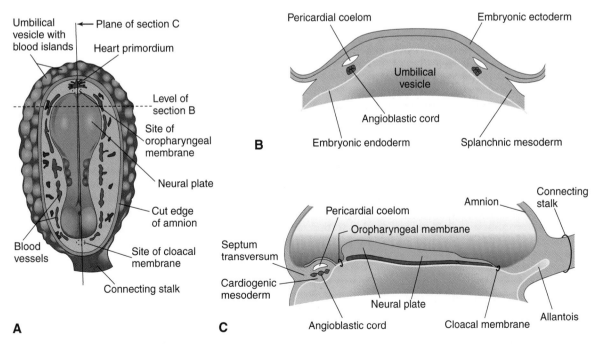

FIGURE 14-1. Early development of the heart. **A,** Dorsal view of an embryo (approximately 18 days). **B,** Transverse section of the embryo, showing angioblastic cords and their relationship to the pericardial coelom. **C,** Longitudinal section through the embryo, showing the relationship of the angioblastic cords to the oropharyngeal membrane, pericardial coelom, and septum transversum.

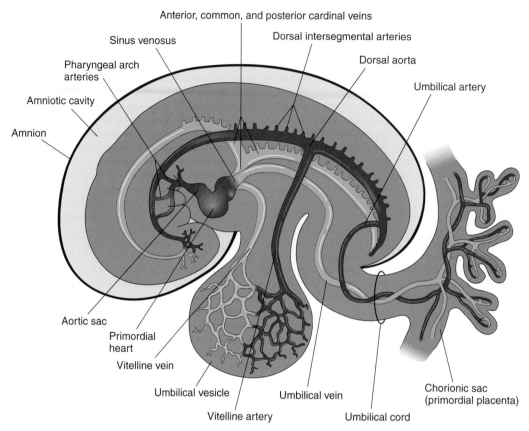

Anterior, common, and posterior cardinal veins
Sinus venosus
Pharyngeal arch arteries
Amniotic cavity
Amnion
Dorsal intersegmental arteries
Dorsal aorta
Umbilical artery
Aortic sac
Primordial heart
Vitelline vein
Umbilical vesicle
Vitelline artery
Umbilical vein
Umbilical cord
Chorionic sac (primordial placenta)

FIGURE 14-2. The embryonic cardiovascular system (at approximately 26 days), showing vessels on the left side only. The umbilical vein carries well-oxygenated blood and nutrients from the chorion (the embryonic part of the placenta) to the embryo. The umbilical arteries carry poorly oxygenated blood and waste products from the embryo to the chorion.

14-3*D* and 14-4*C*). The **superior vena cava** (SVC) forms from the right anterior cardinal vein and the right common cardinal vein. The only adult derivatives of the posterior cardinal veins are the root of the azygos vein and the common iliac veins.

The subcardinal and supracardinal veins gradually replace and supplement the posterior cardinal veins. The **subcardinal veins** appear first (see Fig. 14-3*A*) and form the stem of the left renal vein, the suprarenal veins, the gonadal veins (testicular and ovarian), and a segment of the inferior vena cava (see Fig. 14-3*D*). The **supracardinal veins** become disrupted in the region of the kidneys (see Fig. 14-3*C*). Cranial to this, they become united by an anastomosis that forms the **azygos** and the **hemiazygos veins** (see Figs. 14-3*D* and 14-4*C*). Caudal to the kidneys, the left supracardinal vein degenerates, but the right supracardinal vein becomes the inferior part of the IVC (see Fig. 14-3*D*). The **IVC** forms as blood returning from the caudal part of the embryo is shifted from the left to the right side of the body. The IVC is composed of four main segments (see Fig. 14-3*D*).

Pharyngeal Arch Arteries and Other Branches of the Dorsal Aorta

As the *pharyngeal arches* form during the fourth and fifth weeks of development, they are supplied by arteries—**pharyngeal arch arteries**—that arise from the **aortic sac**

ANOMALIES OF THE VENAE CAVAE

The most common anomaly of the venae cavae is a persistent left SVC. The most common anomaly of the IVC is interruption of its abdominal course; as a result, blood drains from the lower limbs, abdomen, and pelvis to the heart through the azygos system of veins.

and terminate in the **dorsal aortae** (see Fig. 14-2). Initially, the paired dorsal aortae run through the entire length of the embryo. Later, the caudal portions of the paired dorsal aortae fuse to form a single lower thoracic and abdominal aorta. Of the remaining paired dorsal aortae, the right regresses and the left becomes the primary aorta.

Intersegmental Arteries

Thirty or so branches of the dorsal aorta, collectively known as the **intersegmental arteries**, pass between and carry blood to the somites and their derivatives (see Fig. 14-2). The intersegmental arteries in the neck join to form a longitudinal artery on each side, the **vertebral artery**.

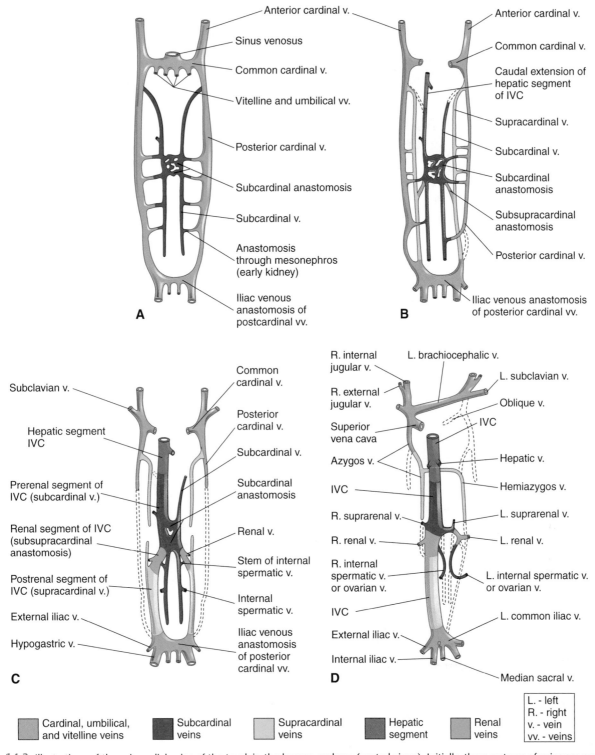

FIGURE 14-3. Illustrations of the primordial veins of the trunk in the human embryo (ventral views). Initially, three systems of veins are present: the umbilical veins from the chorion, the vitelline veins from the umbilical vesicle, and the cardinal veins from the body of the embryo. Next, the subcardinal veins appear, and finally, the supracardinal veins develop. **A,** At 6 weeks. **B,** At 7 weeks. **C,** At 8 weeks. **D,** Adult, showing the transformations that produce the adult venous pattern. (Modified from Arey LB: Developmental Anatomy, rev. 7th ed. Philadelphia, WB Saunders, 1974.)

Most of the original connections of the intersegmental arteries to the dorsal aorta eventually disappear. In the thorax, the intersegmental arteries persist as **intercostal arteries**. Most of the intersegmental arteries in the abdomen become **lumbar arteries**; however, the fifth pair of lumbar intersegmental arteries remains as the **common iliac arteries** (see Fig. 14-3D). In the sacral region, the intersegmental arteries form the lateral sacral arteries. The caudal end of the dorsal aorta becomes the median sacral artery.

FIGURE 14-4. Dorsal views of the developing heart. **A,** During the fourth week (approximately 24 days), the primordial atrium and the sinus venosus, as well as the veins draining into them, are evident. **B,** At 7 weeks, the right sinual horn is enlarged and the venous circulation through the liver is established. (The organs are not drawn to scale.) **C,** At 8 weeks, showing the adult derivatives of the cardinal veins. *Arrows* indicate the flow of blood.

Fate of the Vitelline and Umbilical Arteries

The unpaired ventral branches of the dorsal aorta supply the umbilical vesicle, the allantois, and the chorion (see Fig. 14-2). The **vitelline arteries** supply the umbilical vesicle and, later, the primordial gut, which forms from the incorporated part of the umbilical vesicle. Only three vitelline arteries remain and become:

- The *celiac arterial trunk* to the foregut
- The *superior mesenteric artery* to the midgut
- The *inferior mesenteric artery* to the hindgut

The paired **umbilical arteries** pass through the connecting stalk (primordial umbilical cord) and join the vessels in the chorion. The umbilical arteries carry poorly oxygenated blood to the placenta (see Fig. 14-2). The proximal parts of these arteries become the internal iliac arteries and

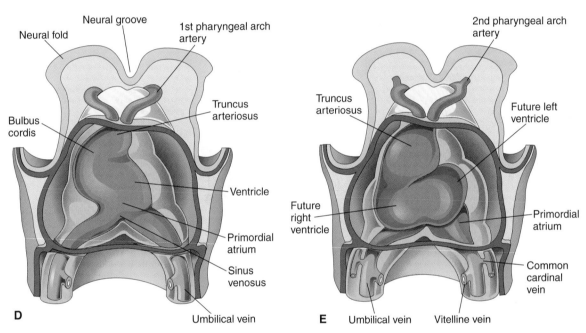

FIGURE 14-5. **A** to **C,** Ventral views of the developing heart and the pericardial region (22–35 days). The ventral pericardial wall has been removed to show the developing myocardium and fusion of the two heart tubes to form a single heart tube. Fusion begins at the cranial ends of the tubes and extends caudally until a single tubular heart is formed. **D** and **E,** As the heart elongates, it bends on itself, forming an S-shaped heart.

the superior vesical arteries, whereas the distal parts are obliterated after birth and become the medial umbilical ligaments.

■ LATER DEVELOPMENT OF THE HEART

As lateral embryonic folding occurs, the heart tubes approach each other and fuse to form a single tube (Figs. 14-5B and C and 14-6D). Fusion of the heart tubes begins at the cranial end and extends caudally. The **primordial myocardium** is formed from the splanchnic mesoderm surrounding the pericardial coelom (see Fig. 14-6B and C). At this stage, the developing heart is composed of a thin, endothelial tube that is separated from a thick, muscular tube (the primordial myocardium) by gelatinous connective tissue called **cardiac jelly** (see Fig. 14-6C and D). The endothelial tube becomes the internal endothelial

lining of the heart, the **endocardium**, and the primordial myocardium becomes the muscular wall of the heart, the **myocardium**. The **epicardium** is derived from the mesothelial cells that arise from the external surface of the sinus venosus (see Fig. 14-6F).

As folding of the head region occurs, the heart and the pericardial cavity appear ventral to the foregut and caudal to the oropharyngeal membrane (Fig. 14-7A to C). Concurrently, the tubular heart elongates and develops alternate dilations and constrictions (see Fig. 14-5C to E): the **bulbus cordis** (composed of the **truncus arteriosus,** the conus arteriosus, and the conus cordis), ventricle, the atrium, and the sinus venosus.

The tubular **truncus arteriosus** (TA) is continuous cranially with the aortic sac (Fig. 14-8A), from which the pharyngeal arch arteries arise. The **sinus venosus** receives the umbilical, vitelline, and common cardinal veins from the chorion, umbilical vesicle, and embryo, respectively

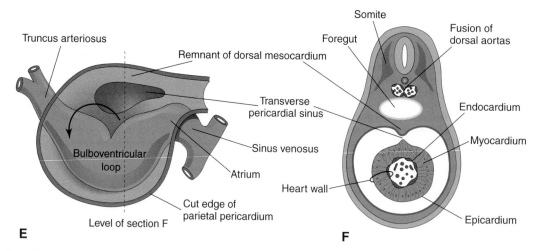

FIGURE 14-6. **A,** Dorsal view of an embryo (approximately 20 days). **B,** Schematic transverse section of the heart region of the embryo illustrated in **A,** showing the two endocardial heart tubes and the lateral folds of the body. **C,** Transverse section of a slightly older embryo, showing the formation of the pericardial cavity and the fusing heart tubes. **D,** Similar section (approximately 22 days), showing the single heart tube suspended by the dorsal mesocardium. **E,** Schematic drawing of the heart (approximately 28 days), showing degeneration of the central part of the dorsal mesocardium and formation of the transverse sinus of the pericardium. The *arrow* shows bending of the primordial heart. **F,** Transverse section of the embryo at the level shown in **E,** showing the layers of the heart wall.

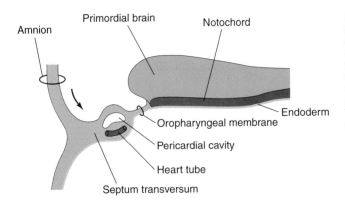

Amnion — Primordial brain — Notochord

Oropharyngeal membrane

Endoderm

Pericardial cavity

Heart tube

Septum transversum

A

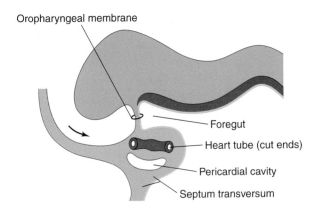

Oropharyngeal membrane

Foregut

Heart tube (cut ends)

Pericardial cavity

Septum transversum

B

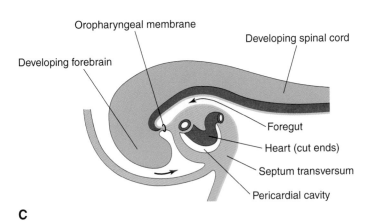

Oropharyngeal membrane

Developing spinal cord

Developing forebrain

Foregut

Heart (cut ends)

Septum transversum

Pericardial cavity

C

FIGURE 14-7. Longitudinal sections through the cranial half of human embryos during the fourth week of development. The effect of the head fold *(arrow)* on the position of the heart and other structures is shown. **A** and **B**, As the head fold develops, the heart tube and the pericardial cavity come to lie ventral to the foregut and caudal to the oropharyngeal membrane. **C,** Note that the positions of the pericardial cavity and the septum transversum have reversed with respect to each other. The septum transversum now lies posterior to the pericardial cavity, where it will form the central tendon of the diaphragm.

(see Fig. 14-8*B*). The arterial and venous ends of the heart are fixed by the pharyngeal arches and the septum transversum, respectively. Because the **bulbus cordis** and the ventricle grow faster than the other regions, the heart bends on itself, forming a U-shaped **bulboventricular loop** (see Fig. 14-6*E*). As the primordial heart bends, the atrium and sinus venosus appear dorsal to the truncus arteriosus, bulbus cordis, and ventricle (see Fig. 14-8*A* and *B*). By this stage, the sinus venosus has developed lateral expansions,

the right and left **horns of the sinus venosus**. As the heart develops, it gradually invaginates the **pericardial cavity** (see Figs. 14-6*C* and D and 14-7*C*). The heart is initially suspended from the dorsal wall by a mesentery, the **dorsal mesocardium**. However, the central part of this mesentery degenerates, forming a communication—the **transverse pericardial sinus**—between the right and left sides of the pericardial cavity (see Fig. 14-6*E* and *F*). At this stage, the heart is attached only at its cranial and caudal ends.

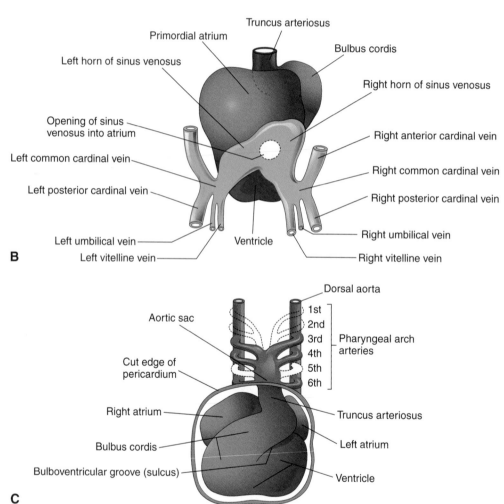

FIGURE 14-8. **A,** Sagittal section of the primordial heart (approximately 24 days), showing blood flowing through it *(arrows).* **B,** Dorsal view of the heart (approximately 26 days), showing the horns of the sinus venosus and the dorsal location of the primordial atrium. **C,** Ventral view of the heart and the pharyngeal arch arteries (approximately 35 days). The ventral wall of the pericardial sac has been removed to show the heart in the pericardial cavity.

Circulation through the Primordial Heart

The initial contractions of the heart originate in muscle. Blood enters the sinus venosus from a number of sites (see Fig. 14-8*A* and *B*), including:

● The embryo through the common cardinal veins
● The placenta through the umbilical veins
● The umbilical vesicle through the vitelline veins

Blood from the sinus venosus enters the primordial atrium; flow from it is controlled by **sinuatrial valves** (see Fig. 14-8*A*). The blood then passes through the **atrioventricular canal** into the **primordial ventricle**. When the ventricle contracts, blood is pumped through the **bulbus cordis** and the **truncus arteriosus** into the **aortic sac,** from which it is distributed to the pharyngeal arch arteries in the pharyngeal arches (see Fig. 14-8*C*). The blood then passes into the dorsal aortas for distribution to the embryo, the umbilical vesicle, and the placenta. Partitioning of the atrioventricular (AV) canal, the primordial atrium, and the ventricle begins at approximately the middle of the fourth week and is essentially completed by the end of the eighth week.

Partitioning of the Atrioventricular Canal

Endocardial cushions form on the dorsal and ventral walls of the AV canal (see Fig. 14-8A). The AV cushions approach each other and fuse, dividing the AV canal into right and

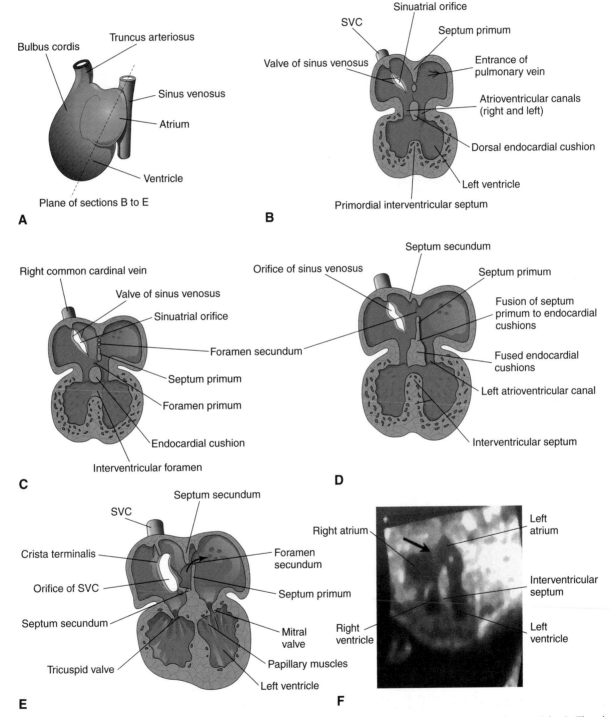

FIGURE 14-9. The developing heart, showing partitioning of the atrioventricular canal, the primordial atrium, and the ventricle. **A,** The plane of sections **B** to **E. B,** At the fourth week of development (approximately 28 days), showing the early appearance of the septum primum, the interventricular septum, and the dorsal endocardial cushion. **C,** Frontal section of the heart (approximately 32 days), showing perforations in the dorsal part of the septum primum. **D,** Frontal section of the heart (approximately 35 days), showing the foramen secundum. **E,** At approximately 8 weeks, the heart is partitioned into four chambers. The *arrow* indicates the flow of well-oxygenated blood from the right to the left atrium. **F,** Sonogram of a second-trimester fetus, showing the four chambers of the heart. Note the septum secundum *(arrow)* and the descending aorta. (**F,** Courtesy of Dr. G.J. Reid, Department of Obstetrics, Gynecology and Reproductive Sciences, University of Manitoba, Women's Hospital, Winnipeg, Manitoba, Canada.)

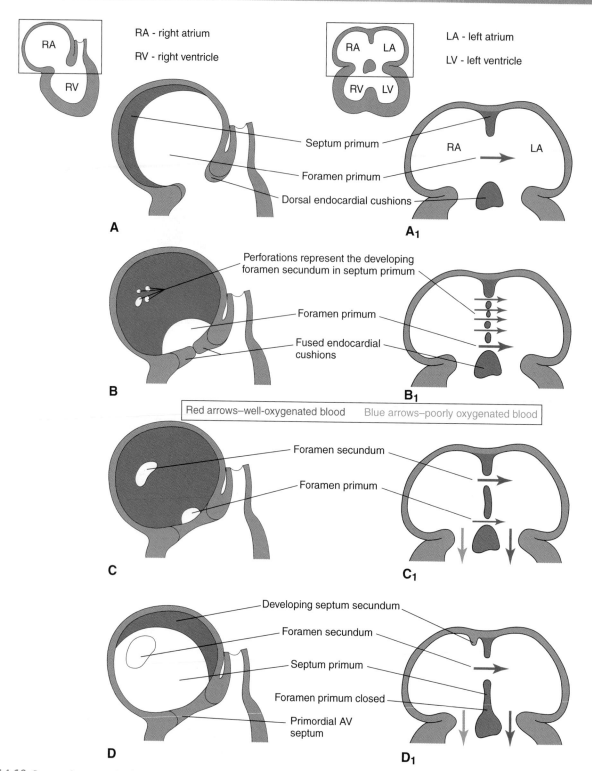

FIGURE 14-10. Progressive stages in the partitioning of the primordial atrium. **A** to **H,** Views of the developing interatrial septum, as viewed from the right side. **A₁** to **H₁,** Frontal sections of the developing interatrial septum. As the septum secundum grows, note that it overlaps the opening in the septum primum (foramen secundum). Observe the valve of the oval foramen in **G₁** and **H₁.** When pressure in the right atrium exceeds that in the left atrium, blood passes from the right to the left side of the heart. When the pressures are equal or higher in the left atrium, the valve formed by the septum primum closes the oval foramen.

left AV canals (Fig. 14-9B). These canals partially separate the primordial atrium from the ventricle, and the cushions function as AV valves. The **endocardial cushions** develop from a specialized matrix related to the myocardium. *Its formation is associated with the expression of transforming growth factor β2 and bone morphogenetic factors 2A and 4.*

Partitioning of the Primordial Atrium

The primordial atrium is divided into right and left atria by the formation and subsequent modification and fusion of two septa, the septum primum and the septum secundum (Figs. 14-9A to E and 14-10).

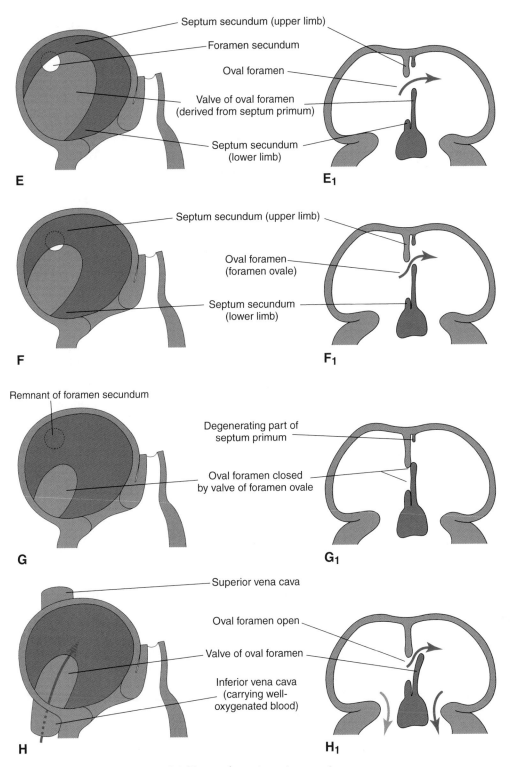

FIGURE 14-10. CONT'D For legend see previous page.

The **septum primum** grows toward the fusing endocardial cushions from the roof of the primordial atrium, partially dividing the atrium into right and left halves. As this curtain-like septum develops, a large opening—the **foramen primum**—forms between its free edge and the endocardial cushions (see Figs. 14-9C and 14-10A to C). The foramen allows shunting of oxygenated blood from the right to the left atrium. The foramen becomes progressively smaller and disappears as the septum primum fuses with the fused endocardial cushions to form the **primordial AV septum** (see Fig. 14-10D and D_1). Before the foramen primum disappears, perforations, produced by apoptosis, appear in the central part of the septum primum. As the septum fuses with the endocardial cushions, the perforations coalesce to form another opening—the **foramen secundum** (see Fig. 14-10*C*). Concurrently, the free edge of the septum primum fuses with the left side of the fused endocardial cushions, obliterating the foramen primum (see Figs. 14-9*D* and 14-10*D*). The foramen secundum ensures shunting of oxygenated blood from the right to the left atrium.

The **septum secundum** grows from the ventrocranial wall of the atrium, immediately to the right of the septum primum (see Fig. 14-10*D₁*). As this thick, crescentic, muscular septum grows during the fifth and sixth weeks, it gradually overlaps the foramen secundum in the septum primum (see Fig. 14-10*E* and *F*). The septum secundum forms an incomplete partition between the atria; the opening in the foramen secundum is called the **oval foramen** (Latin *foramen ovale*). The cranial part of the septum primum, initially attached to the roof of the left atrium, gradually disappears (see Fig. 14-10*G₁* and *H₁*). The remaining part of the septum primum, attached to the endocardial cushions, forms the **valve of the oval foramen**.

Before birth, the oval foramen allows most of the oxygenated blood entering the right atrium from the IVC to pass into the left atrium (see Fig. 14-10*H₁*). It also prevents the passage of blood in the opposite direction because the septum primum closes against the relatively rigid septum secundum (see Fig. 14-10*G₁*). *After birth*, the oval foramen functionally closes due to higher pressure in the left atrium, and the valve of the oval foramen fuses with the septum secundum, forming the oval fossa. As a result, the interatrial septum becomes a complete partition between the atria.

Changes in the Sinus Venosus

Initially, the sinus venosus opens into the posterior wall of the primordial atrium. By the end of the fourth week of development, the right sinual horn becomes larger than the left sinual horn (see Fig. 14-11*A* and *B*). As this occurs, the sinuatrial orifice moves to the right and opens in the part of the primordial atrium that will become the adult right atrium (Fig. 14-12*C*). As the right sinual horn enlarges, it receives all of the blood from the head and neck through the SVC, and from the placenta and the caudal regions of the body through the IVC.

The left sinual horn becomes the **coronary sinus**, and the right sinual horn is incorporated into the wall of the right atrium (see Fig. 14-11*B* and *C*).

The smooth part of the internal wall of the right atrium is called the **sinus venarum** (see Fig. 14-11*B* and *C*). The remainder of the anterior internal surface of the wall of the right atrium, as well as that of the **auricle**, has a rough, trabeculated appearance. These latter two parts are derived from the primordial atrium. The smooth part and the rough part are demarcated internally in the right atrium by a vertical ridge, termed the **crista terminalis**, or terminal crest (see Fig. 14-11*C*), and externally by a shallow groove, the **sulcus terminalis**, or terminal groove

(see Fig. 14-11*B*). The crista terminalis represents the cranial part of the right **sinuatrial valve** (see Fig. 14-11*C*); the caudal part of this valve forms the valves of the IVC and the coronary sinus. The left sinuatrial valve fuses with the septum secundum and is incorporated with it into the interatrial septum.

The Primordial Pulmonary Vein and Formation of the Left Atrium

Most of the wall of the left atrium is smooth because it is formed by the incorporation of the primordial pulmonary vein (see Fig. 14-12*A*). This vein develops as an outgrowth of the dorsal atrial wall, just to the left of the septum primum. As the atrium expands, the primordial pulmonary vein and its main branches are gradually incorporated into the wall of the left atrium (see Fig. 14-12*B*). As a result, four pulmonary veins are formed (see Fig. 14-12*C* and *D*). The small left auricle is derived from the primordial atrium; its internal surface has a rough, trabeculated appearance.

Partitioning of the Primordial Ventricle

Division of the primordial ventricle into two ventricles is first indicated by a median ridge—the **muscular interventricular (IV) septum**—in the floor of the ventricle, near its apex (see Fig. 14-9*B*). This thick, crescentic fold has a concave free edge (Fig. 14-13*A*). Initially, most of its increase in height results from dilation of the ventricles on each side of the muscular IV septum (see Fig. 14-13*B*). The medial walls of the ventricles approach each other and fuse to form the primordium of the *muscular part of the IV septum*. Until the seventh week, there is a crescent-shaped **IV foramen** between the free edge of the IV septum and the fused endocardial cushions (see Fig. 14-15*A* and *B*). The IV foramen permits communication between the right and left ventricles (Figs. 14-13*B* and 14-14*B*). The IV foramen usually closes by the end of the seventh week as the bulbar ridges fuse with the endocardial cushion (see Fig. 14-14*C* to *E*). **Closure of the IV foramen** and formation of the membranous part of the IV septum result from the fusion of tissues from three sources: the right bulbar ridge, the left bulbar ridge, and the endocardial cushion.

The **membranous part of the IV septum** is derived from an extension of tissue from the right side of the endocardial cushion to the muscular part of the IV septum. This tissue merges with the **aorticopulmonary septum** and the thick, muscular part of the IV septum (Fig. 14-15*D*). After closure of the IV foramen and formation of the membranous part of the IV septum, the pulmonary trunk communicates with the right ventricle and the aorta communicates with the left ventricle (see Fig. 14-14*E*). Cavitation of the ventricular walls forms a spongelike mass of muscular bundles. Some bundles remain as the **trabeculae carneae**. Other bundles become the **papillary muscles** and **tendinous cords** (Latin *chordae tendineae*). The tendinous cords run from the papillary muscles to the AV valves (see Fig. 14-15*D*).

■ Left horn of sinus venosus   ▢ Right horn of sinus venosus

A

Primordial atrium

Left anterior cardinal vein

Left common cardinal vein

Future superior vena cava

Right horn of sinus venosus

Site of opening of sinus venosus into right atrium

Left horn of sinus venosus

Inferior vena cava

B

Aorta

Pulmonary artery

Pulmonary veins

Oblique vein of left atrium

Coronary sinus

Superior vena cava

Sinus venarum of right atrium

Sulcus terminalis

Right auricle

Inferior vena cava

Middle cardiac vein

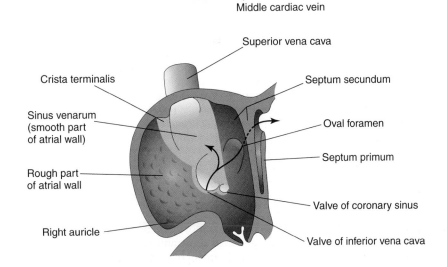

C

Crista terminalis

Sinus venarum (smooth part of atrial wall)

Rough part of atrial wall

Right auricle

Superior vena cava

Septum secundum

Oval foramen

Septum primum

Valve of coronary sinus

Valve of inferior vena cava

FIGURE 14-11. Illustrations of the fate of the sinus venosus. **A,** Dorsal view of the heart (approximately 26 days), showing the primordial atrium and the sinus venosus. **B,** Dorsal view at 8 weeks, after incorporation of the right sinual horn into the right atrium. The left sinual horn has become the coronary sinus. **C,** Internal view of the fetal right atrium, showing the smooth part of the wall of the right atrium (sinus venarum), derived from the right sinual horn, and the crista terminalis and the valves of the inferior vena cava and the coronary sinus, derived from the right sinuatrial valve. The primordial right atrium becomes the right auricle, a conical muscular pouch. *Arrows* indicate the flow of blood.

Partitioning of the Bulbus Cordis and Truncus Arteriosus

During the fifth week, active proliferation of the mesenchymal cells in the walls of the bulbus cordis results in the formation of **bulbar ridges** (Figs. 14-14C and D and 14-16B and C). Similar ridges form in the truncus arteriosus; these are continuous with the bulbar ridges. The bulbar and **truncal ridges** are derived mainly from the neural crest mesenchyme. **Neural crest cells** migrate through the primordial pharynx and the pharyngeal arches to reach the ridges. Bone morphogenetic protein and other signaling systems, such as Wnt and fibroblast growth factor, have been implicated in the induction and migration of neural crest cells. Concurrently, the bulbar and truncal ridges undergo 180-degree spiraling. The spiral orientation of the bulbar and truncal ridges, possibly caused in part by the streaming of blood from the ventricles, results in the formation of a spiral **aorticopulmonary septum** when the ridges fuse (see Fig. 14-16D to G). This septum divides

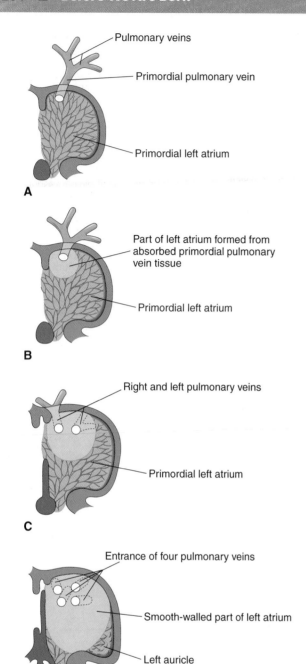

Pulmonary veins

Primordial pulmonary vein

Primordial left atrium

A

Part of left atrium formed from absorbed primordial pulmonary vein tissue

Primordial left atrium

B

Right and left pulmonary veins

Primordial left atrium

C

Entrance of four pulmonary veins

Smooth-walled part of left atrium

Left auricle

D

FIGURE 14-12. Illustrations of absorption of the pulmonary vein into the left atrium. **A,** At 5 weeks, showing the primordial pulmonary vein opening into the primordial left atrium. **B,** Later stage, showing partial absorption of the primordial pulmonary vein. **C,** At 6 weeks, showing the openings of two pulmonary veins into the left atrium as a result of absorption of the primordial pulmonary vein. **D,** At 8 weeks, showing four pulmonary veins with separate atrial orifices. The primordial left atrium becomes the left auricle, a tubular pouch of the atrium. Most of the left atrium is formed by absorption of the primordial pulmonary vein and its branches.

the bulbus cordis and the truncus arteriosus into two arterial channels, the **aorta** and the **pulmonary trunk**. Because of the spiraling of the aorticopulmonary septum, the pulmonary trunk twists around the ascending aorta (see Fig. 14-16*H*).

The **bulbus cordis** is incorporated into the walls of the definitive ventricles in several ways (see Fig. 14-14*A* and *B*):

- In the right ventricle, the bulbus cordis is represented by the **conus arteriosus** (infundibulum), which gives origin to the pulmonary trunk.
- In the left ventricle, the bulbus cordis forms the walls of the **aortic vestibule**, the part of the ventricular cavity just inferior to the aortic valve.

Development of the Cardiac Valves

The semilunar valves develop from three swellings of subendocardial tissue around the orifices of the aorta and pulmonary trunk (Fig. 14-17*B* to *F*). These swellings are hollowed out and reshaped to form three thin-walled cusps. The **AV valves** (tricuspid and mitral valves) develop similarly from localized proliferations of tissue around the AV canals.

Conducting System of the Heart

Initially, the muscle layers of the atrium and the ventricle are continuous. The primordial atrium acts as the interim pacemaker of the heart, but the sinus venosus soon takes over this function. The **sinuatrial node** develops during the fifth week. This node is located in the right atrium, near the entrance of the SVC (see Fig. 14-15*D*). After incorporation of the sinus venosus, cells from its left wall are found in the base of the interatrial septum, near the opening of the coronary sinus. Together with cells from the AV region, they form the **AV node and the AV bundle**, located just superior to the endocardial cushions. The fibers arising from the AV bundle pass from the atrium into the ventricle and split into right and left **bundle branches**, which are distributed throughout the ventricular myocardium (see Fig. 14-15*D*). The sinuatrial node, AV node, and AV bundle are richly supplied by nerves; however, the primordial conducting system is developed before these nerves enter the heart.

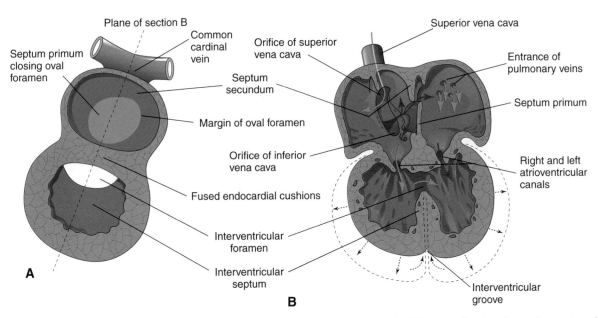

FIGURE 14-13. Illustrations of partitioning of the primordial heart. **A,** Sagittal section late in the fifth week, showing the cardiac septa and foramina. **B,** Frontal section at a slightly later stage, showing the directions of blood flow through the heart *(blue arrows)* and the expansion of the ventricles, indicated by the dotted arrows.

single mechanism is responsible for the sudden, unexpected deaths of apparently healthy infants. A *brain stem developmental abnormality* or maturational delay related to neuroregulation of cardiorespiratory control has been suggested.

■ ANOMALIES OF THE HEART AND GREAT VESSELS

Congenital heart defects (CHDs) occur with a frequency of 6 in 1000 to 8 in 1000 births. Some cases of CHD are caused by single-gene or chromosomal mechanisms; others result from exposure to teratogens, such as the *rubella virus.* Most CHDs are believed to be caused by multiple factors, both genetic and environmental (i.e., multifactorial inheritance). Recent technology, such as real-time, two-dimensional *echocardiography,* has permitted the detection of fetal CHDs as early as the 17th or 18th week of gestation.

DEXTROCARDIA

If the heart tube bends to the left instead of to the right, the heart is displaced to the right (Fig. 14-18) and there is transposition whereby the heart and its vessels are reversed, left to right, as in a mirror image. **Dextrocardia** is the most frequent positional abnormality of the heart. In **dextrocardia with situs inversus** (transposition of the abdominal viscera), the incidence of accompanying cardiac defects is low. In isolated dextrocardia, the abnormal position of the heart is not accompanied by displacement of other viscera. *Transforming growth factor β nodal is involved in looping of the heart tube.* Its role in dextrocardia is uncertain.

ECTOPIA CORDIS

In ectopia cordis, an extremely rare condition, the heart is located outside the thoracic cavity. The most common thoracic form of ectopia cordis results from faulty development of the sternum and pericardium secondary to incomplete fusion of the lateral folds in the formation of the thoracic wall during the fourth week. Death occurs in most cases during the first few days after birth, usually as a result of infection, cardiac failure, or hypoxemia. If no severe cardiac defects are present, surgical therapy usually consists of covering the heart with skin.

ATRIAL SEPTAL DEFECTS

Atrial septal defects (ASDs) occur more frequently in girls than in boys. The most common form of ASD is a patent oval foramen (Figs. 14-19A and 14-20A to D). A small, isolated **patent oval foramen** is of no hemodynamic significance. However, if other defects are present (e.g., pulmonary stenosis, atresia), blood is shunted through the oval foramen into the left atrium, producing **cyanosis**. A probe-patent oval foramen is present in up to 25% of people. In this abnormality, a probe can be passed from one atrium to the other through the superior part of the floor of the oval fossa; the defect is not clinically significant. A **probe patent oval foramen** results from incomplete adhesion between the flap of the valve of the oval foramen and the septum secundum after birth.

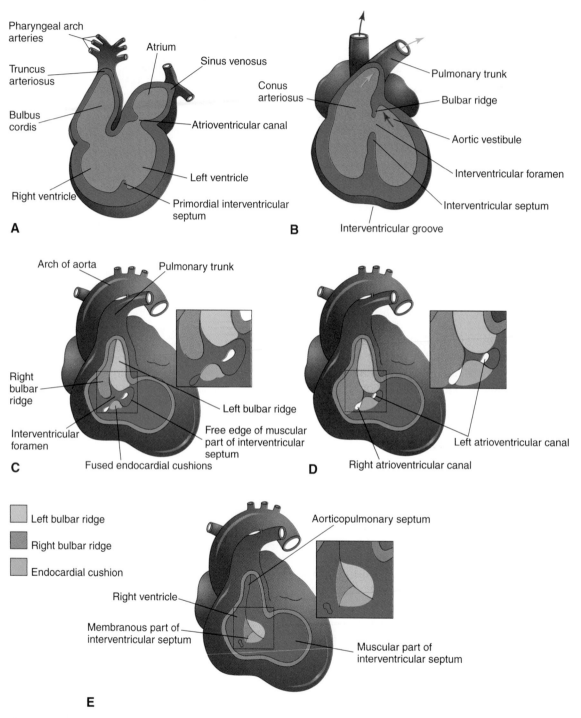

FIGURE 14-14. Illustrations of the incorporation of the bulbus cordis into the ventricles and partitioning of the bulbus cordis and the truncus arteriosus into the aorta and the pulmonary trunk. **A,** Sagittal section at 5 weeks, showing the bulbus cordis as one of the chambers of the primordial heart. **B,** Schematic coronal section at 6 weeks, after the bulbus cordis has been incorporated into the ventricles to become the conus arteriosus (infundibulum) of the right ventricle and the aortic vestibule of the left ventricle. The *arrows* indicate blood flow. **C** to **E,** Closure of the interventricular (IV) foramen and formation of the membranous part of the IV septum. The walls of the truncus arteriosus, the bulbus cordis, and the right ventricle have been removed. **C,** At 5 weeks, showing the bulbar ridges and fused endocardial cushions. **D,** At 6 weeks, showing how the proliferation of subendocardial tissue diminishes the IV foramen. **E,** At 7 weeks, showing the fused bulbar ridges, the membranous part of the IV septum formed by extensions of tissue from the right side of the endocardial cushions, and closure of the IV foramen.

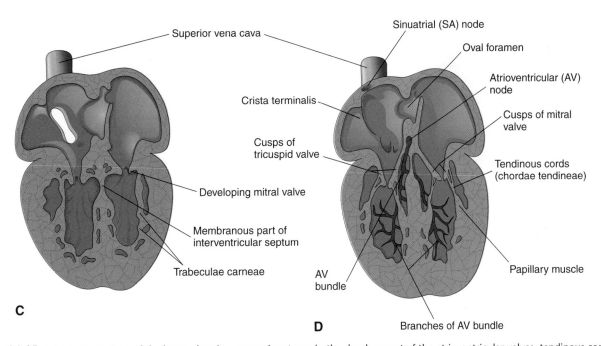

FIGURE 14-15. Schematic sections of the heart, showing successive stages in the development of the atrioventricular valves, tendinous cords (Latin *chordae tendineae*), and papillary muscles. **A,** At 5 weeks. **B,** At 6 weeks. **C,** At 7 weeks. **D,** At 20 weeks, showing the conducting system of the heart.

ATRIAL SEPTAL DEFECTS—CONT'D

There are four clinically significant types of ASD (see Fig. 14-20), of which the first two are relatively common:

- Ostium secundum defect
- Endocardial cushion defect with a foramen primum defect
- Sinus venosus defect
- Common atrium

Ostium secundum ASDs (see Fig. 14-20A to D) occur in the area of the oval fossa and include defects of both the septum primum and the septum secundum. Females with ASDs outnumber males 3 to 1. Ostium secundum ASDs are one of the most common, yet least severe types of CHD. The patent oval foramen usually results from abnormal resorption of the septum primum during the formation of the foramen secundum. If resorption occurs in abnormal locations, the septum primum is fenestrated, or netlike (see Fig. 14-20A). If

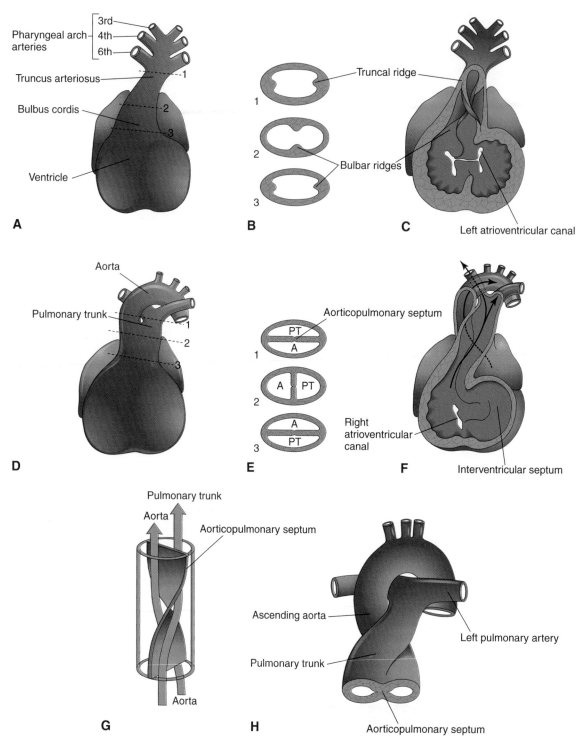

FIGURE 14-16. Partitioning of the bulbus cordis and the truncus arteriosus. **A,** Ventral aspect of the heart at 5 weeks. The *broken lines* and *arrows* indicate the levels of the sections shown in **B. B,** Transverse sections of the truncus arteriosus and the bulbus cordis, showing the truncal and bulbar ridges. **C,** The ventral wall of the heart and the truncus arteriosus has been removed to show these ridges. **D,** Ventral aspect of the heart after partitioning of the truncus arteriosus. The *broken lines* and *arrows* indicate the levels of the sections shown in **E. E,** Sections through the newly formed aorta (A) and the pulmonary trunk (PT) show the aorticopulmonary septum. **F,** At 6 weeks. The ventral wall of the heart and the pulmonary trunk has been removed to show the aorticopulmonary septum. **G,** The spiral form of the aorticopulmonary septum. **H,** The great arteries (ascending aorta and pulmonary trunk) twisting around each other as they leave the heart.

FIGURE 14-17. Development of the semilunar valves of the aorta and the pulmonary trunk. **A,** Section of the truncus arteriosus and the bulbus cordis, showing the valve swellings. **B,** Transverse section of the bulbus cordis. **C,** Similar section after fusion of the bulbar ridges. **D,** Formation of the walls and valves of the aorta and the pulmonary trunk. **E,** Rotation of the vessels has established the adult positions of the valves in relation to each other. **F** and **G,** Longitudinal sections of the aorticoventricular junction, showing successive stages in the hollowing *(arrows)* and thinning of the valve swellings to form the valve cusps. L, left; P, posterior; R, right.

ATRIAL SEPTAL DEFECTS—CONT'D

excessive resorption of the septum primum occurs, the resulting short septum primum does not close the oval foramen (see Fig. 14-20*B*). If an abnormally large oval foramen develops as a result of defective development of the septum secundum, a normal septum primum does not close the abnormal oval foramen at birth (see Fig. 14-20*C*). Large ostium secundum ASDs may also occur because of a combination of excessive resorption

of the septum primum and a large oval foramen (see Fig. 14-20*D*).

Endocardial cushion defects with a patent foramen primum (see Fig. 14-20*E*) are less common forms of ASD. The septum primum does not fuse with the endocardial cushions, resulting in a patent foramen primum. Usually, there is also a cleft in the anterior cusp of the mitral valve.

Sinus venosus ASDs are located in the superior part of the interatrial septum, close to the entry of the SVC (see Fig. 14-20F). These defects result from incomplete absorption of the sinus venosus into the right atrium, abnormal development of the septum secundum, or both. **Common atrium** occurs in patients with all three types of defects: ostium secundum, ostium primum, and sinus venosus.

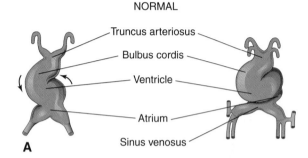

NORMAL

Truncus arteriosus
Bulbus cordis
Ventricle
Atrium
Sinus venosus

A

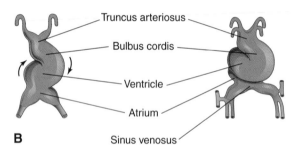

DEXTROCARDIA

Truncus arteriosus
Bulbus cordis
Ventricle
Atrium
Sinus venosus

B

FIGURE 14-18. The primordial heart during the fourth week. **A,** Normal bending to the right *(arrows).* **B,** Abnormal bending to the left *(arrows).*

VENTRICULAR SEPTAL DEFECTS

Ventricular septal defects (VSDs) are the *most common type of CHD*, accounting for approximately 25% of cases. VSDs occur more frequently in males than in females. *Most VSDs involve the membranous part of the IV septum* (Fig. 14-21B). Many small VSDs close spontaneously, usually during the first year of life. Most people with a large VSD have massive left to right shunting of blood. *Muscular VSD is a less common type of defect that may appear anywhere in the muscular part of the IV septum.* **Transposition of the great arteries** (Fig. 14-22) and a rudimentary outlet chamber are present in most infants with this severe type of CHD.

PERSISTENT TRUNCUS ARTERIOSUS

Persistent truncus arteriosus results from failure of the truncal ridges and the aorticopulmonary septum to develop normally and to divide the truncus arteriosus into the aorta and the pulmonary trunk (see Fig. 14-21). The most common type of persistent truncus arteriosus is a **single arterial** trunk that branches to form the pulmonary trunk and the ascending aorta (see Fig. 14-21A and B). In this anomaly, a single arterial trunk, the truncus arteriosus, arises from the heart and supplies the systemic, pulmonary, and coronary circulations. A VSD is always present with truncus arteriosus, and the truncus arteriosus straddles the VSD (see Fig. 14-21B).

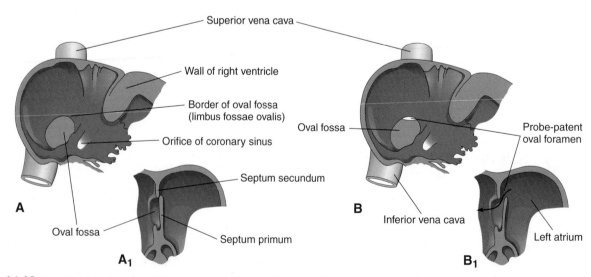

FIGURE 14-19. **A,** Normal postnatal appearance of the right side of the interatrial septum after adhesion of the septum primum to the septum secundum. **A₁,** Section of the interatrial septum, showing the formation of the oval fossa in the interatrial septum. Note that the floor of this fossa is formed by the septum primum. **B** and **B₁,** Similar views of a probe-patent oval foramen resulting from incomplete adhesion of the septum primum to the septum secundum.

FIGURE 14-20. Illustrations of the right aspect of the interatrial septum. The adjacent sketches of sections of the septa show various types of atrial septal defects (ASDs). **A,** Patent oval foramen resulting from resorption of the septum primum in abnormal locations. **B,** Patent oval foramen caused by excessive resorption of the septum primum ("short flap defect"). **C,** Patent oval foramen resulting from an abnormally large oval foramen. **D,** Patent oval foramen resulting from an abnormally large oval foramen and excessive resorption of the septum primum. **E,** Endocardial cushion defect with a primum-type ASD. The adjacent section shows the cleft in the anterior cusp of the mitral valve. **F,** Sinus venosus ASD. The high septal defect resulted from abnormal absorption of the sinus venosus into the right atrium. In **E** and **F**, note that the oval fossa has formed normally. *Arrows* indicate the direction of flow of blood.

TRANSPOSITION OF THE GREAT ARTERIES

Transposition of the great arteries is the most common cause of cyanotic heart disease in newborn infants (see Fig. 14-22). In typical cases, the aorta lies anterior and to the right of the pulmonary trunk and arises anteriorly from the morphologic right ventricle, whereas the pulmonary trunk arises from the morphologic left ventricle. There is also an ASD, with or without an associated patent ductus arteriosus (PDA) and VSD.

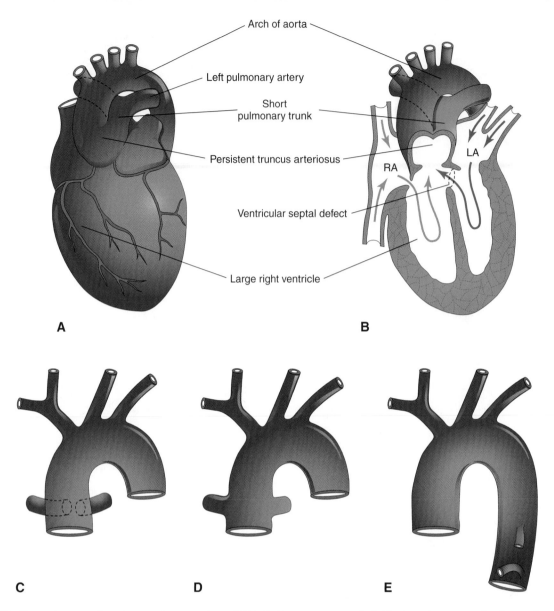

FIGURE 14-21. The main types of persistent truncus arteriosus (PTA). **A,** The common trunk divides into the aorta and a short pulmonary trunk. **B,** Frontal section of the heart shown in **A**. Observe the circulation in this heart *(arrows)* and the VSD. **C,** The right and left pulmonary arteries arise close together from the truncus arteriosus. **D,** The pulmonary arteries arise independently from the sides of the truncus arteriosus. **E,** No pulmonary arteries are present. LA, Left atrium; RA, right atrium.

TRANSPOSITION OF THE GREAT ARTERIES—CONT'D

This defect is believed to result from failure of the conus arteriosus to develop normally during incorporation of the bulbus cordis into the ventricles. Defective neural crest cell migration may also be involved.

UNEQUAL DIVISION OF THE TRUNCUS ARTERIOSUS

Unequal division of the truncus arteriosus (Figs. 14-21 and 14-23A and B) results when partitioning of the truncus arteriosus superior to the valves is disparate, producing one large great artery and one small one. As a result, the aorticopulmonary septum is not aligned with the IV septum, and a VSD results. The larger vessel (aorta or pulmonary trunk) usually straddles the VSD (see Fig. 14-23A and B). In **pulmonary valve stenosis**, the cusps of the pulmonary valve are fused together to form a dome with a narrow central opening (Fig. 14-24). In **infundibular stenosis**, the conus arteriosus of the right ventricle is underdeveloped. The two types of pulmonary stenosis may be concurrent. Depending on the degree of obstruction to blood flow, there is a variable degree of hypertrophy of the right ventricle (see Fig. 14-23B).

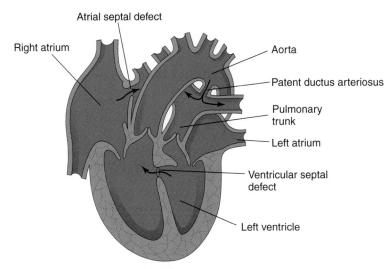

Atrial septal defect
Right atrium
Aorta
Patent ductus arteriosus
Pulmonary trunk
Left atrium
Ventricular septal defect
Left ventricle

FIGURE 14-22. Frontal section of a malformed heart, showing transposition of the great arteries. The ventricular septal defect (VSD) and the atrial septal defect (ASD) allow mixing of the arterial and venous blood. Transposition of the great arteries is the most common single cause of cyanotic heart disease in newborn infants. As is shown here, it is often associated with other cardiac anomalies (VSD and ASD). The *arrows* indicate the flow of blood. For example, when there is an ASD, blood flows from the right atrium to the left atrium.

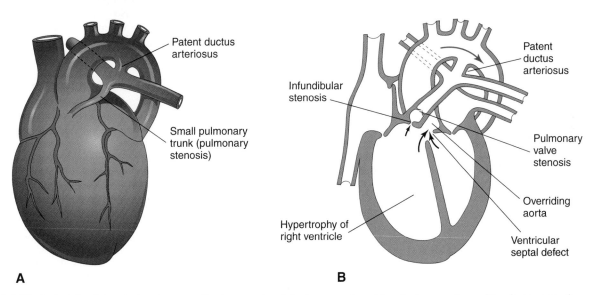

Patent ductus arteriosus
Small pulmonary trunk (pulmonary stenosis)

Infundibular stenosis
Patent ductus arteriosus
Pulmonary valve stenosis
Overriding aorta
Hypertrophy of right ventricle
Ventricular septal defect

A

B

FIGURE 14-23. **A,** An infant's heart, showing a small pulmonary trunk (pulmonary stenosis) and a large aorta resulting from unequal partitioning of the truncus arteriosus. There is also hypertrophy of the right ventricle and a patent ductus arteriosus. **B,** Frontal section of a heart, showing tetralogy of Fallot. Observe the four cardiac defects of this tetralogy: pulmonary valve stenosis, ventricular septal defect, overriding aorta, and hypertrophy of the right ventricle. In this case, infundibular stenosis is also shown. The *arrows* indicate the flow of blood into the great vessels (aorta and pulmonary trunk).

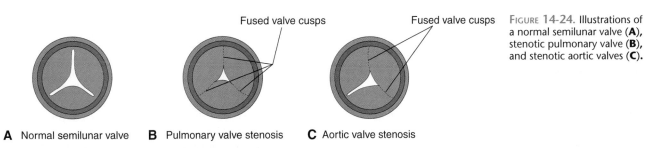

Fused valve cusps
Fused valve cusps

A Normal semilunar valve **B** Pulmonary valve stenosis **C** Aortic valve stenosis

FIGURE 14-24. Illustrations of a normal semilunar valve (**A**), stenotic pulmonary valve (**B**), and stenotic aortic valves (**C**).

TETRALOGY OF FALLOT

The classic group of four cardiac defects known as *tetralogy of Fallot* (see Fig. 14-23A and B) consists of the following:
- Pulmonary stenosis (obstructed right ventricular outflow)
- Ventricular septal defect
- Dextroposition of the aorta (straddling or overriding the aorta)
- Right ventricular hypertrophy

The pulmonary trunk is usually small, and there may be varying degrees of pulmonary artery stenosis as well.

■ DERIVATIVES OF THE PHARYNGEAL ARCH ARTERIES

As the pharyngeal arches develop during the fourth week, they are supplied by **pharyngeal arch arteries** that arise from the *aortic sac* (Fig. 14-25B). The pharyngeal arch arteries terminate in the dorsal aorta on the ipsilateral side. Although six pairs of pharyngeal arch arteries usually develop, they are not all present at the same time (see Fig. 14-6).

Derivatives of the First Pair of Pharyngeal Arch Arteries

The first pair of arteries largely disappears, but remnants of them form parts of the **maxillary arteries**, which supply the ears, teeth, muscles of the eyes and face, and parts of the **external carotid arteries**.

Derivatives of the Second Pair of Pharyngeal Arch Arteries

Dorsal parts of the second pair of pharyngeal arch arteries persist and form the stems of the small **stapedial arteries**, which run through the ring of the stapes.

Derivatives of the Third Pair of Pharyngeal Arch Arteries

Proximal parts of the third pair of pharyngeal arch arteries form the **common carotid arteries**, which supply structures in the head (Fig. 14-26D). Distal parts of the third pair of pharyngeal arch arteries join with the dorsal aortas to form the **internal carotid arteries**, and they supply the ears, the orbits, and the brain and its meninges.

Derivatives of the Fourth Pair of Pharyngeal Arch Arteries

The **left fourth pharyngeal arch artery** forms part of the arch of the aorta (Fig. 14-26C and D). The proximal part of the arch develops from the aortic sac, whereas the distal part is derived from the left dorsal aorta. The **right fourth pharyngeal arch artery** becomes the proximal part of the **right subclavian artery**. The distal part of the subclavian artery forms from the right dorsal aorta and the right seventh intersegmental artery. The left subclavian artery is not derived from a pharyngeal arch artery; it forms from the left seventh intersegmental artery (see Fig. 14-26A). As development proceeds, differential growth shifts the origin of the left subclavian artery cranially. Consequently, it comes to lie close to the origin of the left common carotid artery (see Fig. 14-26D).

Fate of the Fifth Pair of Pharyngeal Arch Arteries

In approximately 50% of embryos, the fifth pair of pharyngeal arch arteries comprises rudimentary vessels that soon degenerate, leaving no vascular derivatives. In other embryos, these arches do not develop.

Derivatives of the Sixth Pair of Pharyngeal Arch Arteries

The **left sixth pharyngeal arch artery** develops as follows (see Fig. 14-26B and C):
● The proximal part of the artery persists as the proximal part of the **left pulmonary artery**.
● The distal part of the artery passes from the left pulmonary artery to the dorsal aorta and forms a prenatal shunt, the **ductus arteriosus**.

The **right sixth pharyngeal arch artery** develops as follows:
● The proximal part of the artery persists as the proximal part of the **right pulmonary artery**.
● The distal part of the artery degenerates.

The transformation of the sixth pair of pharyngeal arch arteries explains why the course of the **recurrent laryngeal nerves** differs on the two sides. These nerves supply the sixth pair of pharyngeal arches and hook around the sixth pair of pharyngeal arch arteries on their way to the developing larynx (Fig. 14-27A). *On the right*, because the distal part of the right sixth pharyngeal arch artery degenerates, the right recurrent laryngeal nerve moves superiorly and hooks around the proximal part of the right subclavian artery, the derivative of the fourth pharyngeal arch artery (see Fig. 14-27B). *On the left*, the left recurrent laryngeal nerve hooks around the ductus arteriosus formed by the distal part of the sixth pharyngeal arch artery. When this arterial shunt involutes after birth, the nerve remains around the **ligamentum arteriosum** (remnant of the ductus arteriosus) and the arch of the aorta (Fig. 14-28C).

■ PHARYNGEAL ARCH ARTERY ANOMALIES

Because of the many changes involved in the transformation of the embryonic pharyngeal arch system of arteries

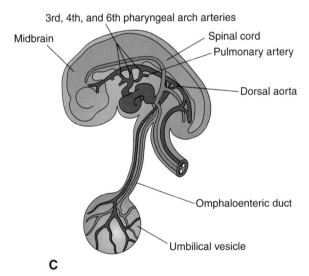

FIGURE 14-25. The pharyngeal arches and pharyngeal arch arteries. **A,** Left side of an embryo (approximately 26 days). **B,** Illustration of this embryo, showing the left pharyngeal arch arteries arising from the aortic sac, running through the pharyngeal arches, and terminating in the left dorsal aorta. **C,** An embryo (approximately 37 days). Note the single dorsal aorta and the mostly degenerated first two pairs of pharyngeal arch arteries.

COARCTATION OF THE AORTA

Aortic coarctation (constriction) occurs in approximately 10% of children and adults with CHDs. Coarctation is characterized by a constriction of the aorta of varying length (see Fig. 14-28). Most constrictions occur distal to the origin of the left subclavian artery, at the entrance of the ductus arteriosus (**juxtaductal coarctation**). A classification system of preductal and postductal coarctations is commonly used; however, in most cases, the coarctation is directly opposite the ductus arteriosus. Coarctation of the aorta occurs twice as often in males as in females. Coarctation of the aorta is caused by genetic factors, environmental factors, or both.

DOUBLE PHARYNGEAL ARCH ARTERY

Double pharyngeal arch artery is a rare anomaly that is characterized by a *vascular ring around the trachea and the esophagus* (Fig. 14-29). The vascular ring results from failure of the distal part of the right dorsal aorta to disappear (see Fig. 14-29A); as a result, right and left arches form. Usually, the right arch of the aorta is the larger one and it passes posterior to the trachea and the esophagus (see Fig. 14-29B).

RIGHT ARCH OF THE AORTA

When the entire right dorsal aorta persists (Fig. 14-30A) and the distal part of the left dorsal aorta involutes, a right pharyngeal arch artery results. There are two main types:
- *Right arch of the aorta without a retroesophageal component* (see Fig. 14-30B). The ductus arteriosus (or ligamentum arteriosum) passes from the right pulmonary artery to the right arch of the aorta.
- *Right arch of the aorta with a retroesophageal component* (see Fig. 14-30C). Originally, a small left arch of the aorta probably involuted, leaving the right arch of the aorta posterior to the esophagus. The ductus arteriosus (or ligamentum arteriosum) attaches to the distal part of the arch of the aorta and forms a ring that may constrict the esophagus and the trachea.

ANOMALOUS RIGHT SUBCLAVIAN ARTERY

The right subclavian artery arises from the distal part of the arch of the aorta and passes posterior to the trachea and the esophagus to supply the right upper limb (Fig. 14-31). A **retroesophageal right subclavian**

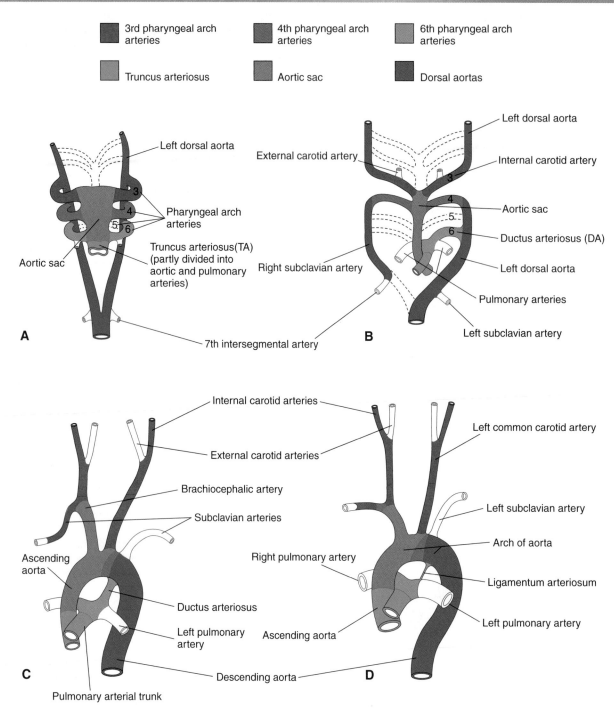

3rd pharyngeal arch arteries   **4th pharyngeal arch arteries**   **6th pharyngeal arch arteries**

Truncus arteriosus   **Aortic sac**   **Dorsal aortas**

FIGURE 14-26. Illustration of the arterial changes that occur during transformation of the truncus arteriosus, aortic sac, pharyngeal arch arteries, and dorsal aortas into the adult arterial pattern. The vessels that are not colored are not derived from these structures. **A,** Pharyngeal arch arteries at 6 weeks. By this stage, the first two pairs of pharyngeal arch arteries have largely disappeared. **B,** Pharyngeal arch arteries at 7 weeks. The parts of the dorsal aortas and pharyngeal arch arteries that normally disappear are indicated with *broken lines.* **C,** Arterial arrangement at 8 weeks. **D,** Arterial vessels of a 6-month-old infant. Note that the ascending aorta and the pulmonary arteries are considerably smaller in **C** than in **D**. This represents the relative flow through these vessels at the different stages of development. Observe the large size of the ductus arteriosus in **C**; it is essentially a direct continuation of the pulmonary trunk. The ductus arteriosus normally becomes functionally closed within the first few days after birth. Eventually, the ductus arteriosus becomes the ligamentum arteriosum, as shown in **D**.

ANOMALOUS RIGHT SUBCLAVIAN ARTERY—CONT'D

artery occurs when the right fourth pharyngeal arch artery and the right dorsal aorta disappear cranial to the seventh intersegmental artery. As a result, the right subclavian artery forms from the right seventh intersegmental artery and the distal part of the right dorsal aorta. As development proceeds, differential growth shifts the origin of the right subclavian artery cranially, until it comes to lie close to the origin of the left subclavian artery.

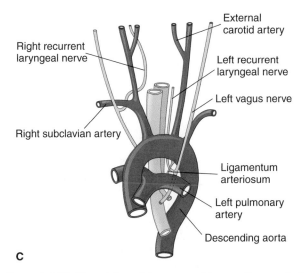

FIGURE 14-27. The relation of the recurrent laryngeal nerves to the pharyngeal arch arteries. **A,** At 6 weeks, showing that the recurrent laryngeal nerves are hooked around the sixth pair of pharyngeal arch arteries. **B,** At 8 weeks, showing that the right recurrent laryngeal nerve is hooked around the right subclavian artery and the left recurrent laryngeal nerve is hooked around the ductus arteriosus and the arch of the aorta. **C,** In a child, the left recurrent laryngeal nerve is hooked around the ligamentum arteriosum and the arch of the aorta.

into the adult arterial pattern, it is understandable why anomalies may occur. Most irregularities result from the persistence of parts of the pharyngeal arch arteries that usually disappear, or from the disappearance of parts that normally persist.

■ FETAL AND NEONATAL CIRCULATION

The fetal circulation (Fig. 14-32) is designed to serve prenatal needs and to permit modifications at birth that establish the neonatal pattern (Fig. 14-33). Prenatally, the lungs do not provide gas exchange and the pulmonary vessels are vasoconstricted. Three shunts are essential in the transitional circulation: the ductus venosus, oval foramen, and ductus arteriosus.

Fetal Circulation

Highly oxygenated, nutrient-rich blood returns from the placenta in the **umbilical vein** (see Fig. 14-32). On approaching the liver, approximately one half of the blood under high pressure passes directly into the **ductus venosus,** a fetal vessel connecting the umbilical vein to the IVC; consequently, the blood bypasses the liver. The other half of the blood in the umbilical vein flows into the sinusoids of the liver and enters the IVC through the **hepatic veins.** Blood flow through the ductus venosus is regulated by a sphincter mechanism close to the umbilical vein. After a short course in the IVC, all of the blood enters the right atrium of the heart. Most blood from the IVC is directed by the inferior border of the septum secundum (**crista dividens**), through the **oval foramen,** and into the left atrium. There, it mixes with the relatively small amount of poorly oxygenated blood returning from the lungs through the pulmonary veins. Fetal lungs use the oxygen from the blood instead of replenishing it. From the left atrium, the blood then passes to the left ventricle and leaves through the ascending aorta.

The arteries to the heart, head, neck, and upper limbs receive well-oxygenated blood. The liver also receives well-oxygenated blood from the umbilical vein. The small amount of well-oxygenated blood from the IVC that remains in the right atrium mixes with poorly oxygenated blood from the SVC and the coronary sinus and passes into the right ventricle. This blood, with medium oxygen content, leaves through the pulmonary trunk. Approximately 10% of the blood goes to the lungs, but most of it passes through the ductus arteriosus into the aorta to the fetal body. It then returns to the placenta through the umbilical arteries (see Fig. 14-32). Because of the high pulmonary vascular resistance in fetal life, pulmonary blood flow is low. Approximately 10% of blood from the ascending aorta enters the descending aorta to supply the viscera and the inferior part of the body. Most of the blood in the descending aorta passes into the umbilical arteries and is returned to the placenta for reoxygenation.

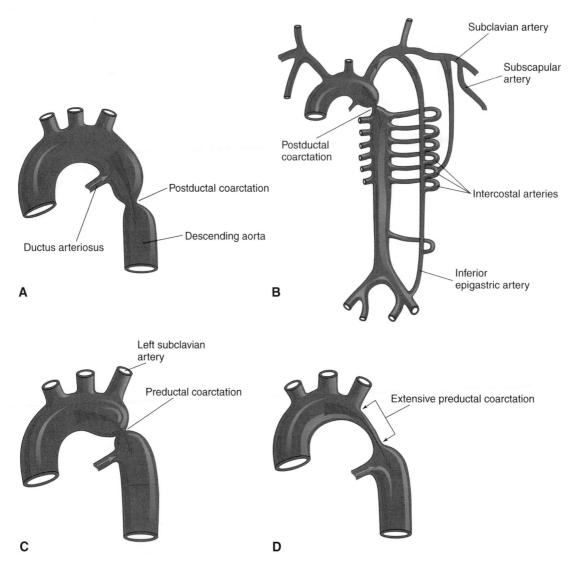

FIGURE 14-28. **A,** Postductal coarctation of the aorta. **B,** Common routes of the collateral circulation that develop in association with postductal coarctation of the aorta. **C** and **D,** Preductal coarctation. *Arrows* indicate flow of blood.

Transitional Neonatal Circulation

Important circulatory adjustments occur at birth, when the circulation of fetal blood through the placenta ceases and the infant's lungs expand and begin to function (see Fig. 14-33). *As soon as the infant is born, the oval foramen, ductus arteriosus, ductus venosus, and umbilical vessels are no longer needed.* The sphincter in the ductus arteriosus constricts, and all blood entering the liver passes through the hepatic sinusoids. Occlusion of the placental circulation causes an immediate decrease in blood pressure in the IVC and the right atrium.

Because of increased pulmonary blood flow, the pressure in the left atrium is higher than in the right atrium. The **increased left atrial pressure closes the oval foramen** by pressing the valve of the foramen against the septum secundum (see Fig. 14-33). The output from the right ventricle then flows entirely into the pulmonary circulation. Because pulmonary vascular resistance is lower than systemic vascular resistance, blood flow in the ductus arteriosus reverses, passing from the aorta to the pulmonary trunk.

The **ductus arteriosus constricts at birth**, but for a few days, there is often a small shunt of blood from the aorta to the pulmonary trunk in healthy, full-term infants. In premature infants and those with persistent hypoxia, the ductus arteriosus may remain open much longer. In full-term infants, oxygen is the most important factor in controlling closure of the ductus arteriosus, and it appears to be mediated by bradykinin and *prostaglandins.*

The **umbilical arteries constrict at birth**, preventing loss of the infant's blood. The umbilical cord is not tied for a minute or so; consequently, blood flow through the umbilical vein continues, transferring fetal blood from the placenta to the infant. *The change from the fetal to the adult pattern of blood circulation is not a sudden occurrence.* Some changes occur with the first breath; others take place over hours and days. During the transitional stage, right to left flow may occur through the oval foramen. The closure of fetal vessels and the oval foramen is

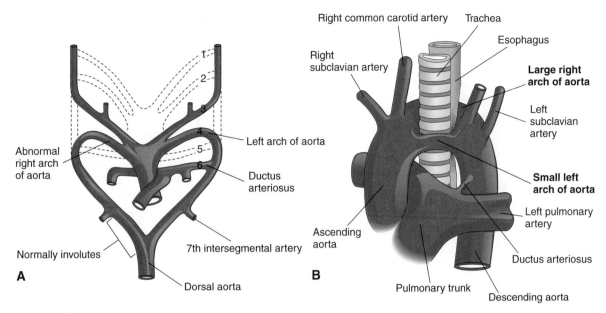

FIGURE 14-29. A, Embryonic pharyngeal arch arteries, showing the embryologic basis of a double arch of the aorta. The distal portion of the right dorsal aorta persists and forms a right pharyngeal arch artery. **B,** A large right arch of the aorta and a small left arch of the aorta arise from the ascending aorta and form a vascular ring around the trachea and the esophagus. Note the compression of the esophagus and the trachea. The right common carotid and subclavian arteries arise separately from the large right arch of the aorta.

initially a functional change. Later, anatomic closure results from the proliferation of endothelial and fibrous tissues.

Derivatives of Fetal Vascular Structures

Because of the changes in the cardiovascular system at birth, certain vessels and structures are no longer required postnatally.

Umbilical Vein and Round Ligament of the Liver

The intra-abdominal part of the *umbilical vein* eventually becomes the *round ligament of the liver* (Latin *ligamentum teres*) (see Fig. 14-33). The umbilical vein remains patent for a considerable period and may be used for blood transfusions during early infancy. These transfusions are often performed to prevent brain damage and death in infants with anemia as a result of erythroblastosis fetalis.

Ductus Venosus and Ligamentum Venosum

The ductus venosus becomes the *ligamentum venosum*; however, its closure is more prolonged than that of the ductus arteriosus. The ligamentum venosum passes through the liver from the left branch of the portal vein to the IVC, to which it is attached (Fig. 14-34).

Umbilical Arteries and Abdominal Ligaments

Most of the intra-abdominal parts of the umbilical arteries become the **medial umbilical ligaments** (see Fig. 14-33); the proximal parts of these vessels persist as the **superior vesical arteries**, which supply the urinary bladder.

Oval Foramen and Oval Fossa

The oval foramen normally closes functionally at birth. Anatomic closure occurs by the third month and results from tissue proliferation and adhesion of the septum primum to the left margin of the septum secundum. The septum primum forms the floor of the oval fossa. The inferior edge of the septum secundum forms a rounded fold, the border of the oval fossa (Latin *limbus fossae ovalis*), which marks the former boundary of the oval foramen (see Fig. 14-19).

Ductus Arteriosus and Ligamentum Arteriosum

Functional closure of the ductus arteriosus is usually completed 10 to 15 hours after birth. Anatomic closure of the ductus arteriosus and formation of the ligamentum arteriosum usually occurs by the 12th postnatal week.

■ DEVELOPMENT OF THE LYMPHATIC SYSTEM

The lymphatic system begins to develop at the end of the sixth week. Lymphatic vessels develop in a manner similar to that described for blood vessels, and they make connections with the venous system. The early lymphatic capillaries join each other to form a network of lymphatics. **Six primary lymph sacs** exist at the end of the embryonic period (Fig. 14-35A):

● Two *jugular lymph sacs* near the junction of the subclavian veins with the anterior cardinal veins (the future internal jugular veins)
● Two *iliac lymph sacs* near the junction of the iliac veins with the posterior cardinal veins
● One *retroperitoneal lymph sac* in the root of the mesentery on the posterior abdominal wall

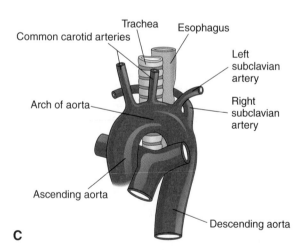

FIGURE 14-30. **A,** Pharyngeal arch arteries showing abnormal involution of the distal portion of the left dorsal aorta. There is also persistence of the entire right dorsal aorta and the distal part of the right sixth pharyngeal arch artery. **B,** Right pharyngeal arch artery without a retroesophageal component. **C,** Right arch of the aorta with a retroesophageal component. The abnormal right arch of the aorta and the ligamentum arteriosum (postnatal remnant of the ductus arteriosus) form a vascular ring that compresses the esophagus and the trachea.

FIGURE 14-31. The possible embryologic basis for an abnormal origin of the right subclavian artery. **A,** The right fourth pharyngeal arch artery and the cranial part of the right dorsal aorta have involuted. As a result, the right subclavian artery forms from the right seventh intersegmental artery and the distal segment of the right dorsal aorta. **B,** As the arch of the aorta forms, the right subclavian artery is carried cranially *(arrows)* with the left subclavian artery. **C,** The abnormal right subclavian artery arises from the aorta and passes posterior to the trachea and the esophagus.

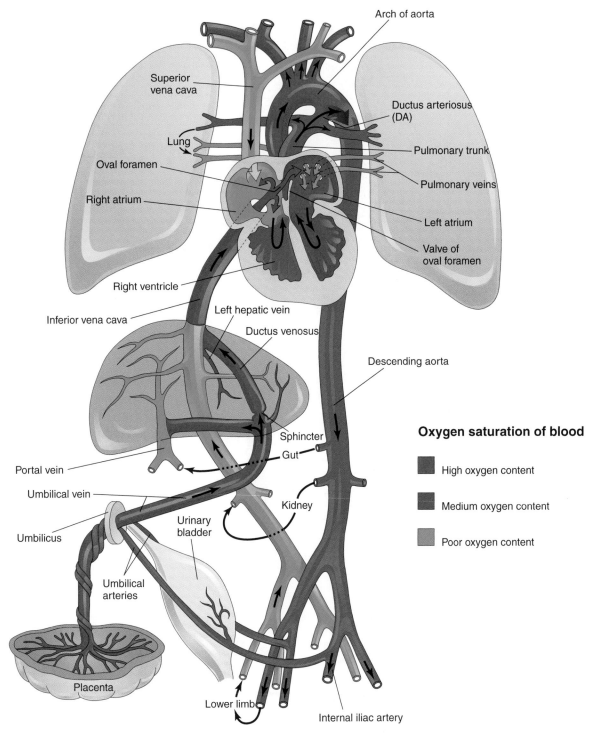

FIGURE 14-32. Fetal circulation. The colors indicate the oxygen saturation of the blood, and the *arrows* show the course of the blood from the placenta to the heart. The organs are not drawn to scale. Observe that three shunts permit most of the blood to bypass the liver and lungs: (1) the ductus venosus, (2) the oval foramen, and (3) the ductus arteriosus. The poorly oxygenated blood returns to the placenta for oxygen and nutrients through the umbilical arteries.

● One *chyle cistern* (Latin *cisterna chyli*) located dorsal to the retroperitoneal lymph sac

Lymphatic vessels soon join the lymph sacs and accompany main veins (1) to the head, neck, and upper limbs from the jugular lymph sacs; (2) to the lower trunk and lower limbs from the iliac lymph sacs; and (3) to the primordial gut from the retroperitoneal lymph sac and the **chyle cistern**. Two large channels (right and left thoracic ducts) connect the jugular lymph sacs with the chyle cistern. Soon, a large anastomosis forms between

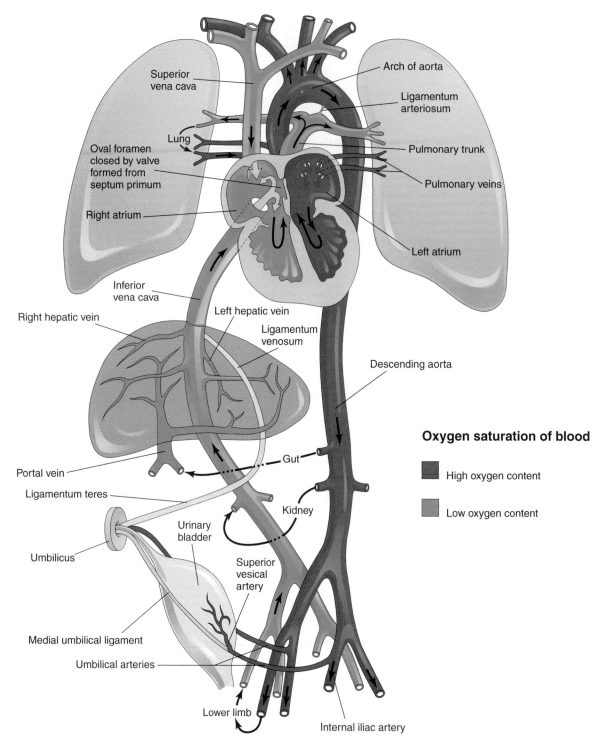

FIGURE 14-33. Neonatal circulation. The adult derivatives of the fetal vessels and structures that become nonfunctional at birth are shown. The *arrows* indicate the course of the blood in the infant. The organs are not drawn to scale. After birth, the three shunts that short-circuited the blood during fetal life cease to function, and the pulmonary and systemic circulations become separated.

these channels (see Fig. 14-35B). The **thoracic duct** develops from:

● The caudal part of the right thoracic duct
● The anastomosis between the thoracic ducts and the cranial part of the left thoracic duct

The **right lymphatic duct** is derived from the cranial part of the right thoracic duct (see Fig. 14-35C). The thoracic duct and the right lymphatic duct connect with the venous system at the venous angle between the internal jugular vein and the subclavian vein.

FIGURE 14-34. Closure of the ductus arteriosus. **A,** The ductus arteriosus of a newborn infant. **B,** Abnormal patent ductus arteriosus in a 6-month-old infant. **C,** The ligamentum arteriosum in a 6-month-old infant.

PATENT DUCTUS ARTERIOSUS

A common anomaly, PDA occurs two to three times more frequently in females than in males (see Fig. 14-34*B*). Functional closure of the ductus arteriosus usually occurs soon after birth; however, if it remains patent, aortic blood is shunted into the pulmonary artery. PDA is the most common congenital anomaly associated with maternal rubella infection during early pregnancy. *Premature infants and infants born at high altitude may also have a PDA; the patency is the result of hypoxia and immaturity.* The embryologic basis of PDA is failure of the ductus arteriosus to involute after birth and form the ligamentum arteriosum. Failure of contraction of the muscular wall of the ductus arteriosus after birth is the primary cause of patency.

ANOMALIES OF THE LYMPHATIC SYSTEM

Congenital anomalies of the lymphatic system are uncommon. There may be diffuse swelling of a part of the body, termed **congenital lymphedema**. This condition may result from dilation of the primordial lymphatic channels or from congenital hypoplasia of the lymphatic vessels. **Cystic hygromas** are large swellings that usually appear in the inferolateral part of the neck and consist of large, single or multilocular, fluid-filled cavities. Hygromas may be present at birth, but they often enlarge and become evident during later infancy. Hygromas are believed to arise from parts of a jugular lymph sac that are pinched off, or from lymphatic spaces that do not establish connections with the main lymphatic channels.

Development of the Lymph Nodes

Except for the superior part of the chyle cistern, the lymph sacs are transformed into groups of lymph nodes during the early fetal period. Mesenchymal cells invade each lymph sac and form a network of lymphatic channels, the primordia of the *lymph sinuses*. Other mesenchymal cells give rise to the capsules and the connective tissue framework of the lymph nodes. The lymphocytes are derived originally from primordial stem cells in the umbilical vesicle mesenchyme and later from the liver and spleen. The lymphocytes eventually enter the bone marrow, where they divide to form *lymphoblasts*. The lymphocytes that appear in the lymph nodes before birth are derived from the thymus, a derivative of the third pair of pharyngeal pouches (see Chapter 10). Small lymphocytes leave the *thymus* and circulate to other lymphoid organs. Later, some mesenchymal cells in the lymph nodes differentiate into lymphocytes.

Development of the Spleen and Tonsils

The spleen develops from an aggregation of mesenchymal cells in the dorsal mesentery of the stomach (see Chapter 12). The **palatine tonsils** develop primarily from the second pair of pharyngeal pouches and the nearby mesenchyme. The tubal tonsils develop from aggregations of lymph nodules around the pharyngeal openings of the pharyngotympanic (auditory) tubes. The **pharyngeal tonsils** (adenoids) develop from an aggregation of lymph nodules in the wall of the nasopharynx. The **lingual tonsil** develops from an aggregation of lymph nodules in the root of the tongue. Lymph nodules also develop in the mucosa of the respiratory and digestive systems.

A

Internal jugular vein

Jugular lymph sac

Inferior vena cava

Retroperitoneal lymph sac

Chyle cistern (cisterna chyli)

Iliac vein

Iliac lymph sac

FIGURE 14-35. Development of the lymphatic system. **A,** Left side of an 7½-week embryo, showing the primary lymph sacs. **B,** Ventral view of the lymphatic system at 9 weeks, showing the paired thoracic ducts. **C,** Later in the fetal period, showing formation of the thoracic duct and the right lymphatic duct.

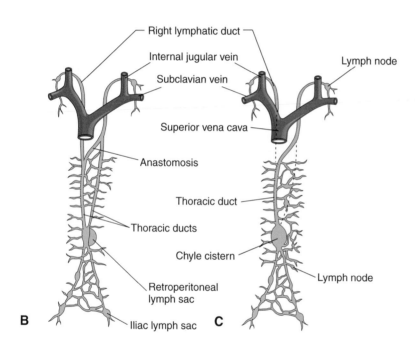

Right lymphatic duct

Internal jugular vein

Lymph node

Subclavian vein

Superior vena cava

Anastomosis

Thoracic duct

Thoracic ducts

Chyle cistern

Lymph node

Retroperitoneal lymph sac

B Iliac lymph sac **C**

CLINICALLY ORIENTED QUESTIONS

1. A pediatrician diagnosed a heart murmur in a newborn infant. What does this mean? What causes this condition, and what does it indicate?

2. Are congenital anomalies of the heart common? What is the most common congenital heart defect in children?

3. What are the causes of congenital anomalies of the cardiovascular system? Can drugs taken by the mother during pregnancy cause congenital cardiac defects? One mother who drank heavily during her pregnancy had a child with a heart defect. Could her drinking have caused her infant's heart defect?

4. Can viral infections cause congenital heart disease? Is it true that if a mother has measles during pregnancy, her infant will have an abnormality of the cardiovascular system? Is it true that women can be given a vaccine that will protect their infants against certain viruses?

5. An infant had its aorta arising from the right ventricle and its pulmonary artery arising from the left ventricle. The infant died during the first week. What is this anomaly called, and how common is this disorder? Can the condition be corrected surgically? If so, how is this done?

6. During a routine examination of identical twin sisters in their forties, it was found that one of them had a reversed heart. Is this a serious heart anomaly? How common is this among identical twins, and what causes this condition to develop?

The answers to these questions are at the back of the book.

THE MUSCULOSKELETAL SYSTEM

■ SKELETAL SYSTEM

As the notochord and the neural tube form, the *intra-embryonic mesoderm* lateral to these structures thickens to form two longitudinal columns of **paraxial mesoderm** (Fig. 15-1*A* and *B*). Toward the end of the third week, these dorsolateral columns located in the trunk become segmented into blocks—the **somites** (see Fig. 15-1*C*). Each somite differentiates into two parts (see Fig. 15-1*D* and *E*):

● The ventromedial part is the **sclerotome**; its cells form the vertebrae and the ribs.

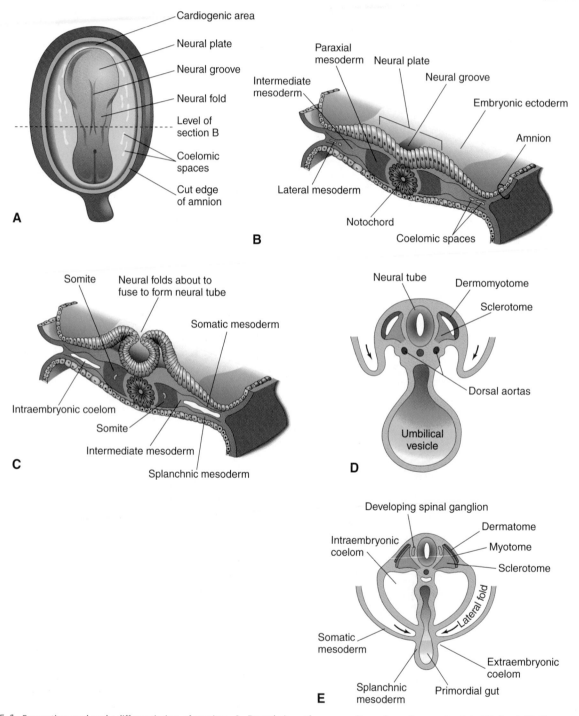

FIGURE 15-1. Formation and early differentiation of somites. **A,** Dorsal view of a presomite embryo (approximately 18 days). **B,** Transverse section of the embryo shown in **A,** illustrating the paraxial mesoderm from which the somites are derived. **C,** Transverse section of an embryo at approximately 22 days, at which time early somites have appeared. **D,** Transverse section of an embryo at approximately 24 days. Note the folding of the embryo in the horizontal plane *(arrows)*. The dermomyotome region of the somite gives rise to the dermatome and myotome. **E,** Transverse section of an embryo at approximately 26 days, showing the dermatome, myotome, and sclerotome regions of the somite. The *arrows* in **D** and **E** indicate movement of the lateral body folds.

- The dorsolateral part is the **dermomyotome;** cells from its *myotome region* form myoblasts (primordial muscle cells), whereas those from its *dermatome* region form the dermis (fibroblasts).

Mesodermal cells give rise to loosely organized embryonic connective tissue called the *mesenchyme*. Most mesenchyme in the head region is derived from the neural crests and forms the bones and connective tissue of the craniofacial structures. *Homeobox (Hox) genes* play an essential role in the migration and subsequent differentiation of the neural crest cells.

■ DEVELOPMENT OF BONE AND CARTILAGE

Most flat bones develop in the mesenchyme within pre-existing membranous sheaths; this type of osteogenesis is called **intramembranous bone formation.** Mesenchymal models of most limb bones are transformed into cartilaginous bone models, which later become ossified by **endochondral bone formation.** Bone morphogenetic proteins 5 and 7 and growth and differentiation factor 5, members of the tumor growth factor-β superfamily, as well as other signaling molecules, have been implicated as endogenous regulators of chondrogenesis and skeletal development.

Histogenesis of Cartilage

Cartilage develops from the mesenchyme and first appears in embryos during the fifth week. In areas where cartilage is to develop, the mesenchyme condenses to form **chondrification centers.** The mesenchymal cells differentiate into **chondroblasts,** which secrete collagenous fibrils and the extracellular matrix. Subsequently, collagenous fibers, elastic fibers, or both are deposited in the intercellular substance, or matrix. *Three types of cartilage* are distinguishable according to the type of matrix that is formed:

- *Hyaline cartilage,* the most widely distributed type (e.g., in joints)
- *Fibrocartilage* (e.g., in the intervertebral discs)
- *Elastic cartilage* (e.g., in the auricle of the ear)

Histogenesis of Bone

Bone develops primarily in two types of connective tissue—the mesenchyme and the cartilage—but it can also develop in other connective tissues. Like cartilage, bone consists of cells and an organic intercellular substance, called **bone matrix,** which comprises collagen fibrils embedded in an amorphous component.

Studies of the cellular and molecular events that occur during embryonic bone formation suggest that osteogenesis and chondrogenesis are programmed early in development and are independent events under the influence of vascular events.

Intramembranous Ossification

The mesenchyme condenses and becomes highly vascular; some cells differentiate into **osteoblasts** (bone-forming

FIGURE 15-2. Light micrograph of intramembranous ossification (×132). The trabeculae of the bone are being formed by osteoblasts lining their surface *(arrows).* Observe that osteocytes are trapped in the lacunae *(arrowheads)* and that primordial osteons are beginning to form. The osteons (canals) contain blood capillaries. (From Gartner LP, Hiatt JL: Color Textbook of Histology, 2nd ed. Philadelphia, WB Saunders, 2001.)

cells) and begin to deposit unmineralized matrix—osteoid (Fig. 15-2). Calcium phosphate is then deposited in the **osteoid tissue** as it is organized into bone. Bone osteoblasts are trapped in the matrix and become **osteocytes.** Spicules of bone soon become organized and coalesce into lamellae (layers). Concentric lamellae develop around the blood vessels, forming haversian systems. Some osteoblasts remain at the periphery of the bone and continue to lay down layers, forming plates of compact bone on the surfaces. Between the surface plates, the intervening bone remains spiculated, or spongy. This spongy environment is somewhat accentuated by the action of **osteoclasts,** which reabsorb bone. In the interstices of the spongy bone, the mesenchyme differentiates into **bone marrow.** During fetal and postnatal life, continuous remodeling of bone occurs by the coordinated action of osteoclasts and osteoblasts.

Endochondral Ossification

Endochondral intracartilaginous ossification is a type of bone formation that occurs in pre-existing cartilaginous models (Fig. 15-3A to E). In a long bone, the **primary center of ossification** appears in the **diaphysis**—the part of the bone between its ends—which forms the **shaft** of the bone (see Fig. 15-3B). Here, the cartilage cells hypertrophy, the matrix becomes calcified, and the cells die. Concurrently, a thin layer of bone is deposited under the **perichondrium** surrounding the diaphysis; thus, the perichondrium becomes the **periosteum** (see Fig. 15-3A and B). Invasion of the vascular connective tissue by the blood vessels

Cartilage Model of Bone

Cartilage Calcified cartilage Bone Arteries

A
- Enlarged area
- Mesenchymal cell
- Perichondrium
- Chondroblast
- Cartilage matrix

B
- Diaphysial (primary) center of ossification
- Periosteal capillary
- Uncalcified hyaline cartilage
- Calcified hyaline cartilage
- Chondrocyte
- Periosteum
- Subperiosteal bone

C
- Epiphysial (secondary) center of ossification
- Epiphysial artery
- Epiphysis
- Diaphysis
- Epiphysis

D
- Nutrient artery
- Epiphysial center of ossification

Intracartilaginous Ossification

E
- Epiphyseal artery
- Epiphysial cartilage plate
- Metaphysial artery
- Medullary cavity of long bone
- Nutrient artery

FIGURE 15-3. **A** to **E**, Schematic longitudinal sections, showing endochondral (intracartilaginous) ossification in a developing long bone.

surrounding the periosteum breaks up the cartilage. Some invading cells differentiate into **hemopoietic cells**, which are responsible for the formation of blood cells in the bone marrow. This process continues toward the **epiphyses**, or ends of the bone. The spicules of bone are remodeled by the action of osteoclasts and osteoblasts. *Lengthening of the long bones occurs at the diaphysial-epiphysial junction.* The

lengthening of bone depends on the **epiphysial cartilage plates** (growth plates), whose chondrocytes proliferate and participate in endochondral bone formation (see Fig. 15-3*D* and *E*). Toward the diaphysis, the cartilage cells hypertrophy and the matrix becomes calcified. Spicules are isolated from each other by vascular invasion from the marrow or **medullary cavity**. Bone is deposited on

RICKETS

Rickets is a disease that occurs in children with vitamin D deficiency. This vitamin is required for calcium absorption by the intestine. The resulting calcium deficiency causes disturbances in ossification of the epiphysial cartilage plates and orientation of cells at the metaphysis. The limbs are shortened and deformed, with severe bowing of the bones.

these spicules by osteoblasts; resorption of this bone keeps the spongy bone masses relatively constant in length and enlarges the medullary cavity.

Ossification of the limb bones makes demands on the maternal supply of calcium and phosphorus beginning at approximately 8 weeks. At birth, the diaphyses are largely ossified, but most of the ends of the bone, or epiphyses, are still cartilaginous. Most **secondary ossification centers** appear in the epiphyses during the first few years after birth. The epiphysial cartilage cells hypertrophy, and there is invasion by vascular connective tissue. Ossification spreads radially. The articular cartilage and the **epiphysial cartilage plate** remain cartilaginous. On completion of growth, this plate is replaced by spongy bone, the epiphyses and the diaphysis are united, and no further elongation of the bone occurs. In most bones, the epiphyses have fused with the diaphysis by approximately 20 years of age. Growth in the diameter of a bone results from deposition of bone at the periosteum and from resorption on the medullary surface. The rate of deposition and resorption is balanced to regulate the thickness of the compact bone and the size of the medullary cavity. The internal reorganization of bone continues throughout life.

■ DEVELOPMENT OF THE JOINTS

Joints begin to develop with the appearance of the **interzonal mesenchyme** during the sixth week (Fig. 15-4A), and they resemble adult joints by the end of the eighth week.

Fibrous Joints

During the development of fibrous joints, the interzonal mesenchyme between the developing bones differentiates into dense fibrous tissue (see Fig. 15-4D). The sutures of the cranium are an example of fibrous joints.

Cartilaginous Joints

During the development of cartilaginous joints, the interzonal mesenchyme between the developing bones differentiates into **hyaline cartilage** (e.g., the costochondral joints) or **fibrocartilage** (see Fig. 15-4C) (e.g., the pubic symphysis).

FIGURE 15-4. Development of joints during the sixth and seventh embryonic weeks. **A,** Condensed mesenchyme continues across the gap, or interzone, between the developing bones, enclosing some interzonal mesenchyme between them. This primordial joint may differentiate into a synovial joint (**B**), a cartilaginous joint (**C**), or a fibrous joint (**D**).

Synovial Joints

During the development of the synovial joints (e.g., the knee joint), the interzonal mesenchyme between the developing bones differentiates as follows (see Fig. 15-4B):
● Peripherally, it forms the capsular and other ligaments.
● Centrally, it disappears, and the resulting space becomes the joint (synovial) cavity.
● Where it lines the joint capsule and the articular surfaces, it forms the synovial membrane, which secretes the synovial fluid.

■ DEVELOPMENT OF THE AXIAL SKELETON

The axial skeleton is composed of the cranium (skull), the vertebral column, the ribs, and the sternum. During the fourth week, cells in the sclerotomes surround the neural tube (primordium of the spinal cord) and the notochord, the structure around which the primordia of the vertebrae develop. This positional change of the sclerotomal cells is effected by differential growth of the surrounding structures, not by the migration of sclerotomal cells.

Development of the Vertebral Column

During the precartilaginous stage, mesenchymal cells from the sclerotomes are found in three main areas (Fig. 15-5*A*):
● Around the notochord
● Surrounding the neural tube
● In the body wall

In a frontal section of a 4-week embryo, the **sclerotomes** appear as paired condensations of mesenchymal cells around the notochord (see Fig. 15-5*B*). Each sclerotome consists of loosely arranged cells cranially and densely packed cells caudally. Some densely packed cells move cranially, opposite the center of the myotome, where they form the **intervertebral (IV) disc** (see Fig. 15-5*C* and *D*). These cells express *Pax-1*, a paired box gene. The remaining densely packed cells fuse with the loosely arranged cells of the immediately caudal sclerotome to form the mesenchymal **centrum**, the primordium of the body of a vertebra. Thus, each centrum develops from two adjacent sclerotomes and becomes an intersegmental structure. The nerves now lie in close relationship to the IV discs, and the intersegmental arteries lie on each side of the vertebral bodies. In the thorax, the dorsal **intersegmental arteries** become the **intercostal arteries**. *Recent studies suggest that the development of the vertebral column is regulated by homeobox (Hox) and paired box (Pax) genes.*

Where it is surrounded by the developing vertebral bodies, the **notochord** degenerates and disappears. Between the vertebrae, the notochord expands to form the gelatinous center of the IV disc, the **nucleus pulposus** (see Fig. 15-5*D*). This nucleus is later surrounded by circularly arranged fibers that form the **anulus fibrosus**. The nucleus pulposus and the anulus fibrosus together constitute the IV disc. The mesenchymal cells that surround the neural tube form the **neural arch**, the primordium of the vertebral arch (Figs. 15-5*C* and 15-6*D*). The mesenchymal cells in the body wall form the **costal processes**, which form the ribs in the thoracic region.

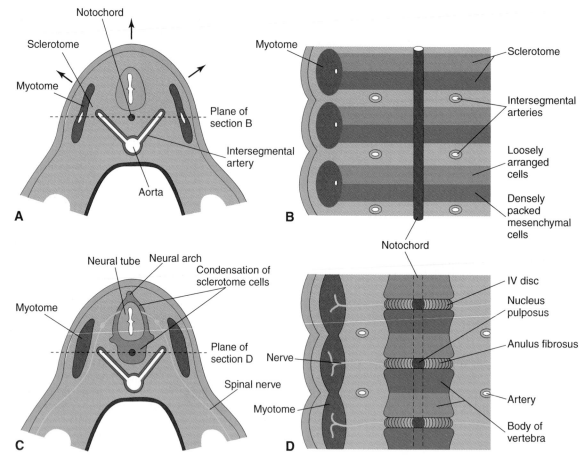

FIGURE 15-5. **A,** Transverse section through a 4-week embryo. The *arrows* indicate the dorsal growth of the neural tube and the simultaneous dorsolateral movement of the somite remnant, which leaves behind a trail of sclerotomal cells. **B,** Frontal section of the same embryo as in **A,** showing that the condensation of sclerotomal cells around the notochord consists of a cranial area of loosely packed cells and a caudal area of densely packed cells. **C,** Transverse section through a 5-week embryo. Note the condensation of sclerotomal cells around the notochord and the neural tube, which forms a mesenchymal vertebra. **D,** Frontal section, showing that the vertebral body forms from the cranial and caudal halves of two successive sclerotomal masses. The intersegmental arteries now cross the bodies of the vertebrae, and the spinal nerves lie between the vertebrae. The notochord is degenerating, except in the region of the intervertebral disc, where it forms the nucleus pulposus.

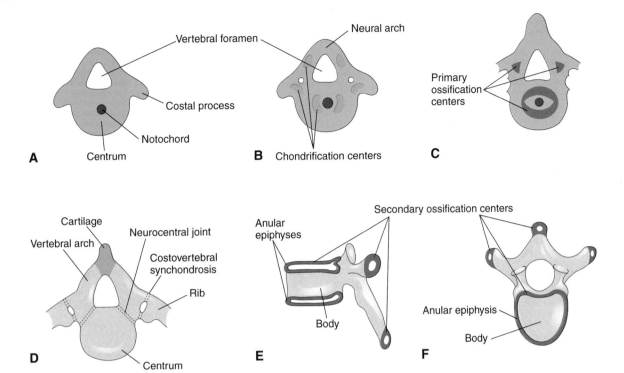

FIGURE 15-6. Stages of vertebral development. **A,** Mesenchymal vertebra at 5 weeks. **B,** Chondrification centers in a mesenchymal vertebra at 6 weeks. The neural arch is the primordium of the vertebral arch. **C,** Primary ossification centers in a cartilaginous vertebra at 7 weeks. **D,** Thoracic vertebra, consisting of three bony parts, at birth. Note the cartilage between the halves of the vertebral arch and between the arch and the centrum (neurocentral joint). **E** and **F,** Two views of a typical thoracic vertebra at puberty, showing the location of the secondary centers of ossification.

CHORDOMA

Remnants of the notochord may persist and give rise to a chordoma. Approximately one third of these slowly growing, malignant tumors involve the base of the cranium and extend to the nasopharynx. Chordomas infiltrate bone and are difficult to remove; few patients survive longer than 5 years. Chordomas may also develop in the lumbosacral region.

Cartilaginous Stage of Vertebral Development

During the sixth week, chondrification centers appear in each mesenchymal vertebra (see Fig. 15-6A and B). At the end of the embryonic period, the two centers in each centrum fuse to form a cartilaginous centrum. Concomitantly, the centers in the neural arches fuse with each other and the centrum. The spinous and transverse processes develop from extensions of chondrification centers in the vertebral arch. Chondrification spreads until a cartilaginous vertebral column is formed.

Bony Stage of Vertebral Development

Ossification begins during the embryonic period. There are two **primary ossification centers**—ventral and dorsal (see Fig. 15-6C), which soon fuse to form one center. Primary

centers are also present by the end of the embryonic period in each half of the vertebral arch.

Ossification becomes evident in the neural arches during the eighth week. At birth, each vertebra consists of three bony parts connected by cartilage (see Fig. 15-6D). The bony halves of the **vertebral arch** usually fuse during the first 3 to 5 years of life. The arches first unite in the lumbar region, and union progresses cranially. The vertebral arch articulates with the **centrum** at cartilaginous **neurocentral joints**. These articulations permit the vertebral arches to grow as the spinal cord enlarges. These joints disappear when the vertebral arch fuses with the centrum during the third to sixth years. Five **secondary ossification centers** appear in the vertebrae after puberty:

- One at the tip of the spinous process
- One at the tip of each transverse process
- Two *anular epiphyses*, one on the superior rim and one on the inferior rim of the vertebral body (see Fig. 15-6E and F)

The **vertebral body** is a composite of the anular epiphyses and the mass of bone between them. All secondary centers unite with the rest of the vertebrae at approximately 25 years of age. Variations in the ossification of vertebrae occur in C_1 (atlas), C_2 (axis), and C_7 vertebrae, and in the lumbar vertebrae, the sacrum, and the coccyx.

Development of the Ribs

The ribs develop from the mesenchymal **costal processes** of the thoracic vertebrae (see Fig. 15-6A). They become cartilaginous during the embryonic period and ossify during the fetal period. The original site of union of the costal processes with the vertebrae is replaced by **costovertebral synovial joints** (see Fig. 15-6D). Seven pairs of ribs (**true ribs**) attach by their own cartilages to the sternum. Five pairs of ribs (**false ribs**) attach to the sternum through the cartilage of another rib or ribs. The last two pairs of ribs (**floating ribs**) do not attach to the sternum.

Development of the Sternum

A pair of vertical mesenchymal bands, called **sternal bars**, develop ventrolaterally in the body wall. Chondrification occurs in these bars as they move medially. They *fuse craniocaudally in the median plane* to form cartilaginous models of the manubrium, sternebrae (segments of the sternal body), and xiphoid process. Fusion at the inferior end of the sternum is sometimes incomplete; as a result, the xiphoid process in these infants is bifid or perforated. Centers of ossification appear craniocaudally in the sternum before birth, except the ossification center for the xiphoid process, which appears during childhood.

Development of the Cranium

The cranium develops from the mesenchyme around the developing brain. The cranium consists of:
● The **neurocranium**, a protective case for the brain
● The **viscerocranium**, the skeleton of the face

Cartilaginous Neurocranium

Endochondral ossification of the **chondrocranium** forms the bones of the base of the cranium. The ossification pattern of these bones has a definite sequence, beginning with the occipital bone, the body of the sphenoid, and the ethmoid bone. The **parachordal cartilage**, or basal plate, forms around the cranial end of the notochord (Fig. 15-7A) and fuses with the cartilages derived from the sclerotome regions of the occipital somites. This cartilaginous mass contributes to the **base of the occipital bone;** later, extensions grow around the cranial end of the spinal cord and form the boundaries of the foramen magnum (see Fig. 15-7C). The **hypophysial cartilage** forms around the developing pituitary gland and fuses to form the body of the sphenoid bone (see Fig. 15-7B). The trabeculae cranii fuse to form the body of the ethmoid bone, and the ala orbitalis forms the lesser wing of the sphenoid bone. **Otic**

capsules develop around the otic vesicles, the primordia of the internal ears (see Chapter 18), and form the petrous and mastoid parts of the temporal bone. **Nasal capsules** develop around the nasal sacs (see Chapter 10) and contribute to the formation of the ethmoid bone.

Membranous Neurocranium

Intramembranous ossification occurs in the mesenchyme at the sides and top of the brain, forming the **calvaria** (cranial vault). During fetal life, the flat bones of the calvaria are separated by dense connective tissue membranes that form fibrous joints, the **sutures** (Fig. 15-8). Six large fibrous areas—known as the **fontanelles**—are present where several sutures meet. The softness of the bones and their loose connections at the sutures enable the calvaria to undergo changes of shape (**molding of the fetal cranium**) during birth. The frontal bones become flat, the occipital bone is drawn out, and one parietal bone slightly overrides the other one. Within a few days after birth, the shape of the calvaria returns to normal.

Cartilaginous Viscerocranium

The cartilaginous viscerocranium is derived from the cartilaginous skeleton of the first two pairs of pharyngeal arches (see Chapter 10).
● The dorsal end of the *first pharyngeal arch cartilage* forms the malleus and the incus.
● The dorsal end of the *second pharyngeal arch cartilage* forms the stapes and the styloid process of the temporal bone. Its ventral end ossifies to form the lesser horn and the superior part of the body of the hyoid bone.
● The *third, fourth, and sixth pharyngeal arch cartilages* form only in the ventral parts of the arches. The third pharyngeal arch cartilages give rise to the greater horns and the inferior part of the body of the hyoid bone.
● The *fourth and sixth pharyngeal arch cartilages* fuse to form the laryngeal cartilages, except for the epiglottis.

Membranous Viscerocranium

Intramembranous ossification occurs in the maxillary prominence of the first pharyngeal arch (see Chapter 10) and subsequently forms the squamous temporal, maxillary, and zygomatic bones. The squamous temporal bones become part of the neurocranium. The mandibular prominence forms the mandible. Some endochondral ossification occurs in the median plane of the chin and in the mandibular condyle.

Newborn Cranium

The cranium of a neonate is large in proportion to the rest of the skeleton, and the face is relatively small compared with the calvaria. The small facial region of the cranium is the result of several factors:
● The small size of the jaws
● The virtual absence of paranasal (air) sinuses
● Underdevelopment of the facial bones

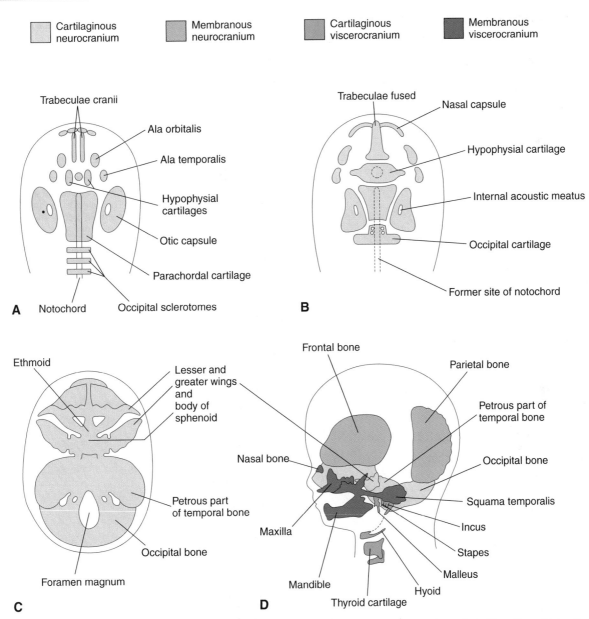

Cartilaginous neurocranium

Membranous neurocranium

Cartilaginous viscerocranium

Membranous viscerocranium

FIGURE 15-7. Stages in the development of the cranium. The base of the developing cranium, viewed superiorly (**A** to **C**), and laterally (**D**). **A,** At 6 weeks, showing the various cartilages that will fuse to form the chondrocranium. **B,** At 7 weeks, after fusion of some of the paired cartilages. **C,** At 12 weeks, showing the cartilaginous base of the cranium, or chondrocranium, formed by the fusion of various cartilages. **D,** At 20 weeks, indicating the derivation of the bones of the fetal cranium.

Postnatal Growth of the Cranium

The fibrous sutures permit the brain and the calvaria (roof of the cranium) to enlarge during infancy and childhood. The increase in size is greatest during the first 2 years of life, but the calvaria continues to expand to conform to brain growth until approximately 16 years, after which its size usually increases slightly for 3 to 4 years because of thickening of its bones.

There is also rapid growth of the face and jaws, coinciding with eruption of the primary (deciduous) teeth. These facial changes are more marked after the secondary (permanent) teeth erupt (see Chapter 18). There is concurrent enlargement of the frontal and facial regions, associated with the increase in the size of the paranasal sinuses. Growth of these sinuses is important in adding resonance to the voice.

KLIPPEL-FEIL SYNDROME (BREVICOLLIS)

The main features of *Klippel-Feil syndrome* are a short neck, a low hairline, and restricted neck movements. In most cases, the number of cervical vertebral bodies is fewer than normal. In some cases, there is a lack of segmentation of several elements of the cervical region of the vertebral column. The number of cervical nerve roots may be normal, but they are small, as are the intervertebral foramina. Persons with this syndrome are often otherwise normal, but the association of this anomaly with other congenital anomalies is not uncommon.

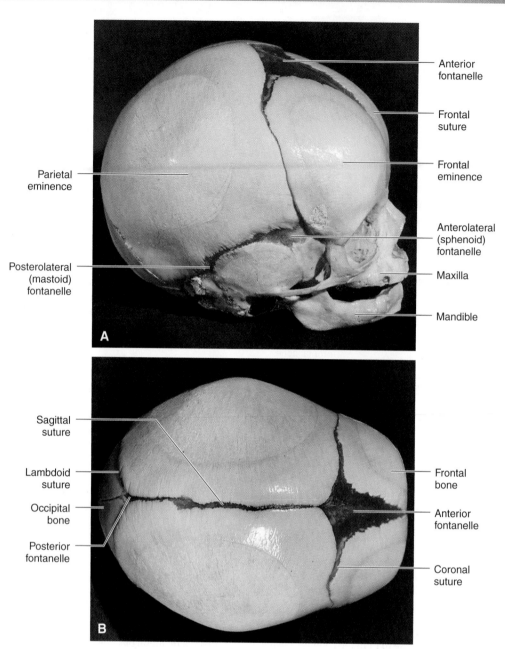

Parietal eminence

Posterolateral (mastoid) fontanelle

Anterior fontanelle

Frontal suture

Frontal eminence

Anterolateral (sphenoid) fontanelle

Maxilla

Mandible

A

Sagittal suture

Lambdoid suture

Occipital bone

Posterior fontanelle

Frontal bone

Anterior fontanelle

Coronal suture

B

FIGURE 15-8. Fetal cranium, showing the bones, fontanelles, and connecting sutures. **A,** Lateral view. **B,** Superior view. The posterior and anterolateral fontanelles disappear within 2 or 3 months after birth because of the growth of the surrounding bones, but they remain as sutures for several years. The posterolateral fontanelles disappear in a similar manner by the end of the first year, and the anterior fontanelle disappears by the end of the second year. The halves of the frontal bone normally begin to fuse during the second year, and the frontal (metopic) suture is usually obliterated by the eighth year. The other sutures disappear during adult life.

SPINA BIFIDA

Failure of the halves of the vertebral arch to fuse results in a defect called **spina bifida** (see Fig. 15-6C; see also Chapter 16).

ACCESSORY RIBS

Accessory ribs, usually rudimentary, result from the development of costal processes from the cervical or lumbar vertebrae (see Fig. 15-6A). The most common type of accessory rib is a **lumbar rib**, but it is clinically insignificant. **Cervical ribs** occur in 0.5% to 1% of people (Fig. 15-9A). A **cervical rib** is attached to the seventh cervical vertebra and may be unilateral or bilateral. Pressure of a cervical rib on the brachial plexus of nerves or the subclavian artery often produces neurovascular symptoms.

FUSED RIBS

Fusion of ribs occasionally occurs posteriorly when two or more ribs arise from a single vertebra. Fused ribs are often associated with a hemivertebra.

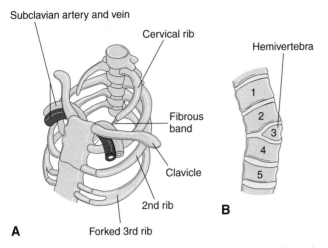

A

B

FIGURE 15-9. Vertebral and rib abnormalities. **A,** Cervical and forked ribs. Observe that the left cervical rib has a fibrous band that passes posterior to the subclavian vessels and attaches to the sternum. **B,** Anterior view of the vertebral column, showing a hemivertebra. The right half of the third thoracic vertebra is absent. Note the associated lateral curvature (scoliosis) of the vertebral column.

FIGURE 15-10. Anterior (**A**) and posterior (**B**) views of a 20-week fetus with severe defects, including acrania (absence of the calvaria), cervical rachischisis (extensive clefts in the vertebral arches), cerebral regression (meroencephaly), iniencephaly (defect in the occiput—back of the cranium), and a sacral dimple. (Courtesy of R. Del Bigio, Department of Pathology [Neuropathology], University of Manitoba, Winnipeg, Manitoba, Canada.)

HEMIVERTEBRA

Developing vertebral bodies have two chondrification centers that soon unite. A hemivertebra results from failure of one of the chondrification centers to appear and subsequent failure of half of the vertebra to form (see Fig. 15-9B). These vertebral defects produce **scoliosis** (lateral curvature) of the vertebral column.

RACHISCHISIS

The term *rachischisis* (cleft vertebral column) refers to vertebral abnormalities in a complex group of anomalies (**axial dysraphic disorders**) that primarily affect axial structures (Fig. 15-10). In affected infants, the neural folds do not fuse, either because of faulty induction by the underlying notochord or because of the action of teratogenic agents on the neuroepithelial cells in the neural folds. The neural and vertebral defects may be extensive, or they may be restricted to a small area.

ACRANIA

In acrania, the calvaria is absent, and extensive defects of the vertebral column are often present (see Fig. 15-10). Acrania is associated with **meroencephaly (anencephaly)**. Partial absence of the brain occurs in approximately 1 in 1000 births and is incompatible with life. Meroencephaly occurs when the cranial end of the neural tube does not close during the fourth week of development, resulting in subsequent failure of the calvaria to form.

CRANIOSYNOSTOSIS

Several cranial deformities result from premature closure of the cranial sutures. Prenatal closure results in the most severe abnormalities. The cause of craniosynostosis is unclear, but genetic factors appear to be important. *Homeobox gene (MSX2 and ALX4) mutations have been implicated in cases of craniosynostosis* and other cranial defects. These abnormalities are much more common in males than in females, and they are often associated with other skeletal anomalies. The type of cranial deformation produced depends on which sutures close prematurely. If the sagittal suture closes early, the cranium becomes elongated and wedge-shaped, a condition known as **scaphocephaly** (Fig. 15-11A). This type of cranial deformity constitutes approximately half of the cases of craniosynostosis. Another 30% of cases involve premature closure of the coronal suture, which results in a high, tower-like cranium, a condition known as **brachycephaly** (see Fig. 15-11B). If the coronal suture closes prematurely on one side only, the cranium is twisted and asymmetrical, resulting in a condition known as **plagiocephaly**. Premature closure of the metopic suture results in a deformity of the frontal bone and other anomalies, known collectively as **trigonocephaly**.

MICROCEPHALY

Infants with microcephaly are born with a normal-sized or slightly small calvaria. The fontanelles close during early infancy, and the sutures close during the first year. Microcephaly is the result of abnormal development

MICROCEPHALY—CONT'D

of the central nervous system that causes the brain, and consequently, the cranium to fail to grow. Usually, persons with microcephaly are severely mentally retarded (see Chapter 16).

■ DEVELOPMENT OF THE APPENDICULAR SKELETON

The appendicular skeleton consists of the pectoral and pelvic girdles and the limb bones. During the sixth week, the **mesenchymal bone models** undergo chondrification to form **hyaline cartilage bone models** (Fig. 15-12D and E). The clavicle initially develops by intramembranous ossification; later, growth cartilages form at both ends. The models of the pectoral girdle and the upper limb bones appear slightly before those of the pelvic girdle and the lower limbs; the bone models appear in a proximodistal sequence. *Patterning in the developing limbs is regulated by Hox genes.* The molecular mechanisms of these *Hox* genes as they relate to limb morphogenesis remain uncertain.

Endochondral ossification begins in the long bones by the eighth week (see Fig. 15-3B and C). By 12 weeks, primary ossification centers have appeared in nearly all limb bones (Fig. 15-13). The clavicles begin to ossify before any other bones in the body, followed by the femora. Virtually all **primary centers of ossification** (diaphysial) are present at birth.

The secondary ossification centers of the bones at the knee are the first to appear in utero. The secondary centers for the distal end of the femur and the proximal end of the tibia usually appear during the last month of intrauterine life (34–38 weeks). The secondary centers of the other bones appear after birth. The bone formed from the primary center in the diaphysis does not fuse at the **epiphyseal plate** with that formed from the secondary centers in the epiphyses until the bone grows to its adult length. This delay enables lengthening of the bone to continue until the final size is reached.

BONE AGE

Bone age is a good index of general maturation. A radiologist can determine the bone age of a person by assessing the ossification centers using two criteria:

- The time of appearance of calcified material in the diaphysis, epiphysis, or both is specific for each diaphysis and epiphysis and for each bone and sex.
- The disappearance of the dark line representing the epiphysial cartilage plate indicates that the epiphysis has fused with the diaphysis.

Fusion of the diaphysial-epiphysial centers, which occurs at specific times for each epiphysis, happens 1 to 2 years earlier in females than in males. In the fetus, ultrasonography is used for the evaluation and measurement of bones.

GENERALIZED SKELETAL MALFORMATIONS

Achondroplasia is a common cause of short stature. It occurs in approximately 1 in 15,000 births. The limbs become bowed and short because of a disturbance of endochondral ossification at the epiphysial cartilage plates, particularly of the long bones, during fetal life (Fig. 15-14). The trunk is usually short, and the head is enlarged, with a bulging forehead and a "scooped-out" nose (flat nasal bone). Achondroplasia is an **autosomal dominant disorder**, and approximately 80% of cases arise from new mutations; the rate increases with paternal age. *The majority of cases are due to a point mutation (f.1,11,12) in the FGFR3 gene*, which results in magnification of the normal inhibiting effect of endochondral ossification, specifically in the zone of chondrocyte proliferation. This results in shortened bone, but does not affect periosteal bone growth.

FIGURE 15-11. Craniosynostosis. **A,** An infant with scaphocephaly resulting from premature closure of the sagittal suture. **B,** An infant with bilateral premature closure of the coronal suture—brachycephaly—resulting in a high, towerlike forehead. (Courtesy of Dr. John A. Jane, Sr., David D. Weaver Professor of Neurosurgery, Department of Neurological Surgery, University of Virginia Health System, Charlottesville, VA.)

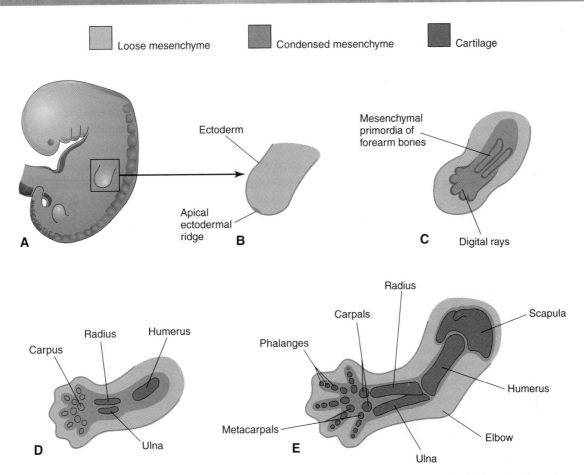

FIGURE 15-12. **A,** Embryo at approximately 28 days, showing the early appearance of a limb bud. **B,** Longitudinal section through an upper limb bud. The apical ectodermal ridge has an inductive influence on the mesenchyme in the limb bud. The apical ectodermal ridge promotes the growth of the mesenchyme and appears to give it the ability to form specific cartilaginous elements. **C,** Upper limb bud at approximately 33 days, showing the mesenchymal primordia of the limb bones. The digital rays are mesenchymal condensations that undergo chondrification and ossification to form the bones of the hand. **D,** Upper limb at 6 weeks, showing the cartilage models of the bones. **E,** Later in the sixth week. Note the completed cartilaginous models of the bones of the upper limb.

HYPERPITUITARISM

Congenital infantile hyperpituitarism, which causes abnormally rapid growth in infancy, is rare. This condition may result in **gigantism** (excessive height and body proportions) or acromegaly in the adult (enlargement of the soft tissues, visceral organs, and bones of the face, hands, and feet). In **acromegaly**, the epiphysial and diaphysial centers of the long bones fuse, thereby preventing elongation of the bones. Both gigantism and acromegaly result from an excessive secretion of growth hormone.

HYPOTHYROIDISM AND CRETINISM

A severe deficiency of fetal thyroid hormone production results in cretinism, a condition characterized by growth retardation, mental deficiency, skeletal abnormalities, and auditory and neurologic disorders. Bone age in an affected individual appears as less than chronologic age because epiphysial development is delayed. Cretinism is very rare, except in areas where iodine is lacking in the soil and water. Agenesis of the thyroid gland also results in cretinism.

■ MUSCULAR SYSTEM

The muscular system develops from the **mesoderm**, except for the muscles of the iris, which develop from the **neuroectoderm**. Myoblasts, which are embryonic muscle cells, are derived from mesenchyme.

Development of Skeletal Muscle

The myoblasts that form the skeletal muscles of the trunk are derived from the mesenchyme in the myotome regions of the somites. The limb muscles develop from **myogenic precursor cells** in the limb buds. Studies show that these cells originate from the ventral **dermomyotome of somites** in response to *molecular signals* from nearby tissues

Parietal bone

Occipital bone

Cervical vertebrae

Scapula

Humerus

Thoracic vertebrae

Femur

Ilium

Frontal bone

Maxilla

Mandible

Metacarpals

Radius

Ulna

Ribs

Metatarsal bone

Tibia

Fibula

FIGURE 15-13. Alizarin-stained, 12-week human fetus. Observe the degree of progression of ossification from the primary centers of ossification, which are endochondral in the appendicular and axial parts of the skeleton, except for most of the cranial bones. Note that the carpus and the tarsus are wholly cartilaginous at this stage, as are the epiphyses of all long bones. (Courtesy of Dr. Gary Geddes, Lake Oswego, OR.)

(Fig. 15-15). The myogenic precursor cells migrate into the limb buds, where they undergo epitheliomesenchymal transformation. The first indication of **myogenesis** (muscle formation) is the elongation of the nuclei and cell bodies of mesenchymal cells as they differentiate into myoblasts. These **primordial muscle cells** soon fuse to form elongated, multinucleated, cylindric structures called **myotubes**. At the molecular level, these events are preceded by gene activation and expression of the MyoD family of muscle-specific basic helix-loop-helix transcription factors (MyoD, myogenin, Myf-5, and MRF4) in the precursor myogenic cells. It has been suggested that signaling molecules from the ventral neural tube (Shh), the notochord (Shh), the dorsal neural tube (Wnt, BMP-4), and the overlying ectoderm (Wnt, BMP-4) regulate the beginning of myogenesis and the induction of the myotome.

Muscle growth during development results from the ongoing fusion of myoblasts and myotubes. **Myofilaments** develop in the cytoplasm of the myotubes during or after fusion of the myoblasts. Soon after that, **myofibrils** and other organelles characteristic of striated muscle cells develop. Because muscle cells are long and narrow, they are called **muscle fibers**. As the myotubes differentiate,

FIGURE 15-14. Achondroplasia in a 1-year-old boy, showing proximal shortening of the lower limbs. (Courtesy of Dr. Prem Sahni, formerly of the Department of Radiology, Children's Hospital, Winnipeg, Manitoba, Canada.)

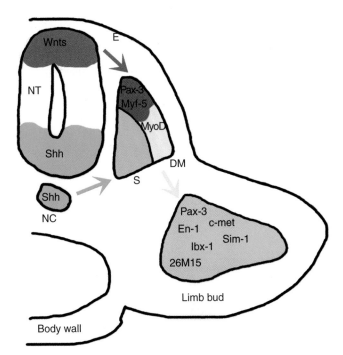

FIGURE 15-15. A model for molecular interactions during myogenesis. Shh and Wnt, produced by the neural tube (NT) and the notochord (NC), induce Pax-3 and Myf-5 in the somites. Either of them can activate the initiation of MyoD transcription and myogenesis. The surface ectoderm (E) is also capable of inducing Myf-5 and MyoD. In addition, Pax-3 regulates the expression of c-met, which is necessary for the migratory ability of the myogenic precursor cells, which also express En-1, Sim-1, lbx-1, and 26M15. DM, dermomyotome; S, sclerotome. (From Kablar B, Rudnicki MA: Skeletal muscle development in the mouse embryo. Histol Histopathol 15:649, 2000.)

they become invested with external laminae, which segregate them from the surrounding connective tissue. Fibroblasts produce the perimysium and epimysium layers of the fibrous sheath; the endomysium is formed by the external lamina, which is derived from the muscle fiber, and by reticular fibers. Most skeletal muscle develops before birth, and almost all remaining muscles are formed by the end of the first year. The increase in the size of a muscle after the first year results from an increase in the diameter of the fibers because of the formation of more myofilaments. Muscles increase in length and width to grow with the skeleton.

Myotomes

Typically, each myotome part of a somite divides into a dorsal **epaxial division** and a ventral **hypaxial division** (Fig. 15-16A and B). Each developing **spinal nerve** also divides and sends a branch to each division, with the **dorsal primary ramus** supplying the epaxial division and the **ventral primary ramus** supplying the hypaxial division. Some muscles—the intercostal muscles, for example—remain segmentally arranged like the somites, but most myoblasts migrate away from the myotome and form nonsegmented muscles.

Derivatives of Epaxial Divisions of Myotomes

Myoblasts from the epaxial divisions of the myotomes form the segmental muscles of the main body axis, the extensor muscles of the neck and vertebral column (Fig. 15-17). The embryonic extensor muscles that are derived from the sacral and coccygeal myotomes degenerate; their adult derivatives are the dorsal sacrococcygeal ligaments.

Derivatives of Hypaxial Divisions of Myotomes

Myoblasts from the hypaxial divisions of the cervical myotomes form the scalene, prevertebral, geniohyoid, and infrahyoid muscles (see Fig. 15-17). The thoracic myotomes form the lateral and ventral flexor muscles of the vertebral column, whereas the lumbar myotomes form the quadratus lumborum muscle. The muscles of the limbs, the intercostal muscles, and the abdominal muscles are also derived from the hypaxial division of the myotomes. The sacrococcygeal myotomes form the muscles of the pelvic diaphragm and probably the striated muscles of the anus and the sex organs.

Pharyngeal Arch Muscles

Myoblasts from the pharyngeal arches form the muscles of mastication and facial expression as well as those of the pharynx and larynx (see Chapter 9). These muscles are innervated by the pharyngeal arch nerves.

Ocular Muscles

The origin of the extrinsic eye muscles is unclear, but they may be derived from mesenchymal cells near the prechordal plate (see Figs. 15-16A and 15-17B). The mesoderm in this area is believed to give rise to three *preotic myotomes* from which myoblasts differentiate. Groups of myoblasts, each supplied by its own cranial nerve (CN) (CN III, CN IV, or CN VI), form the extrinsic muscles of the eye.

Tongue Muscles

Initially, there are four *occipital (postotic) myotomes*; however, the first pair disappears. Myoblasts from the remaining myotomes form the tongue muscles, which are innervated by the hypoglossal nerve (CN XII).

Limb Muscles

The musculature of the limbs develops from myoblasts surrounding the developing bones (see Fig. 15-16B). The **precursor myogenic cells** in the limb buds originate from the somites. These cells are first located in the ventral part of the dermomyotome, and they are epithelial (see Fig. 15-1D). After **epitheliomesenchymal transformation,** the cells migrate into the primordium of the limb.

Development of Smooth Muscle

Smooth muscle fibers differentiate from the **splanchnic mesenchyme** surrounding the endoderm of the primordial

A

B

C

FIGURE 15-16. **A,** Embryo (approximately 41 days), showing the myotomes and the developing muscular system. **B,** Transverse section of the embryo, showing the epaxial and hypaxial derivatives of a myotome. **C,** Similar section of a 7-week embryo, showing the muscle layers formed from the myotomes.

gut and its derivatives (see Fig. 15-1E). The smooth muscle in the walls of many blood and lymphatic vessels arises from the somatic mesoderm. The muscles of the iris (sphincter and dilator pupillae) and the **myoepithelial** cells in the mammary and sweat glands are believed to be derived from mesenchymal cells that originate from the ectoderm.

The first sign of differentiation of smooth muscle is the development of elongated nuclei in spindle-shaped myoblasts. During early development, new myoblasts continue to differentiate from mesenchymal cells, but do not fuse; they remain mononucleated. During later development, the division of existing myoblasts gradually replaces the differentiation of new myoblasts in the production of new smooth muscle tissue. Filamentous, but nonsarcomeric contractile elements develop in their cytoplasm, and the external surface of each differential cell acquires a surrounding external lamina. As smooth muscle fibers develop into sheets or bundles, they receive autonomic innervation; fibroblasts and muscle

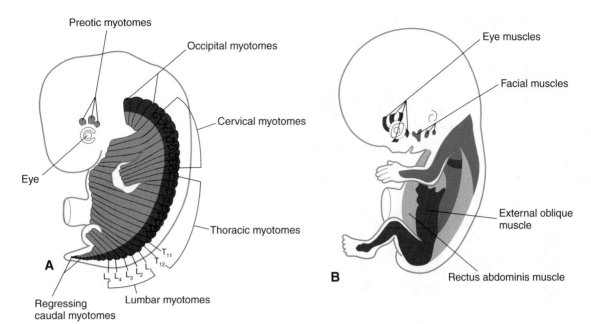

FIGURE 15-17. The developing muscular system. **A,** A 6-week embryo. The myotome regions of the somites give rise to most skeletal muscles. **B,** An 8-week embryo, showing the developing trunk and limb musculature.

cells synthesize and lay down collagenous, elastic, and reticular fibers.

Development of Cardiac Muscle

The lateral splanchnic mesoderm gives rise to the mesenchyme surrounding the developing heart tube (see Chapter 14). **Cardiac myoblasts** differentiate from this primordial myocardium. Heart muscle is recognizable in the fourth week. **Cardiac muscle fibers** arise by the differentiation and growth of single cells, unlike striated skeletal muscle fibers, which develop by the fusion of cells. Growth of cardiac muscle fibers results from the formation of new **myofilaments**. The myoblasts adhere to each other as in developing skeletal muscle, but the intervening cell membranes do not disintegrate; these areas of adhesion give rise to **intercalated discs**. Late in the embryonic period, special bundles of muscle cells develop that have relatively few myofibrils and relatively larger diameters than typical cardiac muscle fibers. These atypical cardiac muscle cells—**Purkinje fibers**—form the conducting system of the heart (see Chapter 14).

VARIATIONS IN MUSCLES

Certain muscles are functionally vestigial, such as those of the external ear and scalp. Some muscles that are present in other primates appear only in some humans (e.g., sternalis muscle). Variations in the form, position, and attachments of muscles are common and are usually functionally insignificant.

ANOMALIES OF MUSCLES

Any muscle in the body may occasionally be absent; common examples are the sternocostal head of the pectoralis major, the palmaris longus, the trapezius, the serratus anterior, and the quadratus femoris. Absence of the pectoralis major, often its sternal part, is usually associated with syndactyly (fusion of digits). These anomalies are part of **Poland syndrome**, which also includes breast and nipple aplasia or hypoplasia, deficiencies of axillary hair and subcutaneous fat, and shortened arms and fingers.

Some muscular anomalies are clinically significant. **Congenital absence of the diaphragm** is usually associated with **pulmonary atelectasis** (incomplete expansion of the lungs or part of a lung) and pneumonitis (pneumonia). The sternocleidomastoid muscle is sometimes injured at birth, resulting in **congenital torticollis**. There is fixed rotation and tilting of the head because of concomitant muscle fibrosis, as well as shortening of the sternocleidomastoid muscle on one side (Fig. 15-18). Although birth trauma is commonly considered a cause of congenital torticollis, this may also result from malpositioning in utero. Genetic factors may also be involved.

ACCESSORY MUSCLES

Accessory muscles occasionally develop. For example, an *accessory soleus muscle* is present in approximately 6% of the population. It has been suggested that the primordium of the soleus muscle may undergo early splitting to form an accessory soleus.

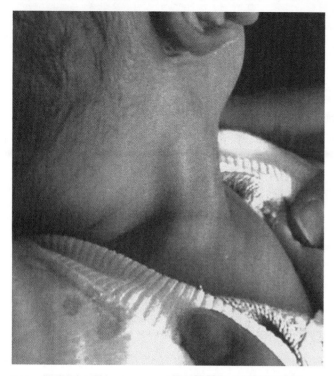

FIGURE 15-18. Congenital muscular torticollis (wry neck), showing extensive involvement of the left sternocleidomastoid muscle, in an infant who was examined at 2 months. (Courtesy of Professor Jack C.Y. Cheng, Department of Orthopaedics & Traumatology, The Chinese University of Hong Kong, Hong Kong, China.)

■ DEVELOPMENT OF THE LIMBS

Early Stages of Limb Development

The **limb buds** first appear as small elevations of the ventrolateral body wall toward the end of the fourth week (Fig. 15-19A). Limb development begins with the activation of a group of mesenchymal cells in the lateral mesoderm. The upper limb buds are visible by day 26 or 27, whereas the lower limb buds appear 1 to 2 days later. Each limb bud consists of a mass of mesenchyme covered by ectoderm (see Fig. 15-12A and B). The mesenchyme is derived from the somatic layer of the lateral mesoderm. The limb buds elongate by the proliferation of the mesenchyme. Although the early stages of limb development are alike for the upper and lower limbs (see Fig. 15-19A and B), there are distinct differences because of their form and function. **The upper limb buds** develop opposite the caudal cervical segments, whereas the **lower limb buds** form opposite the lumbar and upper sacral segments.

At the apex of each limb bud, the ectoderm thickens to form an **apical ectodermal ridge** (AER) (see Fig. 15-12B). The **AER**, a multilayered epithelial structure (Fig. 15-20), interacts with the mesenchyme in the limb bud, promoting outgrowth of the bud. *Expression of endogenous fibroblast growth factors in the AER is involved in this process. The AER exerts an inductive influence on the limb mesenchyme that initiates growth and development of the limbs in a proximodistal axis.* Mesenchymal cells aggregate at the posterior margin of the limb bud to form a **zone of polarizing activity.**

Fibroblast growth factors from the AER activate the zone of polarizing activity, causing expression of the sonic hedgehog gene (Shh), which controls the patterning of the limb along the anteroposterior axis. Expression of Wnt7 from the dorsal epidermis of the limb bud and engrailed-1 (En-1) from the ventral aspect is involved in specifying the dorsoventral axis. Of interest, the AER itself is maintained by inductive signals from Shh and Wnt7. The mesenchyme adjacent to the AER consists of undifferentiated, rapidly proliferating cells, whereas the mesenchymal cells proximal to it differentiate into blood vessels and cartilage bone models. The distal ends of the limb buds eventually flatten into paddle-like hand- and footplates (Fig. 15-21).

By the end of the sixth week of development, mesenchymal tissue in the **handplates** has condensed to form **digital rays** (Figs. 15-21 and 15-22A to C)—finger buds—which outline the pattern of the digits. During the seventh week, similar condensations of mesenchyme form digital rays—*toe buds*—in the **footplates** (see Fig. 15-22E to I). At the tip of each digital ray, a part of the AER induces development of the mesenchyme into the mesenchymal primordia of the bones (phalanges) in the digits. The intervals between the digital rays are occupied by loose mesenchyme. Soon the intervening regions of mesenchyme undergo **apoptosis** (*programmed cell death*), forming *notches between the digital rays* (see Figs. 15-21 and 15-22D and J). As this tissue breakdown progresses, separate digits are produced by the end of the eighth week of development (see Fig. 15-21). Blocking of cellular and molecular events during this process may account for webbing, or fusion, of the fingers or toes, a condition known as **syndactyly** (see Fig. 15-28C and D).

Final Stages of Limb Development

The mesenchyme in the limb bud gives rise to bones, ligaments, and blood vessels (Fig. 15-23). As the limb buds elongate during the early part of the fifth week of development, mesenchymal models of the bones are formed by cellular aggregations (see Fig. 15-23A and B). **Chondrification centers** appear later in the fifth week. By the end of the sixth week, the entire limb skeleton is cartilaginous (see Fig. 15-23C and D). **Osteogenesis of the long bones** begins in the seventh week from primary ossification centers in the diaphyses of the long bones. **Primary ossification centers** are present in all long bones by the 12th week. Ossification of the carpal (wrist) bones begins during the first year after birth.

From the **dermomyotome regions of the somites,** myogenic precursor cells also migrate into the limb bud and later differentiate into **myoblasts**, the precursors of muscle cells. As the long bones form, myoblasts aggregate and form a large muscle mass in each limb bud (see Fig. 15-16B). In general, this muscle mass separates into dorsal (extensor) and ventral (flexor) components.

Early in the seventh week, the limbs extend ventrally and the preaxial and postaxial borders are cranial and caudal, respectively (see Fig. 15-25A and D). The *upper limbs rotate laterally* through 90 degrees on their longitudinal axes; thus, the future elbows point dorsally and the extensor muscles

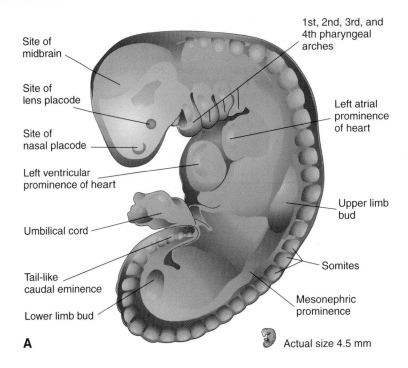

Site of midbrain

Site of lens placode

Site of nasal placode

Left ventricular prominence of heart

Umbilical cord

Tail-like caudal eminence

Lower limb bud

1st, 2nd, 3rd, and 4th pharyngeal arches

Left atrial prominence of heart

Upper limb bud

Somites

Mesonephric prominence

A

Actual size 4.5 mm

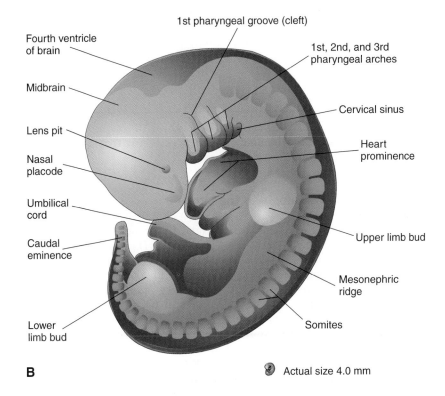

Fourth ventricle of brain

Midbrain

Lens pit

Nasal placode

Umbilical cord

Caudal eminence

Lower limb bud

1st pharyngeal groove (cleft)

1st, 2nd, and 3rd pharyngeal arches

Cervical sinus

Heart prominence

Upper limb bud

Mesonephric ridge

Somites

B

Actual size 4.0 mm

Figure 15-19. A, Lateral view of a human embryo at approximately 28 days. The upper limb buds appear as swellings on the ventrolateral body wall. The lower limb buds are not as well developed. **B,** Lateral view of an embryo at approximately 32 days. The upper limb buds are paddle-shaped, whereas the lower limb buds are flipper-like. (Modified from Nishimura H, Semba R, Tanimura T, Tanaka O: Prenatal Development of the Human with Special Reference to Craniofacial Structures: An Atlas. Washington, DC, National Institutes of Health, 1977.)

lie on the lateral and posterior aspects of the limb. The *lower limbs rotate medially* through almost 90 degrees; thus, the future knees face ventrally and the extensor muscles lie on the anterior aspect of the lower limb (Fig. 15-24*A* to *D*).

The radius and the tibia are homologous bones, as are the ulna and the fibula, just as the thumb and the great toe are homologous digits. **Synovial joints** appear at the beginning of the fetal period, coinciding with functional differentiation of the limb muscles and their innervation.

Cutaneous Innervation of the Limbs

Motor axons arising from the spinal cord enter the limb buds during the fifth week of development and grow into

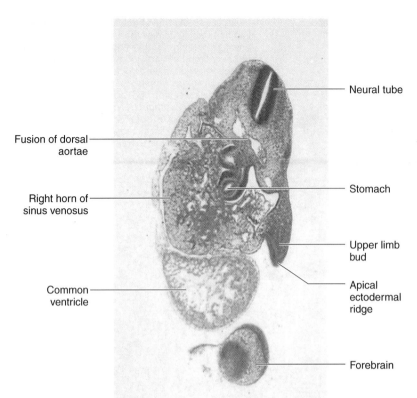

Fusion of dorsal aortae

Right horn of sinus venosus

Common ventricle

Neural tube

Stomach

Upper limb bud

Apical ectodermal ridge

Forebrain

FIGURE 15-20. Oblique section of an embryo at approximately 28 days. Observe the flipperlike upper limb bud lateral to the embryonic heart and the ECR. (From Moore KL, Persaud TVN, Shiota K: Color Atlas of Clinical Embryology, 2nd ed. Philadelphia, WB Saunders, 2000.)

the dorsal and ventral muscle masses. **Sensory axons** enter the limb buds after the motor axons and use them for guidance. **Neural crest cells**, the precursors of Schwann cells, surround the motor and sensory nerve fibers in the limbs and *form the neurolemmal and myelin sheaths* (see Chapter 16).

A **dermatome** is the area of skin supplied by a single spinal nerve and its spinal ganglion. During the fifth week of development, the peripheral nerves grow from the developing **limb plexuses** (brachial and lumbosacral) into the mesenchyme of the limb buds (Fig. 15-25A, B, and E). The spinal nerves are distributed in segmental bands, supplying both the dorsal and the ventral surfaces of the limb buds. As the limbs elongate, the cutaneous distribution of the spinal nerves migrates along the limbs and no longer reaches the surface in the distal part of the limbs. Although the original **dermatomal pattern** changes during growth of the limbs, an orderly sequence of distribution can still be recognized in the adult (see Fig. 15-25C and F). In the upper limb, the areas supplied by C_5 and C_6 adjoin the areas supplied by T_2, T_1, and C_8, but the overlap between them is minimal at the ventral axial line.

Because there is overlapping of **dermatomes**, a particular area of skin is not exclusively innervated by a single segmental nerve. The limb dermatomes may be traced progressively down the lateral aspect of the upper limb and back up its medial aspect. A comparable distribution of dermatomes occurs in the lower limbs and may be traced down the ventral aspect and then

up the dorsal aspect of the lower limb. When the limbs descend, they carry their nerves with them; this explains the oblique course of the nerves arising from the brachial and lumbosacral plexuses.

Blood Supply to the Limbs

The limb buds are supplied by branches of the **intersegmental arteries** (Fig. 15-26A), which arise from the dorsal aorta and form a fine capillary network throughout the mesenchyme. The primordial vascular pattern consists of a **primary axial artery** and its branches (see Fig. 15-26B and C), which drain into a peripheral marginal sinus. Blood in the sinus drains into a peripheral vein. The vascular pattern changes as the limbs develop, chiefly as a result of vessels sprouting from existing vessels (**angiogenesis**). The new vessels coalesce with other sprouts to form new vessels. The primary axial artery becomes the **brachial artery** in the arm and the **ulnar and radial arteries** in the forearm, its terminal branches of the brachial artery (see Fig. 15-26B). As the digits form, the marginal sinus breaks up and the final venous pattern, represented by the basilic and cephalic veins and their tributaries, develops. In the thigh, the primary axial artery is represented by the **deep artery of the thigh** (profunda femoris artery). In the leg, the primary axial artery is represented by the anterior and posterior **tibial arteries** (see Fig. 15-26C).

FIGURE 15-21. Development of the limbs (32–56 days). Note that development of the upper limbs precedes that of the lower limbs.

Flipperlike upper limb bud

Handplate formed

Week 5
32 days

Week 5
35 days

Digital rays appear in handplate

Digital ray

Notch between digital rays; webbed fingers

Upper limbs bend at elbow; fingers are short and slightly webbed

Week 6
44 days

Week 7
48 days

Fingers and toes are distinct and separated

Week 8
56 days

CLEFT HAND AND CLEFT FOOT

In the rare "lobster-claw deformities" known as *cleft hand or cleft foot,* one or more central digits are absent—**ectrodactylyl**—resulting from failure of one or more digital rays to develop (Fig. 15-27A and B). The hand or foot is divided into two parts that oppose each other. The remaining digits are partially or completely fused (**syndactyly**).

CONGENITAL ABSENCE OF THE RADIUS

In some individuals, the radius is partially or completely absent. The hand deviates laterally (radially), and the ulna bows with the concavity on the lateral side of the forearm. This anomaly results from failure of the mesenchymal primordium of the radius to form during the fifth week of development. Absence of the radius is usually caused by genetic factors.

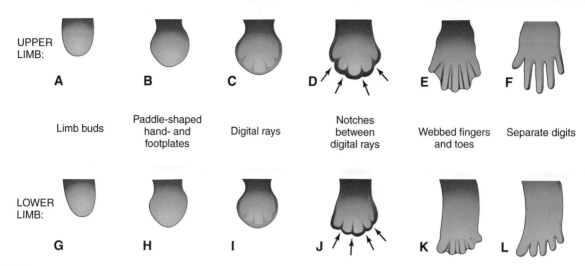

FIGURE 15-22. Development of the hands and feet between the fourth and eighth weeks. The early stages of limb development are similar, except that development of the hands precedes that of the feet by approximately 1 day. **A,** At 27 days. **B,** At 32 days. **C,** At 41 days. **D,** At 46 days. **E,** At 50 days. **F,** At 52 days. **G,** At 28 days. **H,** At 36 days. **I,** At 46 days. **J,** At 49 days. **K,** At 52 days. **L,** At 56 days. The *arrows* in **D** and **J** indicate the tissue breakdown processes that separate the fingers and toes.

BRACHYDACTYLY

Shortness of the digits (fingers or toes) is uncommon and is the result of a reduction in the length of the phalanges. This anomaly is usually inherited as a dominant trait and is often associated with shortness of stature.

POLYDACTYLY

Supernumerary digits are common (Fig. 15-28*A* and *B*). Often, the extra digit is incompletely formed and lacks proper muscular development, rendering it useless. If the hand is affected, the extra digit is most commonly medial or lateral rather than central. In the foot, the extra toe is usually on the lateral side. Polydactyly is inherited as a dominant trait.

SYNDACTYLY

Syndactyly occurs with a frequency of approximately 1 in 2200 births. **Cutaneous syndactyly** (simple webbing of the digits) is the most common limb anomaly (see Fig. 15-28*C*). It occurs more frequently in the foot than in the hand (see Fig. 15-28*C* and *D*). Syndactyly is most frequently observed between the third and fourth fingers and between the second and third toes (see Fig. 15-28*D*). It is inherited as a simple dominant or simple recessive trait. Cutaneous syndactyly results from failure of the webs to degenerate between two or more digits. In some cases, there is fusion of the

bones (synostosis). **Osseous syndactyly** occurs when the notches between the digital rays do not develop during the seventh week; as a result, separation of the digits does not occur.

CONGENITAL TALIPES (CLUBFOOT)

Talipes occurs at a rate of approximately 1 in 1000 births. **Talipes equinovarus**, the most common type (Fig. 15-29), occurs approximately twice as frequently in males as in females. The sole of the foot is turned medially, and the foot is inverted. There is much uncertainty about the cause of talipes. Hereditary factors are involved in some cases, and it appears that environmental factors are involved in most cases. Talipes appears to follow a **multifactorial pattern of inheritance**; hence, any intrauterine position that results in abnormal positioning of the feet may cause talipes if the fetus is genetically predisposed to this deformity.

CONGENITAL DISLOCATION OF THE HIP

Congenital dislocation of the hip occurs with a frequency of approximately 1 in 1500 newborn infants and is more common in females than in males. In these cases, the fibrous capsule of the hip joint is very relaxed, and the acetabulum of the hip bone and the head of the femur are underdeveloped. The actual dislocation almost always occurs after birth.

Ectoderm

A Apical ectodermal ridge (AER)

Loose mesenchyme

Condensed mesenchyme

Cartilage

Ectoderm

Mesenchymal primordia of forearm bones

B

Carpal bone

Humerus

Radius

C Ulna

Radius

Carpus

Phalanges

Scapula

Metacarpals

Humerus

D Ulna

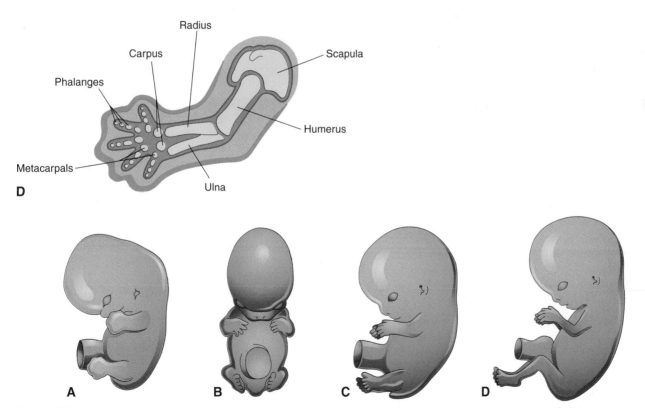

A **B** **C** **D**

FIGURE 15-24. Positional changes of the developing limbs of human embryos. **A,** At approximately 48 days, showing the limbs extending ventrally and the handplates and footplates facing each other. **B,** At approximately 51 days, showing the upper limbs bent at the elbows and the hands curved over the thorax. **C,** At approximately 54 days, showing the soles of the feet facing medially. **D,** At approximately 56 days. Note that the elbows now point caudally and the knees, cranially.

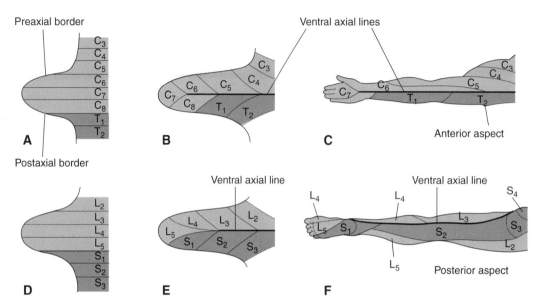

FIGURE 15-25. Development of the dermatomal patterns of the limbs. The axial lines indicate where there is no sensory overlap. **A** and **D,** Ventral aspect of the limb buds early in the fifth week. At this stage, the dermatomal patterns show the primordial segmental arrangement. **B** and **E,** Similar views later in the fifth week, showing the modified arrangement of dermatomes. **C** and **F,** The dermatomal patterns in the adult upper and lower limbs. The primordial dermatomal pattern has disappeared, but an orderly sequence of dermatomes can still be recognized. In **F,** note that most of the original ventral surface of the lower limb lies on the back of the adult limb. This results from the medial rotation of the lower limb that occurs toward the end of the embryonic period. In the upper limb, the ventral axial line extends along the anterior surface of the arm and forearm. In the lower limb, the ventral axial line extends along the medial side of the thigh and knee, to the posteromedial aspect of the leg to the heel.

LIMB ANOMALIES

There are two main types of limb anomalies:
- **Amelia**—complete absence of a limb
- **Meromelia**—partial absence of a limb

Terms such as *hemimelia, peromelia, ectromelia,* and *phocomelia* are also used.

Anomalies of the limbs originate at different stages of development. Suppression of limb bud development during the early part of the fourth week results in amelia (Fig. 15-30A). Arrest or disturbance of the differentiation or growth of the limbs during the fifth week results in **meromelia** (see Fig. 15-30B and C). Some limb defects are caused by the following:

- Genetic factors, such as chromosomal abnormalities associated with trisomy 18 (see Chapter 19)
- Mutant genes, as in brachydactyly or osteogenesis imperfecta; **molecular studies have implicated gene mutation (Hox gene, BMP, Shh, Wnt7, En-1, and others)** in some cases of limb anomalies
- Environmental factors, such as teratogens (e.g., thalidomide)
- A combination of genetic and environmental factors *(multifactorial inheritance),* as in congenital dislocation of the hip
- Vascular disruption and ischemia, as in limb reduction defects

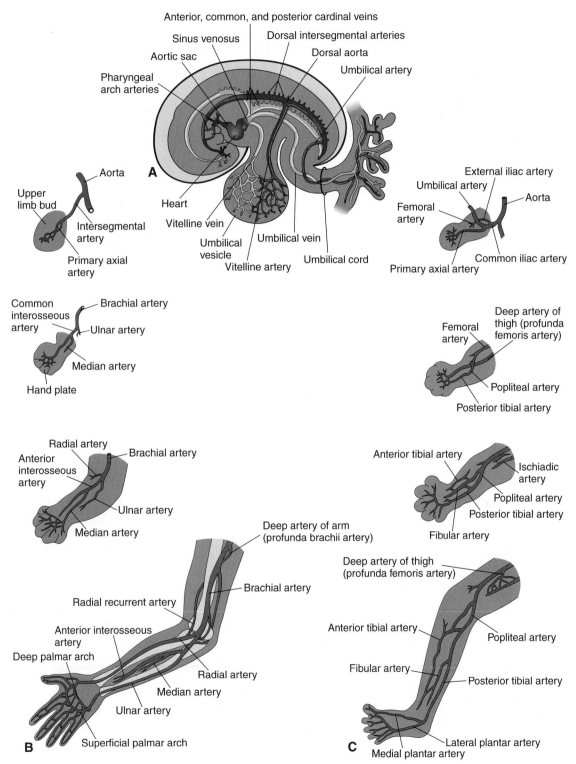

FIGURE 15-26. Development of the limb arteries. **A** and **B,** Development of the arteries in the upper limb. **C,** Development of the arteries in the lower limb.

FIGURE 15-27. Anomalies of the hands and feet. **A,** Ectrodactyly in a child. Note the absence of the central digits of the hands, resulting in split hands (lobster-claw anomaly). **B,** A similar type of defect involving the feet. These limb defects can be inherited in an autosomal dominant pattern. (Courtesy of A.E. Chudley, MD, Section of Genetics and Metabolism, Department of Pediatrics and Child Health, University of Manitoba, Children's Hospital, Winnipeg, Manitoba, Canada.)

FIGURE 15-28. Various types of digital defects. **A,** Polydactyly of the hands. **B,** Polydactyly of the foot. This condition results from the formation of one or more extra digital rays during the embryonic period.

FIGURE 15-28. CONT'D **C** and **D,** Various forms of syndactyly involving the fingers and toes. Cutaneous syndactyly (**C**) is probably caused by incomplete apoptosis (programmed cell death) in the tissues between the digital rays during embryonic life. Syndactyly of the second and third toes is shown in **D**. In osseous syndactyly, the digital rays merge as a result of excessive cell death, causing fusion of the bones. (Courtesy of A.E. Chudley, MD, Section of Genetics and Metabolism, Department of Pediatrics and Child Health, University of Manitoba, Children's Hospital, Winnipeg, Manitoba, Canada.)

FIGURE 15-29. Neonate with bilateral talipes equinovarus deformities (club feet), illustrating the classic type of this anomaly, characterized by inversion and medial rotation of the sole. (Courtesy of A.E. Chudley, MD, Section of Genetics and Metabolism, Department of Pediatrics and Child Health, University of Manitoba, Children's Hospital, Winnipeg, Manitoba, Canada.)

FIGURE 15-30. Limb anomalies caused by thalidomide. **A,** Quadruple amelia (absence of the upper and lower limbs). **B,** Meromelia (partial absence) of the upper limbs. The limbs are represented by rudimentary stumps. **C,** Meromelia in which the rudimentary upper limbs are attached directly to the trunk. (From Lenz W, Knapp K: Foetal malformations due to thalidomide. Ger Med Mon 7:253, 1962.)

CLINICALLY ORIENTED QUESTIONS

1. Occasionally, accessory ribs are associated with the seventh cervical vertebra and the first lumbar vertebra. Are these accessory ribs of clinical importance? What is the embryologic basis of accessory ribs?

2. What vertebral defect can produce scoliosis? Define this condition. What is the embryologic basis of the vertebral defect?

3. What is meant by the term *craniosynostosis*? What results from this developmental abnormality? Give a common example and describe it.

4. A child presented with characteristics of Klippel-Feil syndrome. What are the main features of this condition? What vertebral anomalies are usually present?

5. A newborn infant was born with prune-belly syndrome caused by failure of the abdominal musculature to develop normally. What do you think would cause this congenital anomaly? What urinary anomaly results from abnormal development of the anterior abdominal wall?

6. A boy asked his mother why one of his nipples was much lower than the other one. She was unable to explain this anomaly. How would you explain the abnormally low position of the nipple?

7. An 8-year-old girl asked her doctor why the muscle on one side of her neck was so prominent. What would you tell her? What would happen if this muscle were not treated?

8. After strenuous exercise, a young athlete complained of pain on the posteromedial aspect of his ankle. He was told that he had an accessory calf muscle. Is this possible? If so, what is the embryologic basis of this anomaly?

9. An infant had short limbs. His trunk was normally proportioned, but his head was slightly larger than normal. Both parents had normal limbs, and these problems had never occurred in either of their families. Could the mother's ingestion of drugs during pregnancy have caused these abnormalities? If not, what would be the probable cause of these skeletal disorders? Could they occur again if the couple had more children?

10. A woman is interested in marrying a man who happens to have very short fingers (brachydactyly). He says that two of his relatives have short fingers, but none of his brothers or sisters has them. The woman has normal digits, and so does everyone else in her family. Clearly, heredity is involved, but what are the chances that the couple's children would have brachydactyly if they were to marry?

11. Approximately 1 year ago, a woman was reported to have given birth to a child with no right hand. She had taken a drug that contained doxylamine and dicyclomine to alleviate nausea during the 10th week of her pregnancy (8 weeks after fertilization). The woman is instituting legal proceedings against the company that makes the drug. Does this drug cause limb defects? If it does, could it have caused failure of the child's hand to develop?

12. An infant had syndactyly of the left hand and absence of the left sternal head of the pectoralis major muscle. The infant seemed normal, except that the nipple on the left side was approximately 2 inches lower than the other one. What is the cause of these anomalies? Can they be corrected?

13. What is the most common type of clubfoot? How common is it? What is the appearance of the feet of infants born with this anomaly?

The answers to these questions are at the back of the book.

16

THE NERVOUS SYSTEM

The nervous system consists of three main parts:

- The *central nervous system* (CNS), which includes the brain and the spinal cord
- The *peripheral nervous system* (PNS), which includes neurons (nerve cells) outside the CNS and the cranial and spinal nerves that connect the brain and the spinal cord with the peripheral structures
- The *autonomic nervous system* (ANS), which has parts in both the CNS and the PNS and which consists of neurons that innervate smooth muscle, cardiac muscle, glandular epithelium, or combinations of these tissues

■ ORIGIN OF THE NERVOUS SYSTEM

The nervous system develops from the **neural plate** (Fig. 16-1*A* and *B*). The notochord and the paraxial mesoderm induce the overlying ectoderm to differentiate into the neural plate. Formation of the neural folds, neural tube, and neural crest from the neural plate is shown in Figure 16-1*B* to *F*. The neural tube differentiates into the CNS. The neural crest gives rise to the cells that form most of the PNS and the autonomic nervous system.

Formation of the neural plate and neural tube, a process known as **neurulation**, begins during the early part of the fourth week (22–23 days). Fusion of the neural folds proceeds in cranial and caudal directions until only small areas remain open at both ends (Fig. 16-2*A* and *B*). At these sites, the lumen of the neural tube—the **neural canal**—communicates freely with the amniotic cavity (see Fig. 16-2*C*). The cranial opening—the *rostral neuropore*—closes on approximately the 25th day; the *caudal neuropore* closes 2 days later (see Fig. 16-2*D*). **Closure of the neuropores** coincides with the establishment of a blood vascular circulation for the neural tube. The walls of the neural tube thicken to form the brain and the spinal cord (Fig. 16-3). The neural canal forms the ventricular system of the brain and the central canal of the spinal cord. *The dorsoventral patterning of the neural tube appears to involve the sonic hedgehog (Shh) gene, Pax genes, bone morphogenetic proteins, and dorsalin, a transforming growth factor (TGF-β).*

■ DEVELOPMENT OF THE SPINAL CORD

The neural tube caudal to the fourth pair of somites develops into the spinal cord (see Fig. 16-3). The lateral walls of the neural tube thicken and gradually reduce the size of the neural canal to a small **central canal** (Fig. 16-4*A* to *C*). Initially, the wall of the neural tube is composed of a thick, pseudostratified, columnar neuroepithelium (see Fig. 16-4*D*). These neuroepithelial cells constitute the **ventricular zone** (ependymal layer), which gives rise to all neurons and macroglial cells (e.g., astrocytes, oligodendrocytes) in the spinal cord (Fig. 16-5). Soon, a **marginal zone** composed of the outer parts of the neuroepithelial cells is recognizable (see Fig. 16-4*E*). This zone gradually becomes the white matter of the spinal cord as axons grow into it from nerve cell bodies in the spinal cord, spinal ganglia, and brain. Some neuroepithelial cells in the ventricular zone differentiate into primordial neurons—**neuroblasts**. These embryonic cells form an **intermediate zone** (mantle layer) between the ventricular and marginal zones. Neuroblasts become neurons as they develop cytoplasmic processes (see Fig. 16-5). The primordial supporting cells of the CNS—the **glioblasts** (spongioblasts)—differentiate from the neuroepithelial cells, mainly after neuroblast formation has ceased. The glioblasts migrate from the ventricular zone into the intermediate and marginal zones. Some glioblasts become **astroblasts** and later **astrocytes**, whereas others become oligodendroblasts and eventually **oligodendrocytes** (see Fig. 16-5). When neuroepithelial cells cease producing neuroblasts and glioblasts, they differentiate into ependymal cells, which form the **ependyma** lining the central canal of the spinal cord.

Microglial cells, scattered throughout the gray and white matter, are small cells that are derived from **mesenchymal cells** (see Fig. 16-5). Microglial cells invade the CNS rather late in the fetal period, after it has been penetrated by blood vessels. Microglia originate in the bone marrow and are part of the mononuclear phagocytic cell population. Proliferation and differentiation of neuroepithelial cells in the primordial spinal cord produce thick walls and thin roof and floor plates (see Fig. 16-4*B*). Differential thickening of the lateral walls of the spinal cord soon produces a shallow, longitudinal groove on each side, the **sulcus limitans** (Figs. 16-4*B* and 16-6). This groove separates the dorsal part, the **alar plate** (lamina), from the ventral part, the **basal plate** (lamina). The alar and basal plates produce longitudinal bulges extending through most of the length of the developing spinal cord. This regional separation is of fundamental importance because the alar and basal plates are later associated with afferent and efferent functions, respectively.

Cell bodies in the alar plates form the dorsal gray columns that extend the length of the spinal cord. In transverse sections, these columns are the **dorsal gray horns** (Fig. 16-7). Neurons in these columns constitute afferent nuclei, and groups of these nuclei form the **dorsal gray columns**. As the alar plates enlarge, the **dorsal median septum** forms. Cell bodies in the basal plates form the ventral and lateral gray columns. In transverse sections of the spinal cord, these columns are the **ventral gray horns** and the **lateral gray horns**, respectively. Axons of the ventral horn cells grow out of the cord and form the **ventral roots of the spinal nerves** (see Fig. 16-7). As the basal plates enlarge, they bulge ventrally on each side of the median plane. As this bulging occurs, the *ventral median septum* forms and a deep longitudinal groove—the ventral median fissure—develops on the ventral surface of the cord.

Development of the Spinal Ganglia

The unipolar neurons in the spinal ganglia (dorsal root ganglia) are derived from **neural crest cells** (see Fig. 16-7). The peripheral processes of the **spinal ganglion cells** pass in the spinal nerves to sensory endings in somatic or visceral structures. The central processes enter the spinal cord, constituting the **dorsal roots of the spinal nerves**.

FIGURE 16-1. The neural plate and its folding to form the neural tube. **A,** Dorsal view of an embryo at approximately 18 days, exposed by removing the amnion. **B,** Transverse section of the embryo, showing the neural plate and early development of the neural groove and neural folds. **C,** Dorsal view of an embryo at approximately 22 days. The neural folds have fused opposite the fourth to sixth somites, but are spread apart at both ends. **D** to **F,** Transverse sections of this embryo at the levels shown in **C,** showing the formation of the neural tube and its detachment from the surface ectoderm. Note that some neuroectodermal cells are not included in the neural tube, but remain between it and the surface ectoderm as the neural crest.

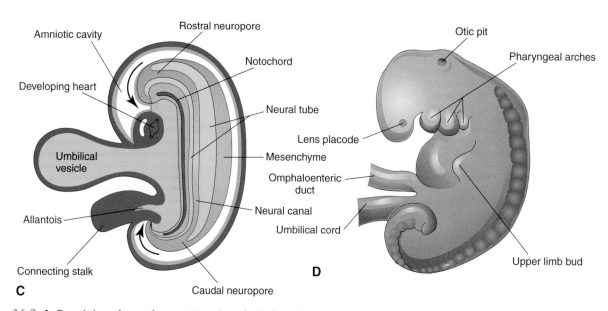

FIGURE 16-2. **A,** Dorsal view of an embryo at approximately 23 days, showing fusion of the neural folds, leading to formation of the neural tube. **B,** Lateral view of an embryo at approximately 24 days, showing the forebrain prominence and closing of the rostral neuropore. **C,** Sagittal section of the embryo, showing the transitory communication of the neural canal with the amniotic cavity *(arrows).* **D,** Lateral view of an embryo at approximately 27 days. Note that the neuropores shown in **B** are closed.

Development of the Spinal Meninges

The mesenchyme surrounding the neural tube condenses to form the primordial meninx (or meninges) (see Fig. 16-4*A, D*, and *E*). The external layer of this membrane gives rise to the dura mater (Fig. 16-8). The internal layer—the pia mater and the arachnoid mater—is derived from neural crest cells. Fluid-filled spaces appear within the leptomeninges that soon coalesce to form the **subarachnoid space** (Fig. 16-9*A*). Embryonic cerebrospinal fluid (CSF) begins to form during the fifth week.

Positional Changes of the Spinal Cord

The spinal cord in the embryo extends the entire length of the vertebral canal (see Fig. 16-8*A*). The spinal nerves pass through the intervertebral foramina opposite their levels of origin. Because the vertebral column and the dura mater grow more rapidly than the spinal cord, the positional relationship to the spinal nerves does not persist. The caudal end of the spinal cord gradually comes to lie at relatively higher levels. At 6 months, it lies at the level of the first sacral vertebra (see Fig. 16-8*B*). The **spinal**

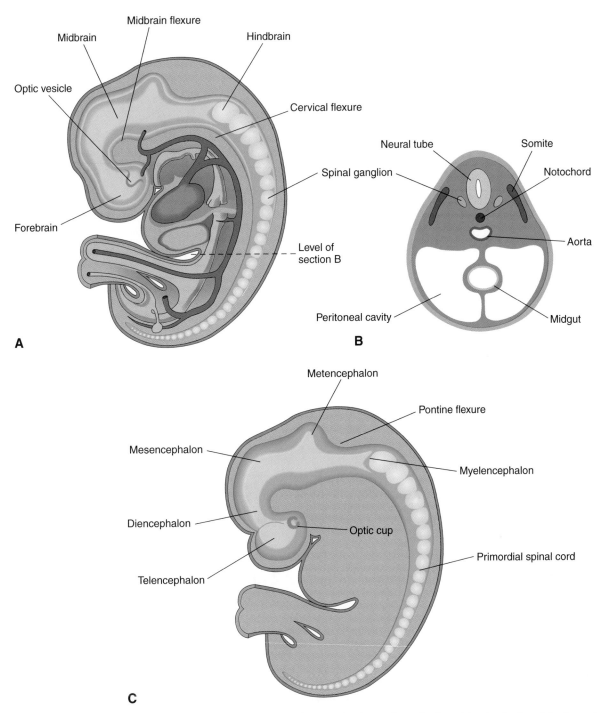

FIGURE 16-3. **A,** Lateral view of an embryo at approximately 28 days, showing the three primary brain vesicles: forebrain, midbrain, and hindbrain. Two flexures demarcate the primary divisions of the brain. **B,** Transverse section of the embryo, showing the neural tube that will develop into the spinal cord in this region. The spinal ganglia derived from the neural crest are also shown. **C,** Lateral view of the central nervous system of a 6-week embryo, showing the secondary brain vesicles and the pontine flexure. The flexure occurs as the brain grows rapidly.

cord in the newborn infant terminates at the level of the second or third lumbar vertebra (see Fig. 16-8C). The **spinal cord in the adult** usually terminates at the inferior border of the first lumbar vertebra (see Fig. 16-8D). As a result, the spinal nerve roots, especially those of the lumbar and sacral segments, run obliquely from the spinal cord to the corresponding level of the vertebral column. The nerve roots inferior to the end of the cord—the **medullary cone** ([Latin [L.] *conus medullaris*)—form a sheaf of nerve roots, the **cauda equina** (L. horse's tail). Although in adults the dura mater and the arachnoid mater usually end at the S₂ vertebra distal to the caudal end of the spinal cord, the pia mater forms a long, fibrous thread, the **terminal filum** (L. *filum terminale*) [see Fig. 16-8C and D]. The terminal filum

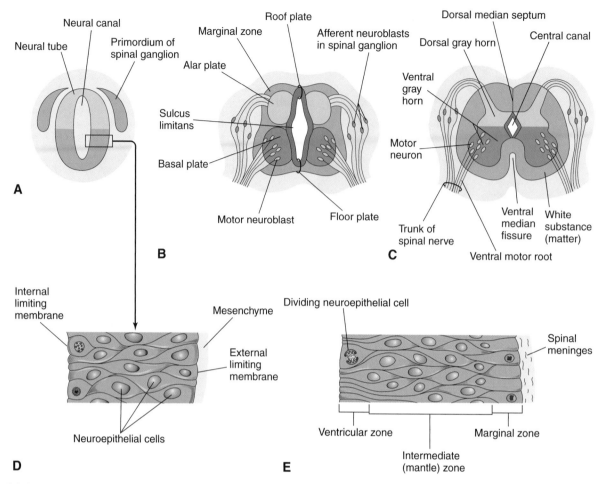

FIGURE 16-4. Development of the spinal cord. **A,** Transverse section of the neural tube of an embryo at approximately 23 days. **B** and **C,** Similar sections in 6- and 9-week embryos, respectively. **D,** Section of the wall of the neural tube shown in **A. E,** Section of the wall of the developing spinal cord, showing its three zones. In **A** to **C,** note that the neural canal of the neural tube is converted into the central canal of the spinal cord.

extends from the medullary cone to the periosteum of the first coccygeal vertebra.

Myelination of Nerve Fibers

Myelin sheaths in the spinal cord begin to form during the late fetal period and continue to form during the first postnatal year. In general, fiber tracts become myelinated at approximately the time they become functional. Motor roots are myelinated before sensory roots. The **myelin sheaths** surrounding the nerve fibers within the spinal cord are formed by **oligodendrocytes**. The myelin sheaths around the axons of peripheral nerve fibers are formed by the plasma membranes of the **neurolemma (Schwann) cells**. These neuroglial cells are derived from **neural crest cells** that migrate peripherally and wrap themselves around the axons of somatic motor neurons and presynaptic autonomic motor neurons as they pass out of the CNS (see Fig. 16-7). These cells also wrap themselves around both the central and the peripheral processes of the somatic and the visceral sensory neurons, as well as around the axons of postsynaptic autonomic motor neurons.

■ CONGENITAL ANOMALIES OF THE SPINAL CORD

Most congenital anomalies of the spinal cord result from defective closure of the neural tube during the fourth week. These **neural tube defects** (NTDs) affect the tissues overlying the spinal cord, including the meninges, neural arches, muscles, and skin (see Fig. 16-9B to D). Anomalies involving the neural arches are referred to as **spina bifida**.

SPINA BIFIDA OCCULTA

Spina bifida occulta results from failure of the embryonic halves of the neural arch to grow normally and fuse in the median plane (see Fig. 16-9A). Spina bifida occulta occurs in vertebra L_5 or S_1 in approximately 10% of otherwise normal people. In its most minor form, the only evidence of its presence may be a small dimple with a tuft of hair arising from it (Fig. 16-10). Spina bifida occulta usually produces no clinical symptoms.

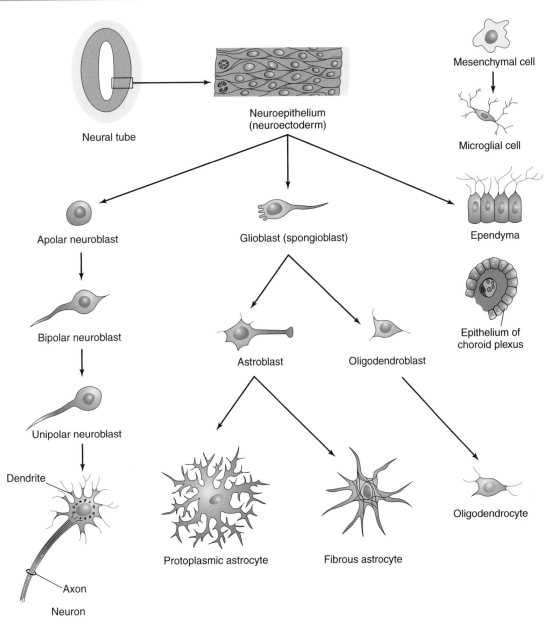

FIGURE 16-5. Histogenesis of cells in the central nervous system. After further development, the multipolar neuroblast *(lower left)* becomes a nerve cell or a neuron. Neuroepithelial cells give rise to all neurons and macroglial cells. Microglial cells are derived from the mesenchymal cells that invade the developing nervous system with the blood vessels.

SPINA BIFIDA CYSTICA

Severe types of spina bifida, involving protrusion of the spinal cord, the meninges, or both through the defects in the vertebral arches, are referred to collectively as **spina bifida cystica** because of the cystlike sac that is associated with these anomalies (Figs. 16-9B to D and 16-11). Spina bifida cystica occurs in approximately 1 in 1000 births. When the sac contains meninges and CSF, the anomaly is called **spina bifida with meningocele** (see Fig. 16-9B). The spinal cord and the spinal roots are in their normal position, but spinal cord abnormalities may be present. If the spinal cord, nerve roots, or both are included in the sac, the anomaly is called **spina bifida with meningomyelocele** (see Figs. 16-9C and 16-11). Meningoceles are rare compared with meningomyeloceles. Spina bifida with meningomyelocele involving several vertebrae is often associated with partial absence of the brain— meroencephaly (anencephaly) (Fig. 16-12).

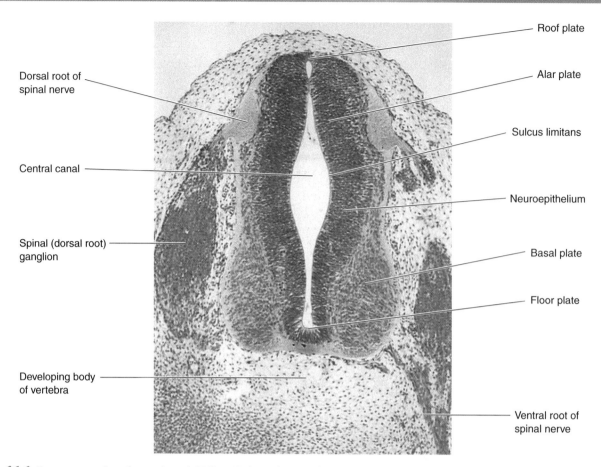

Roof plate

Alar plate

Sulcus limitans

Neuroepithelium

Basal plate

Floor plate

Ventral root of spinal nerve

Dorsal root of spinal nerve

Central canal

Spinal (dorsal root) ganglion

Developing body of vertebra

FIGURE 16-6. Transverse section of an embryo (×100) at 40 days. The ventral root of the spinal nerve is composed of nerve fibers arising from neuroblasts in the basal plate, whereas the dorsal root is formed by nerve processes arising from neuroblasts in the spinal ganglion.

CAUSES OF NEURAL TUBE DEFECTS

Genetic, nutritional, and environmental factors play a role in the production of NTDs. Epidemiologic studies have shown that some vitamins and folic acid supplements taken before or after conception reduce the incidence of NTDs. Certain drugs increase the risk of NTD. For example, valproic acid, an anticonvulsant, causes NTDs in 1% to 2% of pregnant women if given during the fourth week of development, when the neural folds are fusing.

■ DEVELOPMENT OF THE BRAIN

The **neural tube** cranial to the fourth pair of somites develops into the brain. Even before the neural folds are completely fused, three distinct vesicles are recognizable in the rostral end of the developing neural tube. From rostral to caudal, these three **primary brain vesicles** (Fig. 16-13) form the *forebrain* (prosencephalon), the *midbrain* (mesencephalon), and the *hindbrain* (rhombencephalon). By the beginning of the fourth week, the forebrain partially divides into two **secondary brain vesicles**, the *telencephalon* and the

diencephalon. By the fifth week, the hindbrain gives rise to the metencephalon and the myelencephalon (see Fig. 16-13).

Brain Flexures

The embryonic brain grows rapidly and bends ventrally with the head fold. This bending produces the **midbrain flexure** in the midbrain region and the **cervical flexure** at the junction of the hindbrain and the spinal cord (Fig. 16-14A). Later, unequal growth of the brain between these flexures produces the **pontine flexure** in the opposite direction. This flexure results in thinning of the roof of the hindbrain. The **sulcus limitans** extends cranially to the junction of the midbrain and the forebrain, and the alar and basal plates are recognizable only in the midbrain and the hindbrain (see Fig. 16-4B).

Hindbrain

The cervical flexure demarcates the hindbrain from the spinal cord (see Fig. 16-14A). The pontine flexure divides the hindbrain into caudal (myelencephalon) and rostral (metencephalon) parts. The myelencephalon becomes the **medulla oblongata**, or medulla, whereas the metencephalon becomes the **pons** and the **cerebellum**. The cavity of the

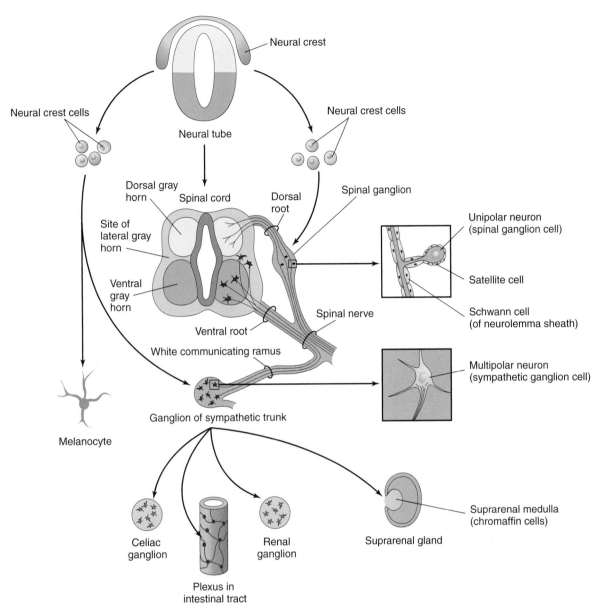

FIGURE 16-7. Derivatives of the neural crest. Neural crest cells also differentiate into the cells in the afferent ganglia of cranial nerves and many other structures. The formation of a spinal nerve is also shown.

hindbrain becomes the fourth ventricle and the central canal in the caudal part of the medulla (see Fig. 16-14B).

Myelencephalon

Neuroblasts from the alar plates in the myelencephalon migrate into the marginal zone and form isolated areas of gray matter known as the **gracile nuclei** medially and the **cuneate nuclei** laterally (see Fig. 16-14B). These nuclei are associated with correspondingly named tracts that enter the medulla from the spinal cord. The ventral area of the medulla contains a pair of fiber bundles—**pyramids**—that consist of corticospinal fibers descending from the developing cerebral cortex.

The rostral part of the myelencephalon (the "open" part of the medulla) is wide and rather flat, especially opposite

the pontine flexure (see Fig. 16-14C and D). As the pontine flexure is formed, the walls of the medulla move laterally and the alar plates come to lie lateral to the basal plates. As the positions of the plates change, the motor nuclei generally develop medial to the sensory nuclei.

Neuroblasts in the basal plates of the medulla, like those in the spinal cord, develop into motor neurons. In the medulla, the neuroblasts form nuclei (groups of nerve cells) and organize into three cell columns on each side (see Fig. 16-14D). From medial to lateral, they are:

● *The general somatic efferent,* represented by neurons of the hypoglossal nerve
● *The special visceral efferent,* represented by neurons innervating muscles derived from the pharyngeal arches (see Chapter 10)
● *The general visceral efferent,* represented by some neurons of the vagus and the glossopharyngeal nerves

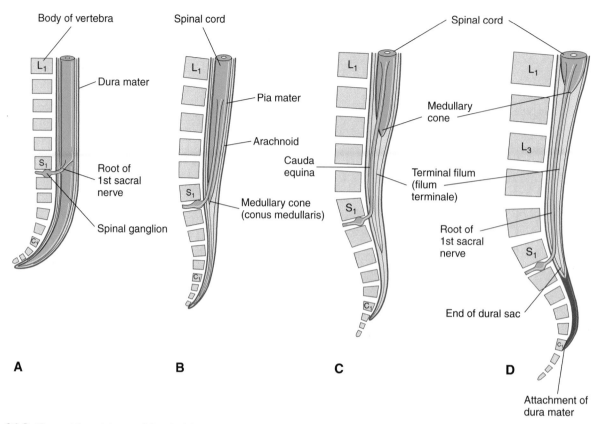

FIGURE 16-8. The position of the caudal end of the spinal cord in relation to the vertebral column and the meninges at various stages of development. The increasing inclination of the root of the first sacral nerve is also shown. **A,** At 8 weeks. **B,** At 24 weeks. **C,** Newborn infant. **D,** Adult.

Neuroblasts of the alar plates of the medulla form neurons that are arranged in four columns on each side (see Fig. 16-14D). From medial to lateral, they are:

- *The general visceral afferent,* receiving impulses from the viscera
- *The special visceral afferent,* receiving taste fibers
- *The general somatic afferent,* receiving impulses from the surface of the head
- *The special somatic afferent,* receiving impulses from the ear

Some neuroblasts from the alar plates migrate ventrally and form the neurons in the **olivary nuclei** (see Fig. 16-14C and D).

Metencephalon

The walls of the metencephalon form the **pons** and the **cerebellum,** and its cavity forms the superior part of the fourth ventricle (Fig. 16-15). As in the rostral part of the myelencephalon, the pontine flexure causes divergence of the lateral walls of the pons, which spreads the gray substance in the floor of the fourth ventricle. Neuroblasts in each basal plate develop into motor nuclei and organize into three columns on each side.

The **cerebellum** develops from the dorsal parts of the alar plates (see Fig. 16-15A and B). Initially, the **cerebellar swellings** project into the fourth ventricle (see Fig. 16-15C).

As the swellings enlarge and fuse in the median plane, they overgrow the rostral half of the fourth ventricle and overlap the pons and the medulla (see Fig. 16-15D). Some neuroblasts in the intermediate zone of the alar plates migrate to the marginal zone and differentiate into the neurons of the **cerebellar cortex.** Other neuroblasts from these plates give rise to the central nuclei, the largest of which is the **dentate nucleus** (see Fig 16-15D). Cells from the alar plates also give rise to the **pontine nuclei,** the cochlear and vestibular nuclei, and the sensory nuclei of the trigeminal nerve.

Nerve fibers connecting the cerebral and cerebellar cortices with the spinal cord pass through the marginal layer of the ventral region of the metencephalon—**the pons** (see Fig. 16-15C and D).

Choroid Plexuses and Cerebrospinal Fluid (CSF)

The thin ependymal roof of the fourth ventricle is covered externally by the *pia mater* (see Fig. 16-15C and D). This vascular membrane, together with the ependymal roof, forms the **tela choroidea.** Because of the active proliferation of the pia mater, the tela choroidea invaginates the fourth ventricle, where it differentiates into the **choroid plexus.** Similar choroid plexuses develop in the roof of the third ventricle and in the medial walls of the lateral ventricles. *The choroid plexuses secrete CSF.* The thin roof of

FIGURE 16-9. Various types of spina bifida. **A,** Spina bifida occulta. Observe the unfused vertebral arch. **B,** Spina bifida with meningocele. **C,** Spina bifida with meningomyelocele. **D,** Spina bifida with myeloschisis. This severe type of spina bifida results from failure of the caudal neuropore to close at the end of the fourth week of development. The types shown in **B** to **D** are referred to collectively as *spina bifida cystica* because of the cystlike sac that is associated with them.

the fourth ventricle evaginates in three locations. These outpouchings rupture to form openings, the **median and lateral apertures**. These apertures permit CSF to enter the **subarachnoid space** from the fourth ventricle.

Midbrain

The midbrain (mesencephalon) undergoes very little change. The neural canal narrows and becomes the **cerebral aqueduct** (see Fig. 16-15D), a canal that connects the third and fourth ventricles. Neuroblasts migrate from the alar plates of the midbrain into the **tectum** (roof), where they aggregate to form four large groups of neurons—the paired **superior and inferior colliculi** (Fig. 16-16B), which are concerned with visual and auditory reflexes, respectively. Neuroblasts from the basal plates appear to give rise to groups of neurons in the **tegmentum** (red nuclei, nuclei of the third and fourth cranial nerves, and reticular nuclei). The **substantia nigra**, a broad layer of gray matter adjacent to the cerebral peduncle (see Fig. 16-16D and E), may also differentiate from the basal plate, but some authorities believe that it is derived from cells in the alar plate that migrate ventrally. Fibers growing from

the cerebrum form the **cerebral peduncles** anteriorly (see Fig. 16-16B). These peduncles become progressively more prominent as additional descending fiber groups (corticopontine, corticobulbar, and corticospinal) pass through the developing midbrain on their way to the brainstem and the spinal cord.

Forebrain

As closure of the rostral neuropore occurs, two lateral outgrowths—**optic vesicles**—appear (see Fig. 16-3A), one on each side of the forebrain. The optic vesicles are the primordia of the retinas and the optic nerves. A second pair of diverticula soon arises more dorsally and rostrally, representing the **telencephalic vesicles** (see Fig. 16-16C). They are the primordia of the **cerebral hemispheres**, and their cavities become the **lateral ventricles**. The rostral, or anterior, part of the forebrain, including the primordia of the cerebral hemispheres, is known as the **telencephalon**, whereas the caudal, or posterior, part of the forebrain is called the **diencephalon**. The cavities of the telencephalon and the diencephalon contribute to the formation of the **third ventricle** (Fig. 16-17D and E).

FIGURE 16-10. A female child with a hairy patch in the lumbosacral region, indicating the site of a spina bifida occulta. (Courtesy of A.E. Chudley, MD, Section of Genetics and Metabolism, Department of Pediatrics and Child Health, Children's Hospital and University of Manitoba, Winnipeg, Manitoba, Canada.)

Diencephalon

Three swellings develop in the lateral walls of the third ventricle; these later become the epithalamus, thalamus, and hypothalamus (see Fig. 16-17C to E). The **thalamus** develops rapidly on each side and bulges into the cavity of the third ventricle, eventually reducing it to a narrow cleft. The **hypothalamus** arises by the proliferation of neuroblasts in the intermediate zone of the diencephalic walls. A pair of nuclei, the **mammillary bodies**, form pea-sized swellings on the ventral surface of the hypothalamus (see Fig. 16-17C). The **epithalamus** develops from the roof and the dorsal part of the lateral wall of the diencephalon.

FIGURE 16-11. The back of a newborn infant with a large lumbar meningomyelocele. The neural tube defect is covered with a thin membrane. (Courtesy of A.E. Chudley, MD, Section of Genetics and Metabolism, Department of Pediatrics and Child Health, Children's Hospital and University of Manitoba, Winnipeg, Manitoba, Canada.)

FIGURE 16-12. **A,** A fetus with meroencephaly (anencephaly). **B,** The neural tube defect was detected by ultrasonography at 18 weeks' gestation. Note the absence of the calvaria and the presence of some brain tissue. (Courtesy of Wesley Lee, MD, Division of Fetal Imaging, Department of Obstetrics and Gynecology, William Beaumont Hospital, Royal Oak, Michigan.)

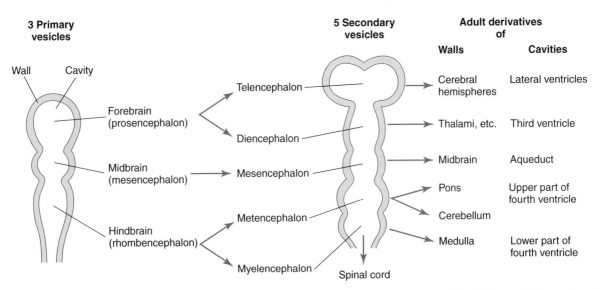

FIGURE 16-13. Brain vesicles, indicating the adult derivatives of their walls and cavities. The rostral part of the third ventricle forms from the cavity of the telencephalon; most of this ventricle is derived from the cavity of the diencephalon.

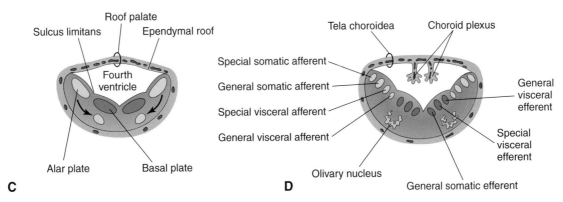

FIGURE 16-14. A, The developing brain at the end of the fifth week, showing the three primary divisions of the brain and the brain flexures. B, Transverse section of the caudal part of the myelencephalon. C and D, Similar sections of the rostral part of the myelencephalon, showing the position and successive stages of differentiation of the alar and basal plates. The *arrows* in C show the pathway taken by the neuroblasts from the alar plates to form the olivary nuclei.

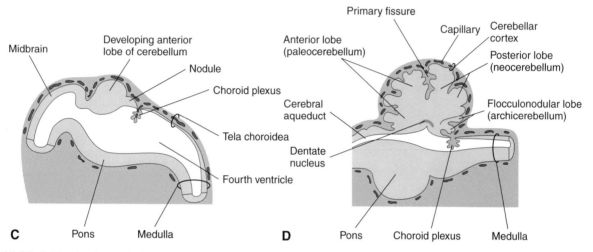

FIGURE 16-15. **A,** The developing brain at the end of the fifth week. **B,** Transverse section of the metencephalon (developing pons and cerebellum), showing the derivatives of the alar and basal plates. **C** and **D,** Sagittal sections of the hindbrain at 6 and 17 weeks, respectively, showing successive stages in the development of the pons and cerebellum.

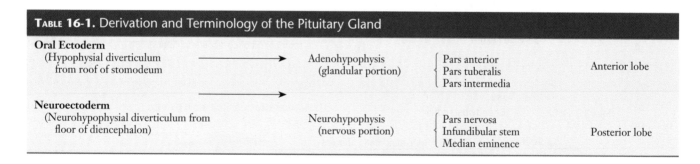

TABLE 16-1. Derivation and Terminology of the Pituitary Gland

Oral Ectoderm (Hypophysial diverticulum from roof of stomodeum	→ Adenohypophysis (glandular portion)	Pars anterior Pars tuberalis Pars intermedia	Anterior lobe
Neuroectoderm (Neurohypophysial diverticulum from floor of diencephalon)	→ Neurohypophysis (nervous portion)	Pars nervosa Infundibular stem Median eminence	Posterior lobe

Initially, the epithalamic swellings are large, but later, they become relatively small. The **pineal gland** (body) develops as a median diverticulum of the caudal part of the roof of the diencephalon (see Fig. 16-17D). Proliferation of the cells in its walls soon converts it into a solid, cone-shaped gland.

The **pituitary gland** (Fig. 16-18 and Table 16-1) is ectodermal in origin. It develops from two sources:

● An upgrowth from the ectodermal roof of the stomodeum—**hypophysial diverticulum**
● A downgrowth from the neuroectoderm of the diencephalon—**neurohypophysial diverticulum**

This double embryonic origin explains why the pituitary gland is composed of two different types of tissue.
● The **adenohypophysis** (glandular part), or anterior lobe, arises from the oral ectoderm.
● The **neurohypophysis** (nervous part), or posterior lobe, originates from the neuroectoderm.

During the fourth week, a **hypophysial diverticulum** projects from the roof of the stomodeum and lies adjacent to the floor (ventral wall) of the diencephalon (see Fig. 16-18A and B). By the fifth week, this pouch has elongated and has become constricted at its attachment to the oral epithelium, giving it a nipple-like appearance (see Fig. 16-18C). By this

FIGURE 16-16. **A,** The developing brain at the end of the fifth week. **B,** Transverse section of the developing midbrain, showing the early migration of cells from the basal and alar plates. **C,** The developing brain at 11 weeks. **D** and **E,** Transverse sections of the developing midbrain at the level of the inferior and superior colliculi, respectively.

stage, it has come into contact with the **infundibulum** (derived from the neurohypophysial diverticulum), a ventral downgrowth of the diencephalon (see Fig. 16-18*C*). The hypophysial diverticulum stalk regresses (see Fig 16-18*D*). The parts of the pituitary gland that develop from the ectoderm of the stomodeum—pars anterior, pars intermedia, and pars tuberalis—form the **adenohypophysis** (see Table 16-1).

Cells of the anterior wall of the hypophysial diverticulum give rise to the **pars anterior** of the pituitary gland. Later, a small extension, the **pars tuberalis**, grows around the infundibular stem. The extensive proliferation of the anterior wall of the hypophysial diverticulum reduces its lumen to a narrow cleft (see Fig. 16-18*E*). Cells in the posterior wall of the hypophysial diverticulum do not proliferate; they give rise to the thin, poorly defined **pars intermedia** (see Fig. 16-18*F*). The part of the pituitary gland that develops from the neuroectoderm of the brain (infundibulum) is the **neurohypophysis**. The infundibulum gives rise to the *median eminence, the infundibular stem, and the pars nervosa.*

PHARYNGEAL HYPOPHYSIS AND CRANIOPHARYNGIOMA

A remnant of the stalk of the hypophysial diverticulum may persist and form a pharyngeal hypophysis in the roof of the oropharynx (Fig. 16-18*E* and *F*). Occasionally, craniopharyngiomas from remnants of the stalk of the hypophysial diverticulum develop in the pharynx or in the basisphenoid (posterior part of the sphenoid bone), but most often, they form in or superior to the sella turcica of the cranium (Fig. 16-19).

Telencephalon

The telencephalon consists of a median part and two lateral diverticula, the **cerebral vesicles** (see Fig. 16-18*A*). These vesicles give rise to the **cerebral hemispheres**, which are identifiable at 7 weeks (Fig. 16-20*A*). The cavity of the median part of the telencephalon forms the extreme

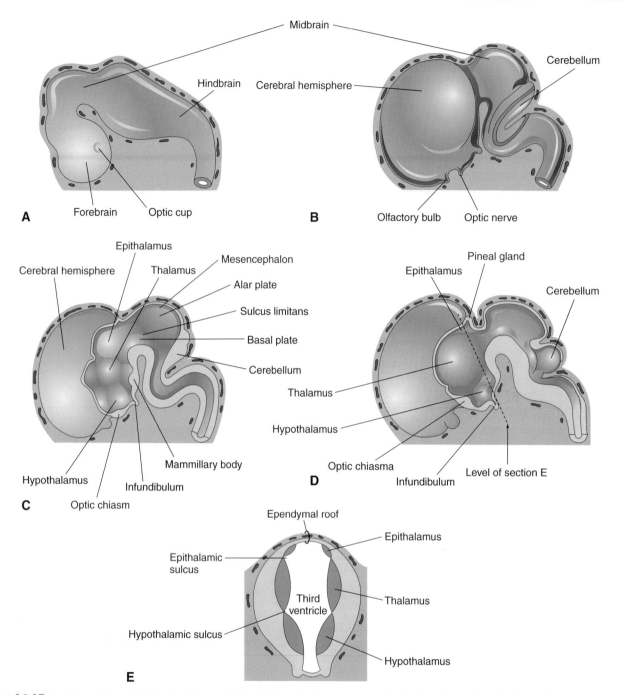

FIGURE 16-17. **A,** External view of the brain at the end of the fifth week of development. **B,** Similar view at 7 weeks. **C,** Median section of the brain, showing the medial surface of the forebrain and midbrain. **D,** Similar section at 8 weeks. **E,** Transverse section of the diencephalon, showing the epithalamus dorsally, the thalamus laterally, and the hypothalamus ventrally.

anterior part of the third ventricle. At first, the cerebral hemispheres are in wide communication with the cavity of the third ventricle through the **interventricular foramina** (see Fig. 16-20B). As the cerebral hemispheres expand, they cover successively the diencephalon, the midbrain, and the hindbrain. The hemispheres eventually meet each other in the midline, flattening their medial surfaces.

The **corpus striatum** appears during the sixth week as a prominent swelling in the floor of each cerebral hemisphere (Fig. 16-21B). As a result, the floor of each hemisphere expands more slowly than its thin cortical wall, and

the cerebral hemispheres become C-shaped (Fig. 16-22). The growth and curvature of the hemispheres also affect the shape of the lateral ventricles. They become roughly C-shaped cavities filled with CSF. The caudal end of each cerebral hemisphere turns ventrally and then rostrally, forming the temporal lobe; in so doing, it carries with it the ventricle (forming the temporal horn) and the **choroid fissure** (see Fig. 16-22). Here, the thin medial wall of the hemisphere is invaginated along the choroid fissure by the vascular pia mater to form the *choroid plexus of the temporal horn* of the lateral ventricle (see Figs. 16-21B and 16-22B).

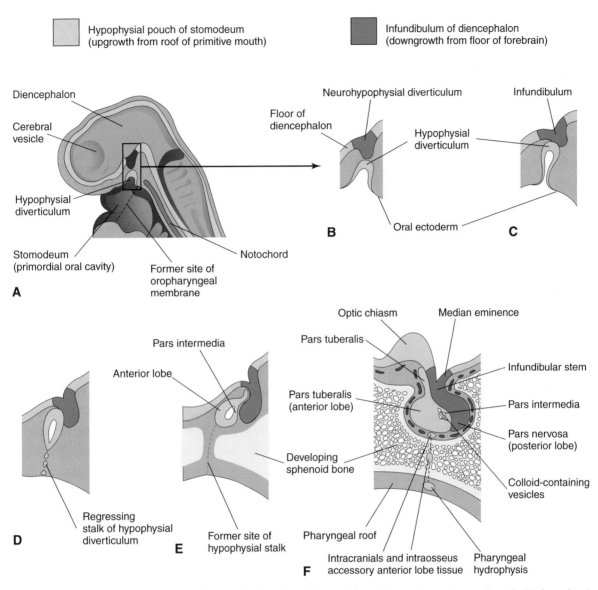

Hypophysial pouch of stomodeum (upgrowth from roof of primitive mouth)

Infundibulum of diencephalon (downgrowth from floor of forebrain)

FIGURE 16-18. Development of the pituitary gland. **A,** Sagittal section of the cranial end of an embryo at approximately 36 days, showing the hypophysial diverticulum (pouch), an upgrowth from the stomodeum, and the neurohypophysial diverticulum, a downgrowth from the forebrain. **B to D,** Successive stages of the developing pituitary gland. By 8 weeks, the diverticulum loses its connection with the oral cavity and is in close contact with the infundibulum and the posterior lobe (neurohypophysis) of the pituitary gland. **E and F,** Later stages, showing proliferation of the anterior wall of the hypophysial diverticulum to form the anterior lobe (adenohypophysis) of the pituitary gland.

As the cerebral cortex differentiates, fibers passing to and from it pass through the **corpus striatum** and divide it into the *caudate and lentiform nuclei.* This fiber pathway—the **internal capsule** (see Fig. 16-21*C*)—becomes C shaped as the hemisphere assumes this form. The **caudate nucleus** becomes elongated and C-shaped, conforming to the outline of the lateral ventricle (see Fig. 16-22*A* to *C*). Its pear-shaped head and elongated body lie in the floor of the frontal horn and the body of the lateral ventricle; its tail makes a U-shaped turn to gain the roof of the temporal horn.

Cerebral Commissures

As the cerebral cortex develops, groups of fibers—**commissures**—connect corresponding areas of the cerebral hemispheres with one another (see Fig. 16-21). The most important commissures cross in the **lamina terminalis,** the rostral end of the forebrain. This lamina extends from the roof plate of the diencephalon to the optic chiasm. The **anterior commissure** connects the olfactory bulb and the related brain areas of one hemisphere with those of the opposite side. The **hippocampal commissure** connects the hippocampal formations. The anterior and hippocampal commissures connect phylogenetically older parts of the brain and are the first to form. The **corpus callosum** (see Fig. 16-21*A*), the largest cerebral commissure, connects the neocortical areas. The rest of the lamina terminalis becomes stretched to form the **septum pellucidum,** a thin plate of brain tissue. At birth, the corpus callosum extends over the roof of the diencephalon. The **optic chiasm,** which develops in

FIGURE 16-19. Magnetic resonance image of a large craniopharyngioma *(arrow)*. (Courtesy of Dr. R. Shane Tubbs and Dr. W. Jerry Oakes, Children's Hospital, Birmingham, Alabama.)

the ventral part of the lamina terminalis (Fig. 16-21*A*), consists of fibers from the medial halves of the retinas that cross to join the optic tract of the opposite side.

Initially, the surface of the hemispheres is smooth (Fig. 16-23); however, as growth proceeds, **sulci** (grooves) and **gyri** (convolutions) develop (see Fig. 16-23). The sulci and gyri permit a considerable increase in the surface area of the cerebral cortex without requiring an extensive increase in cranial size. As each cerebral hemisphere grows, the cortex covering the external surface of the corpus striatum grows relatively slowly and is soon overgrown. This buried cortex,

hidden from view in the depths of the lateral sulcus (fissure) of the cerebral hemisphere, is known as the **insula**.

■ CONGENITAL ANOMALIES OF THE BRAIN

Because of the complexity of its embryologic history, abnormal development of the brain is common (occurring with a frequency of approximately 3 in 1000 births). Most major congenital anomalies of the brain result from defective closure of the rostral neuropore during the fourth week of development (Fig. 16-24) and involve the overlying tissues (meninges and calvaria). The factors causing neural tube defects (NTDs) are genetic, nutritional, or environmental.

CRANIUM BIFIDUM

Defects in the formation of the cranium (cranium bifidum) are often associated with congenital anomalies of the brain, meninges, or both. Defects of the cranium usually involve the median plane of the calvaria. The defect is often in the squamous part of the occipital bone and may include the posterior part of the foramen magnum. When the defect is small, usually only the meninges herniate, and the anomaly is called a *cranial meningocele.* Cranium bifidum associated with herniation of the brain, the meninges, or both occurs in approximately 1 in 2000 births. When the cranial defect is large, the meninges and part of the brain herniate, forming a meningoencephalocele (see Fig. 16-24*A* and *B*). If the protruding brain contains part of the ventricular system, the anomaly is called a *meningohydroencephalocele* (see Fig. 16-23*C*).

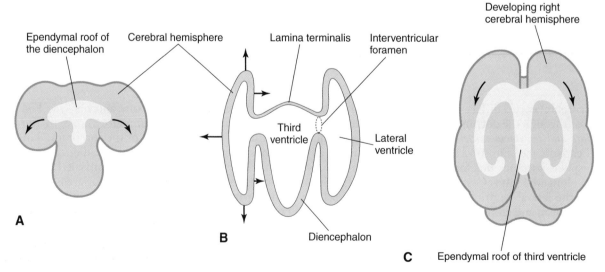

FIGURE 16-20. **A,** Dorsal surface of the forebrain, showing how the ependymal roof of the diencephalon is carried out to the dorsomedial surface of the cerebral hemispheres. **B,** The forebrain, showing how the developing cerebral hemispheres grow from the lateral walls of the forebrain and expand in all directions until they cover the diencephalon. The rostral wall of the forebrain, the lamina terminalis, is very thin. **C,** The forebrain, showing how the ependymal roof is finally carried into the temporal lobes as a result of the C-shaped growth pattern of the cerebral hemispheres. The *arrows* indicate some of the directions in which the hemispheres expand.

FIGURE 16-21. **A,** Medial surface of the forebrain of a 10-week embryo, showing the diencephalic derivatives, the main commissures, and the expanding cerebral hemispheres. **B,** Transverse section of the forebrain at the level of the interventricular foramina, showing the corpus striatum and the choroid plexuses of the lateral ventricles. **C,** Similar section at approximately 11 weeks, showing division of the corpus striatum into the caudate and lentiform nuclei by the internal capsule. The developing relationship of the cerebral hemispheres to the diencephalon is also shown.

MEROENCEPHALY AND EXENCEPHALY

Meroencephaly (anencephaly) is a severe anomaly of the brain that results from failure of the rostral neuropore to close during the fourth week of development. As a result, the forebrain primordium is abnormal and development of the calvaria is defective (see Fig. 16-12). In such cases, most of the infant's brain extrudes from the cranium, a condition known as *exencephaly*. Because of the abnormal structure and vascularization of the embryonic exencephalic brain, the nervous tissue undergoes degeneration, leaving a spongy, vascular mass consisting mostly of hindbrain structures. Although this NTD is often called *anencephaly* (Greek *an*, without + *enkephalos*, brain), a rudimentary brain stem and functioning neural tissue are always present. For this reason, *meroencephaly* (Greek *meros*, part) is a better name for this anomaly. Meroencephaly is a common lethal anomaly, occurring at a rate of at least 1 in 1000 births. It is more common in females than in males. Meroencephaly is usually associated with a multifactorial pattern of inheritance. Polyhydramnios (excess amniotic fluid) is often associated with this anomaly, possibly because the fetus lacks the neural control for swallowing amniotic fluid.

A

B

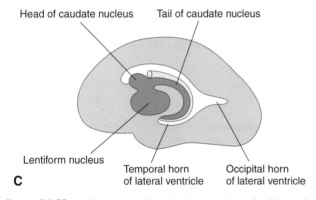

C

FIGURE 16-22. Medial surface of the developing right cerebral hemisphere, showing the development of the lateral ventricle, choroid fissure, and corpus striatum. **A,** At 13 weeks. **B,** At 21 weeks. **C,** At 32 weeks.

MICROCEPHALY

In microcephaly, the calvaria and the brain are small, but the face is of normal size. Affected infants are grossly mentally retarded because the brain is underdeveloped. Some cases of microcephaly appear to be genetic (autosomal recessive); others are caused by environmental factors, such as cytomegalovirus infection in utero (see Chapter 19). Exposure during the fetal period to large amounts of ionizing radiation, infectious agents, and certain drugs (as with maternal alcohol abuse) is a contributing factor in some cases.

HYDROCEPHALUS

Hydrocephalus results from impaired circulation and absorption of CSF or, in unusual cases, from increased production of CSF by a choroid plexus adenoma. An excess of CSF is present in the ventricular system of the brain (Fig. 16-25). Impaired circulation of CSF often results from congenital aqueductal stenosis (narrow cerebral aqueduct). Blockage of CSF circulation results in dilation of the ventricles proximal to the obstruction and increased pressure on the cerebral hemispheres. This squeezes the brain between the ventricular fluid and the calvaria. In infants, the internal pressure results in an accelerated rate of expansion of the brain and the calvaria because the fibrous sutures of the calvaria are not fused. All ventricles are enlarged if the apertures of the fourth ventricle or the subarachnoid spaces are blocked, whereas only the lateral and third ventricles are dilated when the cerebral aqueduct is obstructed. Hydrocephalus resulting from obliteration of the subarachnoid cisterns or malfunction of the arachnoid villi is known as *nonobstructive, or communicating, hydrocephalus.* Hydrocephalus may be associated with spina bifida cystica.

16 weeks   22 weeks   27 weeks   40 weeks

FIGURE 16-23. Lateral and medial surfaces of human fetal brains at 16, 22, 27, and 40 weeks' gestation. As the brain enlarges, the gyral pattern of the cerebral hemispheres becomes more complex. Note that, in the younger brains, the leptomeninges and associated blood vessels are not shown. (Courtesy of Dr. Marc R. Del Bigio, Department of Pathology [Neuropathology], University of Manitoba and Health Sciences Centre, Winnipeg, Manitoba, Canada.)

FIGURE 16-24. Cranium bifidum (bony defect in the cranium) and herniation of the brain and meninges. **A,** Infant with a large meningoencephalocele in the occipital area. **B,** Meningoencephalocele consisting of a protrusion of part of the cerebellum that is covered by meninges and skin. **C,** Meningohydroencephalocele consisting of a protrusion of part of the occipital lobe that contains part of the posterior horn of a lateral ventricle. (**A,** Courtesy of A.E. Chudley, MD, Section of Genetics and Metabolism, Department of Pediatrics and Child Health, Children's Hospital and University of Manitoba, Winnipeg, Manitoba, Canada.)

FIGURE 16-25. **A,** An infant with hydrocephalus and a bilateral cleft palate. Hydrocephalus often produces thinning of the bones of the calvaria, prominence of the forehead, and atrophy of the cerebral cortex and white substance. **B,** Axial magnetic resonance imaging scan (transverse section through the brain) of a fetus with X-linked hydrocephalus at approximately 29 weeks' gestation, showing the massively enlarged ventricles and thinned cortex. (Courtesy of Dr. E.H. Whitby, Magnetic Resonance Imaging Unit, University of Sheffield, UK.)

HOLOPROSENCEPHALY

Holoprosencephaly results from a failure of cleavage of the forebrain. It occurs in approximately 1 in 15,000 to 1 in 20,000 live births. Most affected infants die within 6 months. Infants with this condition have a small, undivided forebrain and often a large, single, fused ventricle. Defects in forebrain development usually induce facial anomalies. This severe spectrum of congenital anomalies is attributable to genetic and environmental factors that cause extensive cell death in the median plane of the embryonic disc during the third week.

ARNOLD-CHIARI MALFORMATION

Arnold-Chiari malformation is the most common congenital anomaly involving the cerebellum (Fig. 16-26). A tonguelike projection of the medulla and inferior displacement of the vermis of the cerebellum herniate through the foramen magnum into the vertebral canal. The condition results in a type of communicating hydrocephalus in which there is interference with the absorption of CSF; as a result, the entire ventricular system is distended. Arnold-Chiari malformation occurs in approximately 1 in 1000 births and is frequently associated with spina bifida with meningomyelocele, spina bifida with myeloschisis, and hydrocephalus. The cause of Arnold-Chiari malformation is uncertain; however, the posterior cranial fossa is abnormally small in some infants.

FIGURE 16-26. Arnold-Chiari type II malformation in a 23-week fetus. In situ exposure of the hindbrain shows cerebellar tissue well below the foramen magnum (arrow). (Courtesy of Dr. Marc R. Del Bigio, Department of Pathology [Neuropathology], University of Manitoba, Winnipeg, Manitoba, Canada.)

■ DEVELOPMENT OF THE PERIPHERAL NERVOUS SYSTEM

The PNS consists of cranial, spinal, and visceral nerves and cranial, spinal, and autonomic ganglia. All of the sensory cells (somatic and visceral) of the PNS are derived from **neural crest cells**. The cell bodies of these sensory cells are located outside the CNS. The cell body of each afferent neuron is closely invested by a capsule of modified Schwann cells, called *satellite cells* (see Fig. 16-7), which are derived from neural crest cells. This capsule is continuous with the neurolemma sheath of Schwann cells that surrounds the axons of afferent neurons.

Neural crest cells in the developing brain migrate to form sensory ganglia only in relation to the trigeminal (cranial nerve [CN] V), facial (CN VII), vestibulocochlear (CN VIII), glossopharyngeal (CN IX), and vagus (CN X) nerves. Neural crest cells also differentiate into multipolar neurons of the *autonomic ganglia* (see Fig. 16-7), including ganglia of the sympathetic trunks that lie along the sides of the vertebral bodies; collateral or prevertebral ganglia in the plexuses of the thorax and abdomen (e.g., cardiac,

celiac, and mesenteric plexuses); and parasympathetic, or terminal ganglia in or near the viscera (e.g., submucosal, or Meissner, plexus). Paraganglia—**chromaffin cells**—are also derived from the neural crest. The term *paraganglia* includes several widely scattered groups of cells that are similar in many ways to the medullary cells of the suprarenal glands. The cell groups largely lie retroperitoneally, often in association with sympathetic ganglia. The carotid and aortic bodies also have small islands of chromaffin cells associated with them. These widely scattered groups of chromaffin cells constitute the **chromaffin system**.

Spinal Nerves

Motor nerve fibers arising from the spinal cord begin to appear at the end of the fourth week (see Fig. 16-4). The nerve fibers arise from cells in the *basal plates* of the developing spinal cord and emerge as a continuous series of rootlets along its ventrolateral surface. The fibers destined for a particular developing muscle group become

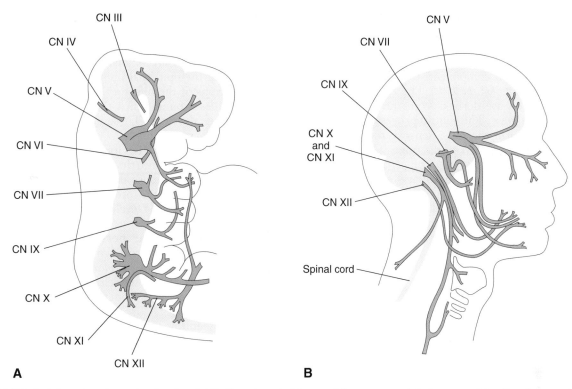

FIGURE 16-27. **A,** A 5-week embryo, showing the distribution of most of the cranial nerves, especially those supplying the pharyngeal arches. **B,** The head and neck of an adult, showing the general distribution of most of the cranial nerves.

arranged in a bundle, forming a **ventral nerve root** (Figs. 16-6 and 16-7). The nerve fibers of the **dorsal nerve root** are formed by axons derived from neural crest cells that migrate to the dorsolateral aspect of the spinal cord, where they differentiate into the cells of the **spinal ganglion** (see Fig. 16-7). The central processes of the neurons in the spinal ganglion form a single bundle that grows into the spinal cord, opposite the apex of the dorsal horn of gray matter (see Fig. 16-4B and C). The distal processes of the spinal ganglion cells grow toward the ventral nerve root and eventually join it to form a **spinal nerve** (see Fig. 16-7).

As each limb bud develops, the nerves from the spinal cord segments opposite to it elongate and grow into the limb. The nerve fibers are distributed to its muscles, which differentiate from myogenic cells that originate from the somites (see Chapter 15). The skin of the developing limbs is also innervated in a segmental manner.

Cranial Nerves

Twelve pairs of cranial nerves form during the fifth and sixth weeks. They are classified into three groups according to their embryologic origins.

Somatic Efferent Cranial Nerves

The hypoglossal (CN XII), abducent (CN VI), and trochlear (CN IV) nerves, as well as the greater part of the oculomotor (CN III) nerves, are homologous with the ventral roots of the spinal nerves (Fig. 16-27A). The cells of origin of these nerves are located in the *somatic efferent*

column (derived from the basal plates) of the brain stem. Their axons are distributed to the muscles derived from the head myotomes (preotic and occipital; see Fig. 15-17).

The **hypoglossal nerve** (CN XII) develops by fusion of the ventral root fibers of three or four occipital nerves (see Fig. 16-27A). Sensory roots, corresponding to the dorsal roots of the spinal nerves, are absent. The somatic motor fibers originate from the *hypoglossal nucleus*. These fibers leave the ventrolateral wall of the medulla in several groups—the hypoglossal nerve roots—converging to form the common trunk of CN XII (see Fig. 16-27B). They grow rostrally and eventually innervate the muscles of the tongue, which are derived from the occipital myotomes (see Fig. 15-16A).

The **abducent nerve** (CN VI) arises from nerve cells in the basal plates of the metencephalon. It passes from its ventral surface to the posterior of the three preotic myotomes from which the lateral rectus muscle of the eye is believed to originate.

The **trochlear nerve** (CN IV) arises from nerve cells in the somatic efferent column in the posterior part of the midbrain. Although a motor nerve, it emerges from the brain stem dorsally and then passes ventrally to supply the superior oblique muscle of the eye.

The **oculomotor nerve** (CN III) supplies the superior, inferior, and medial recti and the inferior oblique muscles of the eye.

Nerves of the Pharyngeal Arches

Cranial nerves V, VII, IX, and X supply the embryonic pharyngeal arches; thus, the structures that develop from these arches are innervated by these cranial nerves (see Fig. 16-27A and Table 10-1).

The **trigeminal nerve** (CN V) is the nerve of the first pharyngeal arch, but it has an ophthalmic division that is not a pharyngeal arch component. *Cranial nerve V is the principal sensory nerve for the head.* The cells of the large trigeminal ganglion are derived from the most anterior part of the neural crest. The central processes of the cells in this ganglion form the large sensory root of CN V, which enters the lateral part of the pons. The peripheral processes of the cells in this ganglion separate into three large divisions (ophthalmic, maxillary, and mandibular nerves). Their sensory fibers supply the skin of the face as well as the lining of the mouth and nose. The *motor fibers of CN V* arise from cells in the most anterior part of the *special visceral efferent* column in the metencephalon. These fibers pass to the muscles of mastication and to other muscles that develop in the mandibular prominence of the first pharyngeal arch (see Table 10-1). The mesencephalic nucleus of CN V differentiates from cells in the midbrain.

The **facial nerve** (CN VII) is the nerve of the second pharyngeal arch. It consists mostly of motor fibers that arise principally from a nuclear group in the *special visceral efferent column* in the caudal part of the pons. These fibers are distributed to the *muscles of facial expression* and to other muscles that develop in the mesenchyme of the second pharyngeal arch (see Table 10-1). The small general visceral efferent component of CN VII terminates in the peripheral autonomic ganglia of the head. The sensory fibers of CN VII arise from the cells of the *geniculate ganglion*. The central processes of these cells enter the pons; the peripheral processes pass to the greater superficial petrosal nerve and, via the chorda tympani nerve, to the taste buds in the anterior two thirds of the tongue.

The **glossopharyngeal nerve** (CN IX) is the nerve of the third pharyngeal arch. Its motor fibers arise from the special and, to a lesser extent, the general visceral efferent columns of the anterior part of the myelencephalon. CN IX forms from several rootlets that arise from the medulla just caudal to the developing internal ear. All of the fibers from the special visceral efferent column are distributed to the stylopharyngeus muscle, which is derived from the mesenchyme in the third pharyngeal arch (see Table 10-1). The general efferent fibers are distributed to the otic ganglion from which postsynaptic fibers pass to the parotid and posterior lingual glands. The *sensory fibers of CN IX* are distributed as general sensory and special visceral afferent fibers (taste fibers) to the posterior part of the tongue.

The **vagus nerve** (CN X) is formed by fusion of the nerves of the fourth and sixth pharyngeal arches (see Table 10-1). The nerve of the fourth pharyngeal arch becomes the superior laryngeal nerve, which supplies the cricothyroid muscle and the constrictor muscles of the pharynx. The nerve of the sixth pharyngeal arch becomes the recurrent laryngeal nerve, which supplies various laryngeal muscles.

The **spinal accessory nerve** (CN XI) arises from the cranial five or six cervical segments of the spinal cord (see Fig. 16-26). The spinal accessory nerve supplies the sternocleidomastoid and trapezius muscles.

Special Sensory Nerves

The **olfactory nerve** (CN I) arises from the olfactory bulb. The olfactory cells are bipolar neurons that differentiate from cells in the epithelial lining of the primordial nasal sac. The axons of the olfactory cells are collected into 18 to 20 bundles around which the cribriform plate of the ethmoid bone develops. These unmyelinated nerve fibers end in the olfactory bulb.

The **optic nerve** (CN II) is formed by more than 1 million nerve fibers that grow into the brain from neuroblasts in the primordial retina. Because the optic nerve develops from the evaginated wall of the forebrain, it actually represents a fiber tract of the brain. Development of the optic nerve is described in Chapter 17.

The **vestibulocochlear nerve** (CN VIII) consists of two kinds of sensory fiber in two bundles; these fibers are known as *the vestibular and cochlear nerves.* The **vestibular nerve** originates in the semicircular ducts, whereas the **cochlear nerve** proceeds from the cochlear duct, in which the **spiral organ** (of Corti) develops (see Chapter 17). The bipolar neurons of the vestibular nerve have their cell bodies in the vestibular ganglion. The central processes of these cells terminate in the vestibular nuclei in the floor of the fourth ventricle. The bipolar neurons of the cochlear nerve have their cell bodies in the spiral ganglion. The central processes of these cells end in the ventral and dorsal *cochlear nuclei* in the medulla.

■ DEVELOPMENT OF THE AUTONOMIC NERVOUS SYSTEM

Functionally, the autonomic system can be divided into sympathetic (thoracolumbar) and parasympathetic (craniosacral) parts.

Sympathetic Nervous System

During the fifth week of development, neural crest cells in the thoracic region migrate along each side of the spinal cord, where they form paired cellular masses (ganglia) dorsolateral to the aorta (see Fig. 16-7). All of these segmentally arranged **sympathetic ganglia** are connected in a bilateral chain by longitudinal nerve fibers. These ganglionated cords—**sympathetic trunks**—are located on each side of the vertebral bodies. Some neural crest cells migrate ventral to the aorta and form neurons in the **preaortic ganglia**, such as the celiac and mesenteric ganglia (see Fig. 16-7). Other neural crest cells migrate to the area of the heart, lungs, and gastrointestinal tract, where they form terminal ganglia in sympathetic organ plexuses, located near or within these organs.

After the sympathetic trunks have formed, axons of sympathetic neurons located in the **intermediolateral cell column** (lateral horn) of the thoracolumbar segments of the spinal cord pass through the ventral root of a spinal nerve and a **white communicating ramus** (L. *ramus communicans*) to a paravertebral ganglion (see Fig. 16-7). There, they may synapse with neurons or ascend or descend in the sympathetic trunk to synapse at other levels. Other presynaptic fibers pass through the paravertebral ganglia without synapsing, forming splanchnic nerves to the viscera. The postsynaptic fibers course through a **gray communicating ramus**, passing from a sympathetic ganglion into a spinal nerve; hence, the sympathetic trunks are composed of ascending and descending fibers.

Parasympathetic Nervous System

The presynaptic parasympathetic fibers arise from neurons in the nuclei of the brain stem and in the sacral region of the spinal cord. The fibers from the brain stem leave through the oculomotor (CN III), facial (CN VII), glossopharyngeal (CN IX), and vagus (CN X) nerves. The postsynaptic neurons are located in the peripheral ganglia or in plexuses near or within the structure being innervated (e.g., pupil of the eye, salivary glands).

CLINICALLY ORIENTED QUESTIONS

1. Are neural tube defects hereditary? A woman had an infant with spina bifida cystica, and her daughter had an infant with meroencephaly. Is the daughter likely to have another child with a neural tube defect? Can meroencephaly and spina bifida be detected early in fetal life?

2. An infant was born with no cerebral hemispheres, but a normal-appearing head. The infant exhibited excessive sleepiness, continuous crying when awake, and feeding problems. What is this condition called? What is its embryologic basis? Do affected children usually survive?

3. Some say that pregnant women who are heavy drinkers may have infants who exhibit mental and growth retardation. Is this true? There are reports of women who get drunk during pregnancy, yet have infants who seem to be normal. Is there a safe threshold for alcohol consumption during pregnancy?

4. A woman was told that cigarette smoking during pregnancy probably caused the slight mental retardation of her infant. She is not a heavy smoker. Was the woman correctly informed?

5. Do all types of spina bifida cause loss of motor function in the lower limbs? What treatments are there for infants with spina bifida cystica?

The answers to these questions are at the back of the book.

THE EYE AND EAR

■ DEVELOPMENT OF THE EYE AND RELATED STRUCTURES

Early eye development results from a series of inductive signals and is first evident at the beginning of the fourth week, when **optic grooves** appear in the neural folds at the cranial end of the embryo (Fig. 17-1*A* and *B*). As the neural folds fuse, the optic grooves evaginate to form hollow diverticula—**optic vesicles**—which project from the wall of the forebrain into the adjacent mesenchyme

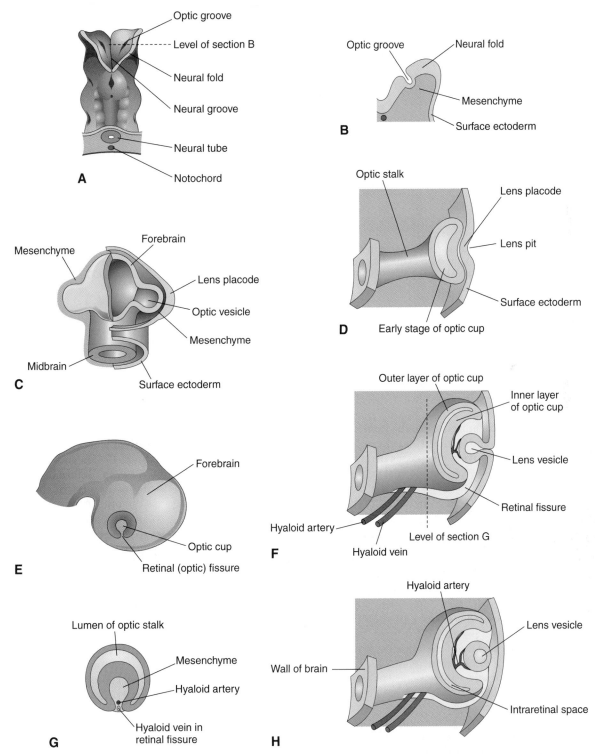

FIGURE 17-1. Early stages of eye development. **A,** Dorsal view of the cranial end of an embryo at approximately 22 days, showing the optic grooves, the first indication of eye development. **B,** Transverse section of a neural fold, showing the optic groove. **C,** Forebrain of an embryo (approximately 28 days). **D, F,** and **H,** The developing eye, showing successive stages in the development of the optic cup and the lens vesicle. **E,** Lateral view of an embryo (approximately 32 days), showing the external appearance of the optic cup. **G,** Transverse section of the optic stalk, showing the retinal fissure and its contents.

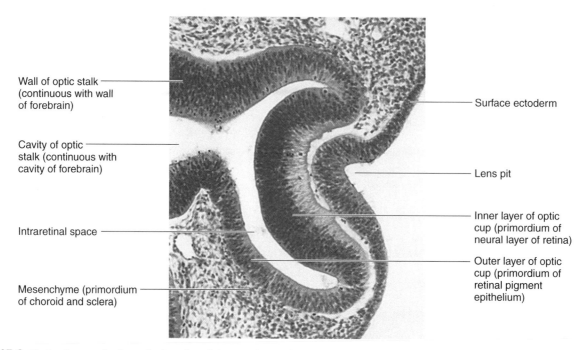

Wall of optic stalk (continuous with wall of forebrain)

Cavity of optic stalk (continuous with cavity of forebrain)

Intraretinal space

Mesenchyme (primordium of choroid and sclera)

Surface ectoderm

Lens pit

Inner layer of optic cup (primordium of neural layer of retina)

Outer layer of optic cup (primordium of retinal pigment epithelium)

FIGURE 17-2. Photomicrograph of a sagittal section of the eye of an embryo (×200) at approximately 32 days. Observe the primordium of the lens (invaginated lens placode), the walls of the optic cup (primordium of the retina), and the optic stalk (primordium of the optic nerve). (From Moore KL, Persaud TVN, Shiota K: Color Atlas of Clinical Embryology, 2nd ed. Philadelphia, WB Saunders, 2000.)

(see Fig. 17-1C). Formation of the optic vesicles is induced by the mesenchyme adjacent to the developing brain. As the optic vesicles enlarge, their connections with the forebrain narrow to form hollow **optic stalks** (see Fig. 17-1D).

The surface ectoderm adjacent to the optic vesicles thickens to form **lens placodes**, the primordia of the lenses (see Fig. 17-1C). An inductive signal passes from the optic vesicles, stimulating the surface ectodermal cells to form the **lens primordia**. These placodes invaginate and sink deep to the surface ectoderm, forming **lens pits** (Figs. 17-1D and 17-2). The edges of the lens pits approach each other and fuse to form spherical **lens vesicles** (see Fig. 17-1F and H), which soon lose their connection with the surface ectoderm. As the lens vesicles develop, the optic vesicles invaginate to form double-walled **optic cups** (see Figs. 17-1H and 17-2), with the lens becoming infolded by the rim of the optic cup (Fig. 17-3A). By this stage, the lens vesicles have entered the cavities of the optic cups (Fig. 17-4). Linear grooves—**retinal (optic) fissures**—develop on the ventral surface of the optic cups and along the optic stalks (see Figs. 17-1E to H and 17-3A to D). The retinal fissures contain vascular mesenchyme from which the hyaloid blood vessels develop. The **hyaloid artery** supplies the inner layer of the optic cup, the lens vesicle, and the mesenchyme in the optic cup (see Figs. 17-1H and 17-3). As the edges of the retinal fissure fuse, the hyaloid vessels are enclosed within the **primordial optic nerve** (Fig. 17-3C to F). Distal parts of the hyaloid vessels eventually degenerate, but proximal parts persist as the **central artery** and **vein of the retina** (Fig. 17-5D).

Development of the Retina

The retina develops from the walls of the *optic cup* (see Figs. 17-1 and 17-2). The outer, thinner layer of the optic cup becomes the **retinal pigment epithelium**, whereas the inner, thicker layer differentiates into the **neural retina**. The two retinal layers are separated by an **intraretinal space** (see Figs. 17-1H and 17-4), which is the original cavity of the *optic cup*. Before birth, this space gradually disappears as the two layers of the retina fuse (see Fig. 17-5D). Because the optic cup is an outgrowth of the forebrain, the layers of the optic cup are continuous with the wall of the brain (see Fig. 17-1H). Under the influence of the developing lens, the inner layer of the optic cup proliferates to form a thick **neuroepithelium** (see Fig. 17-4). Subsequently, the cells of the inner layer closest to the pigmented retina differentiate into the **neural retina**, the light-sensitive region of the retina (see Fig. 17-4). This region contains photoreceptors (rods and cones) and the cell bodies of neurons (e.g., ganglion cells). Because the optic vesicle invaginates as it forms the optic cup, the neural retina is "inverted"; that is, light-sensitive parts of the photoreceptor cells are adjacent to the retinal pigment epithelium. As a result, light must pass through the thickest part of the retina before reaching the receptors; however, because the retina is thin and transparent, it does not form a barrier to light. The axons of the ganglion cells in the superficial layer of the neural retina grow proximally in the wall of the optic stalk to the brain (see Fig. 17-3A). The cavity of the **optic stalk** is gradually obliterated as the axons of the ganglion cells form the **optic nerve** (see Fig. 17-3F).

FIGURE 17-3. Closure of the retinal fissure and formation of the optic nerve. **A, C,** and **E,** Views of the inferior surface of the optic cup and the optic stalk, showing progressive stages in the closure of the retinal fissure. **C₁,** Longitudinal section of a part of the optic cup and the optic stalk, showing the axons of the ganglion cells of the retina growing through the optic stalk to the brain. **B, D,** and **F,** Transverse sections of the optic stalk, showing successive stages in the closure of the retinal fissure and formation of the optic nerve. Note that the lumen of the optic stalk is gradually obliterated as the axons of the ganglion cells accumulate in the inner layer of the optic stalk.

CONGENITAL ANOMALIES OF THE EYE

Because of the complexity of eye development, anomalies or birth defects occur. The type and the severity of the anomaly depend on the embryonic stage at which development is disrupted. Several environmental teratogens (agents or factors that cause birth defects) can cause congenital eye defects (see Chapter 19).

CONGENITAL RETINAL DETACHMENT

Congenital detachment of the retina occurs when the inner and outer layers of the optic cup do not fuse during the fetal period to form the retina and obliterate the intraretinal space (see Figs. 17-3 and 17-5). The separation of the neural and the pigmented layers may be partial or complete. Retinal detachment may

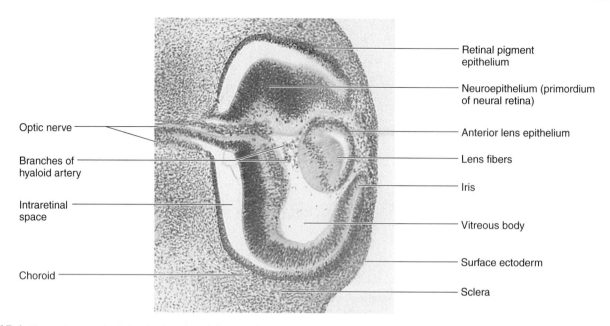

FIGURE 17-4. Photomicrograph of a sagittal section of the eye of an embryo (×100) at approximately 44 days. Observe that the posterior wall of the lens vesicle forms the lens fibers. The anterior wall does not change appreciably as it becomes the anterior lens epithelium. (From Nishimura H [ed]: Atlas of Human Prenatal Histology. Tokyo, Igaku-Shoin, 1983.)

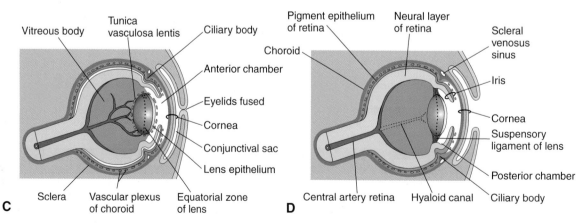

FIGURE 17-5. Sagittal sections of the eye, showing the successive developmental stages of the lens, retina, iris, and cornea. **A**, At 5 weeks. **B**, At 6 weeks. **C**, At 20 weeks. **D**, Newborn infant. Note that the layers of the optic cup fuse to form the retinal pigment epithelium and the neural retina and that they extend anteriorly as the double epithelium of the ciliary body and its iris.

result from unequal rates of growth of the two retinal layers; as a result, the layers of the optic cup are not in perfect apposition. Although separated from the retinal pigment epithelium, the neural retina retains its blood supply (central artery of the retina). Normally, the retinal pigment epithelium becomes firmly fixed to the choroid, but its attachment to the neural retina is not firm; hence, retinal detachment may follow a blow to the eyeball. In such cases, fluid accumulates between the layers and vision is impaired.

COLOBOMA OF THE RETINA

Retinal coloboma is a defect that is characterized by a localized gap in the retina, usually inferior to the optic disc. The defect is bilateral in most cases. A typical coloboma results from defective closure of the retinal fissure.

COLOR OF THE IRIS

The iris is typically light blue or gray in most newborn infants. It acquires its definitive color as pigmentation occurs after birth. It is the concentration and distribution of pigment-containing cells, called *chromatophores,* in the loose vascular connective tissue of the iris that determines eye color. If the melanin pigment is confined to the pigmented epithelium on the posterior surface of the iris, the eye appears blue. If melanin is also distributed throughout the connective tissue of the iris, the eye appears brown.

Myelination of the optic nerve fibers begins late in the fetal period and is complete by the 10th week after birth.

Development of the Ciliary Body

The ciliary body is the wedge-shaped extension of the **choroid** (see Fig. 17-5C and D). Its medial surface projects toward the lens, forming the **ciliary processes**. The pigmented part of the ciliary epithelium is derived from the outer layer of the optic cup and is continuous with the retinal pigment epithelium. The nonpigmented part of the ciliary epithelium represents the anterior prolongation of the neural retina, in which no neural elements develop. The smooth **ciliary muscle** that is responsible for focusing the lens and the connective tissue in the ciliary body develops from the mesenchyme located at the edge of the optic cup in the region between the anterior scleral condensation and the ciliary pigment epithelium.

Development of the Iris

The iris develops from the rim of the optic cup, which grows inward and partially covers the lens (see Fig. 17-5D). The two layers of the optic cup remain thin in this area. The epithelium of the iris represents both layers of the optic cup; it is continuous with the double-layered epithelium of the ciliary body and with the retinal pigment epithelium and the neural retina. The connective tissue framework of the iris is derived from neural crest cells that migrate into the iris. The **dilator pupillae** and **sphincter pupillae muscles** of the iris are derived from the *neuroectoderm of the optic cup*. These smooth muscles result from a transformation of epithelial cells into smooth muscle cells.

COLOBOMA OF THE IRIS

In infants with coloboma of the iris, a defect in the inferior sector of the iris or the pupillary margin gives the pupil a keyhole appearance (Fig. 17-6). The coloboma may be limited to the iris, or it may extend deeper and involve the ciliary body and retina. A typical coloboma *results from failure of closure of the retinal fissure* during the sixth week. The defect may be genetically determined, or it may be caused by environmental factors. A simple coloboma of the iris is frequently hereditary and is transmitted as an autosomal dominant characteristic.

Development of the Lens

The lens develops from the **lens vesicle**, a derivative of the surface ectoderm (see Fig. 17-1). Lens formation involves the expression of L-Maf (lens-specific Maf) and other transcription factors in the lens placode and vesicle. The anterior wall of the lens vesicle becomes the subcapsular **lens epithelium** (see Fig. 17-5C). The nuclei of the tall columnar cells that form the posterior wall of the lens vesicle undergo dissolution. These cells lengthen considerably to form highly transparent epithelial cells, the **primary lens fibers**. As these fibers grow, they gradually obliterate the cavity of the lens vesicle (Figs. 17-5A to C and 17-7). The rim of the lens is known as the **equatorial zone** because it is located midway between the anterior and the posterior poles of the lens. The cells in the equatorial zone are cuboidal; as they elongate, they lose their nuclei and become **secondary lens fibers** (Fig. 17-8). These fibers are added to the external sides of the primary lens fibers. Although secondary lens fibers continue to form during adulthood and the lens increases in diameter as a result, the primary lens fibers must last a lifetime. The developing lens is supplied with blood by the distal part of the **hyaloid artery** (see Figs. 17-4 and 17-5); however, it becomes avascular in the fetal period, when this part of the artery degenerates (see Fig. 17-5D). After this occurs, the lens depends on diffusion from the aqueous humor in the anterior chamber of the eye, which bathes its anterior surface, and from the vitreous humor in other parts. The developing lens is invested by a vascular mesenchymal layer, the **tunica vasculosa lentis**. The anterior part of this capsule is the **pupillary membrane** (see Fig. 17-5*B* and *C*). The part of the hyaloid artery that supplies the tunica vasculosa lentis disappears during the late fetal period. As a result, the tunica vasculosa lentis and the pupillary membrane degenerate (see Fig. 17-5*C*); however, the lens capsule produced by the anterior lens epithelium and the lens fibers persists. The **lens capsule** represents a greatly thickened basement membrane and has a lamellar structure. The former site of the hyaloid artery is indicated by the **hyaloid canal** in the vitreous body (see Fig. 17-5*D*); this canal is usually inconspicuous in the living eye.

The **vitreous body** forms within the cavity of the optic cup (see Fig. 17-5*C*). It is composed of **vitreous humor**, an avascular mass of transparent, gel-like, intercellular substance.

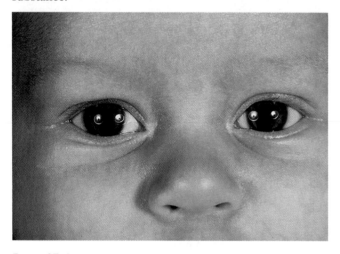

FIGURE 17-6. Bilateral coloboma of the right iris. Observe the defect in the inferior part of the iris (at the 6 o'clock position). The defect is in the area of closure of the retinal fissure. (Courtesy of A.E. Chudley, MD, Section of Genetics and Metabolism, Department of Pediatrics and Child Health, Children's Hospital, University of Manitoba, Winnipeg, Manitoba, Canada.)

PERSISTENCE OF THE HYALOID ARTERY

The distal part of the hyaloid artery normally degenerates as its proximal part becomes the central artery of the retina. If part of the hyaloid artery persists distally, it may appear as a freely moving, nonfunctional vessel or as a wormlike structure projecting from the optic disc. Sometimes the hyaloid artery remnant may appear as a fine strand traversing the vitreous body. In other cases, the remnant may form a cyst.

Development of the Aqueous Chambers

The **anterior chamber of the eye** develops from a cleftlike space that forms in the mesenchyme located between the developing lens and the cornea (see Fig. 17-5*A* and *B*). The **posterior chamber of the eye** develops from a space that forms in the mesenchyme posterior to the developing iris and anterior to the developing lens (see Fig. 17-5*D*). After the lens is established, it induces the surface ectoderm to develop into the epithelium of the cornea and the conjunctiva. When the pupillary membrane disappears and the pupil forms, the anterior and posterior chambers of the eye communicate with each other through the **scleral venous sinus**. This sinus encircles the anterior chamber and allows aqueous humor to flow from the anterior chamber of the eye to the venous system.

Development of the Cornea

The cornea, induced by the lens vesicle, is formed from three sources:

● The external corneal epithelium, derived from the **surface ectoderm**
● The **mesenchyme,** derived from the **mesoderm**

FIGURE 17-7. Photomicrograph of a sagittal section of the eye of an embryo (×50) at approximately 56 days. Observe the developing neural retina and the retinal pigment epithelium. Note the large intraretinal space between the two layers of the retina. (From Moore KL, Persaud TVN, Shiota K: Color Atlas of Clinical Embryology, 2nd ed. Philadelphia, WB Saunders, 2000.)

● **Neural crest cells** that migrate from the lip of the optic cup and become transformed into the corneal endothelium

CONGENITAL GLAUCOMA

Abnormal elevation of intraocular pressure in newborn infants usually results from abnormal development of the drainage mechanism of aqueous humor during the fetal period. *Intraocular tension* increases because of an imbalance between the production of aqueous humor and its outflow. This imbalance may result from abnormal development of the *scleral venous sinus* (see Fig. 17-5D). Congenital glaucoma is usually genetically heterogeneous, but the condition may result from rubella infection during early pregnancy (see Fig. 19-16B).

CONGENITAL CATARACTS

In congenital cataracts, the lens is opaque and frequently appears grayish white. Blindness results. Many lens opacities are inherited, with dominant transmission being more common than recessive, or sex-linked, transmission. Some congenital cataracts are caused by teratogenic agents—particularly the **rubella virus** (see Fig. 19-16A)—that affect the early development of the lenses. The lenses are vulnerable to the rubella virus between the fourth and seventh weeks, when primary lens fibers are forming. Physical agents, such as **radiation**, can also damage the lens and produce cataracts (see Chapter 19).

Development of the Choroid and Sclera

The mesenchyme surrounding the optic cup differentiates into an inner, vascular layer—the **choroid**—and an outer, fibrous layer—the **sclera** (see Figs. 17-5C and 17-7). At the rim of the optic cup, the choroid forms the cores of the **ciliary processes**, consisting chiefly of capillaries supported by delicate connective tissue.

Development of the Eyelids

The eyelids develop during the sixth week from the mesenchyme derived from the neural crest and from two folds of skin that grow over the cornea (see Fig. 17-5B).

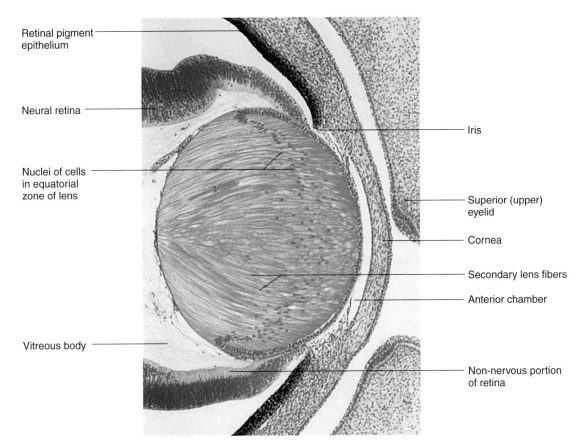

FIGURE 17-8. Photomicrograph of a sagittal section of a portion of the developing eye of an embryo (×280) at approximately 56 days. Observe that the lens fibers have elongated and obliterated the cavity of the lens vesicle. Note that the inner layer of the optic cup has thickened greatly to form the neural retina. Also observe the thick outer layer of retinal pigment epithelium. (From Moore KL, Persaud TVN, Shiota K: Color Atlas of Clinical Embryology, 2nd ed. Philadelphia, WB Saunders, 2000.)

The eyelids adhere to one another at approximately the 10th week, and remain so until the 26th to 28th weeks (see Fig. 17-5*C*). The **palpebral conjunctiva** lines the inner surface of the eyelids. The **eyelashes** and the **glands** in the eyelids are derived from the surface ectoderm (see Chapter 18). The connective tissue and the **tarsal plates** develop from mesenchyme in the developing eyelids. The *orbicularis oculi muscle* is derived from the mesenchyme in the second pharyngeal arch (see Chapter 10).

Development of the Lacrimal Glands

The lacrimal glands are derived from a number of solid buds from the surface ectoderm. The buds branch and canalize to form the **nasolacrimal ducts** and the alveoli of the glands. The lacrimal glands are small at birth and do not function fully until approximately 6 weeks; hence, the newborn infant does not produce tears when crying.

CONGENITAL PTOSIS OF THE EYELID

Drooping of the superior (upper) eyelids at birth is relatively common. Congenital ptosis may result from dystrophy of the levator palpebrae superioris muscle. Ptosis occurs more rarely as a result of prenatal injury or dystrophy of the superior division of the **oculomotor nerve** (cranial nerve III) that supplies this muscle. Congenital ptosis may be transmitted as an autosomal dominant trait.

COLOBOMA OF THE EYELID

Most palpebral colobomas are characterized by a small notch in the superior eyelid. Coloboma of the inferior (lower) eyelid is rare. **Palpebral colobomas** appear to result from developmental disturbances in the formation of the eyelids.

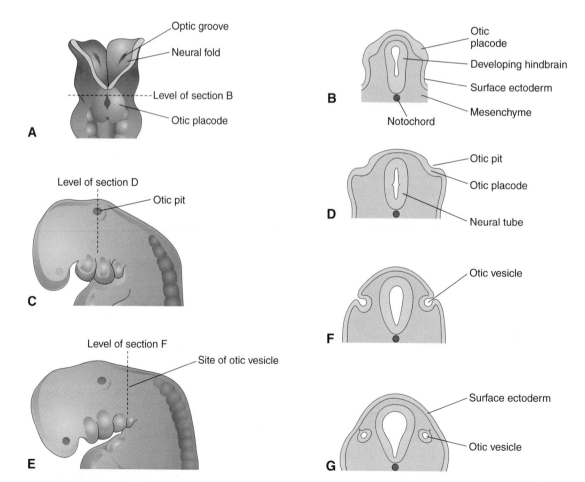

FIGURE 17-9. Early development of the internal ear. **A,** Dorsal view of a 4-week embryo (at approximately 22 days). **B, D, F,** and **G,** Schematic coronal sections, showing successive stages in the development of the otic vesicles. **C** and **E,** Lateral views of the cranial region of embryos at approximately 24 and 28 days, respectively.

■ DEVELOPMENT OF THE EAR

The ear is composed of external, middle, and internal anatomic parts. The external and middle parts of the ear regulate the transference of sound waves from the exterior to the internal ear; this process converts the sound waves into nerve impulses. The internal ear is concerned with both hearing and balance.

Development of the Internal Ear

The internal ear is the first of the three parts of the ear to develop. Early in the fourth week, a thickening of the surface ectoderm—the **otic placode**—appears on each side of the embryo at the level of the caudal part of the hindbrain (Fig. 17-9A and B). Inductive influences from the notochord and the paraxial mesoderm stimulate the surface ectoderm to form the **otic placodes**. *Fibroblast growth factor 3 (FGF-3)* may play a role in this process. Each otic placode soon invaginates and sinks deep to the surface ectoderm into the underlying mesenchyme, forming an **otic pit** (see Fig. 17-9C and D). The edges of the otic pit come together and fuse to form an **otic vesicle** (see Fig. 17-9E to G). The otic vesicle then loses its connection with the surface ectoderm, and a diverticulum grows from the

otic vesicle and elongates to form the **endolymphatic duct** and **sac** (Fig. 17-10A to E). Two regions of the otic vesicle are now recognizable:

● A dorsal **utricular part** from which the endolymphatic duct, the utricle, and the semicircular ducts arise
● A ventral **saccular part**, which gives rise to the saccule and the cochlear duct, in which the spiral organ (of Corti) is located

Three disclike diverticula grow out from the utricular part of the **primordial membranous labyrinth**. The central parts of these diverticula fuse and disappear (see Fig. 17-10B to E). The peripheral unfused parts of the diverticula become the **semicircular ducts**, which are attached to the utricle and are later enclosed in the **semicircular canals** of the **bony labyrinth**. Localized dilatations, the **ampullae**, develop at one end of each semicircular duct. Specialized receptor areas, called **cristae ampullares**, differentiate in these ampullae as well as in the utricle and the saccule.

From the ventral saccular part of the otic vesicle, a tubular diverticulum—the **cochlear duct**—grows and coils to form the **membranous cochlea** (see Fig. 17-10C to E). A connection of the cochlea with the saccule, the **ductus reuniens**, soon forms. The **spiral organ** (of Corti) differentiates from cells in the wall of the cochlear duct (see Fig. 17-10F to I). Ganglion cells of the vestibulocochlear nerve (cranial nerve VIII) migrate along the coils of the

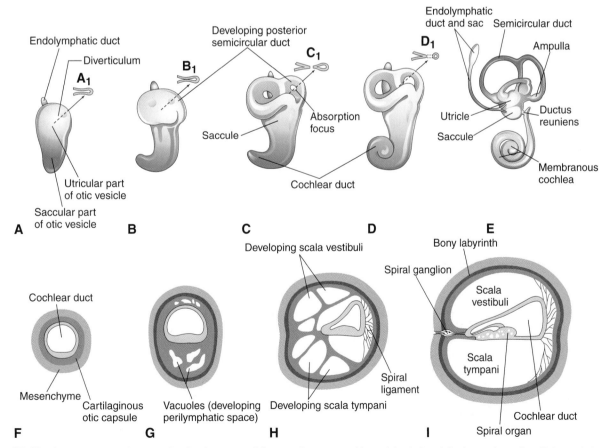

FIGURE 17-10. The otic vesicle, showing the development of the membranous and bony labyrinths of the internal ear. **A to E,** Lateral views, showing successive stages in the development of the otic vesicle into the membranous labyrinth from the fifth to eighth weeks. **A₁ to D₁,** Development of a semicircular duct. **F to I,** Sections through the cochlear duct, showing successive stages in the development of the spiral organ and the perilymphatic space from the eighth to 20th weeks.

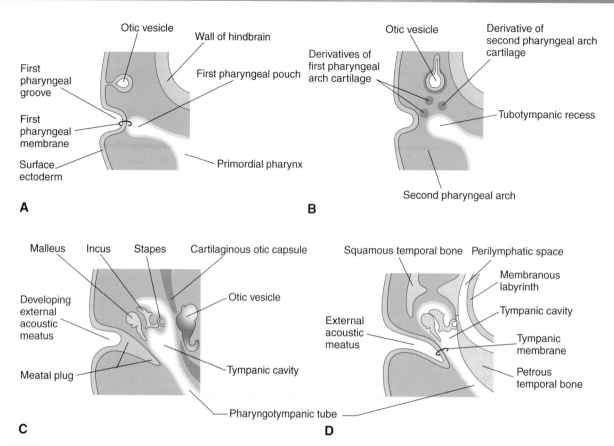

FIGURE 17-11. Development of the external and middle parts of the ear. **A,** At 4 weeks, showing the relation of the otic vesicle to the pharyngeal apparatus. **B,** At 5 weeks, showing the tubotympanic recess and the pharyngeal arch cartilages. **C,** At a later stage, showing the tubotympanic recess (primordium of the tympanic cavity and the mastoid antrum) beginning to envelop the ossicles. **D,** Final stage of ear development, showing the relation of the middle ear to the perilymphatic space and the external acoustic meatus.

membranous cochlea and form the **spiral ganglion**. Nerve processes extend from this ganglion to the spiral organ, where they terminate on **hair cells**. The cells in the spiral ganglion retain their embryonic bipolar condition; that is, they do not become unipolar like spinal ganglion cells.

Inductive influences from the otic vesicle stimulate the mesenchyme around the otic vesicle to differentiate into a **cartilaginous otic capsule** (see Fig. 17-10F). *Transforming growth factor β₁ may play a role in modulating epithelial-mesenchymal interaction in the internal ear and directing the formation of the otic capsule.* As the membranous labyrinth enlarges, vacuoles appear in the cartilaginous otic capsule that soon coalesce to form the **perilymphatic space**. The membranous labyrinth is now suspended in perilymph (fluid in the perilymphatic space). The perilymphatic space related to the cochlear duct develops two divisions, the **scala tympani** and the **scala vestibuli** (Fig. 17-10H and I). The cartilaginous otic capsule later ossifies to form the **bony labyrinth** of the internal ear. The internal ear reaches its adult size and shape by the middle of the fetal period (20–22 weeks).

Development of the Middle Ear

Development of the **tubotympanic recess** (Fig. 17-11B) from the first pharyngeal pouch is described in Chapter 10. The proximal part of the tubotympanic recess forms the **pharyngotympanic tube** (auditory tube). The distal part of the tubotympanic recess expands and becomes the **tympanic cavity** (see Fig. 17-11C), which gradually envelops the **auditory ossicles** (malleus, incus, and stapes), their tendons and ligaments, and the chorda tympani nerve. All of these structures receive a more or less complete epithelial investment. An epithelial-type organizer, located at the tip of the tubotympanic recess, probably plays a role in the early development of the middle ear cavity by inducing *programmed cell death*—apoptosis. The malleus and the incus develop from the cartilage of the first pharyngeal arch, whereas the stapes develops from the cartilage of the second arch. The **tensor tympani**, the muscle attached to the malleus, is derived from the mesenchyme in the first pharyngeal arch, and the **stapedius muscle** is derived from the second pharyngeal arch. During the late fetal period, expansion of the tympanic cavity gives rise to the **mastoid antrum**, located in the temporal bone. The mastoid antrum is almost adult size at birth; however, *no mastoid cells are present in newborn infants.* By 2 years, the mastoid cells are well developed and produce conic projections of the temporal bones, the mastoid processes. The middle ear continues to grow through puberty.

Development of the External Ear

The **external acoustic meatus** develops from the dorsal part of the first pharyngeal groove. The ectodermal cells at the bottom of this tube proliferate to form a solid epithelial

CONGENITAL DEAFNESS

Approximately 1 in 1000 newborn infants have significant hearing loss. Congenital deafness may be the result of maldevelopment of the sound-conducting apparatus of the middle and external ears, or of the neurosensory structures in the internal ear. Most types of congenital deafness are caused by genetic factors. *Rubella infection* during the critical period of development of the internal ear can cause maldevelopment of the spiral organ (of Corti) and deafness. Congenital fixation of the stapes results in conductive deafness in an otherwise normal ear. Failure of differentiation of the anular ligament, which attaches the base of the stapes to the oval window, results in fixation of the stapes to the bony labyrinth.

AURICULAR ANOMALIES

Minor auricular deformities are common and may serve as indicators of a specific pattern of congenital anomalies. For example, the auricles are often low-set and abnormal in shape in infants with chromosomal syndromes, such as trisomy 18 (see Chapter 19), and in infants affected by maternal ingestion of certain drugs (e.g., trimethadione).

AURICULAR APPENDAGES

Auricular appendages (skin tags) are common and result from the development of accessory auricular hillocks (Fig. 17-13). The appendages usually appear anterior to the auricle, more often unilaterally than bilaterally. The appendages, often with narrow pedicles, consist of skin, but may also contain some cartilage.

MICROTIA

Microtia (small auricle) results from suppressed development of the auricular hillocks (see Fig. 17-13). This anomaly often serves as an indicator of associated anomalies, such as atresia of the external acoustic meatus and abnormalities of the middle ear.

plate, the **meatal plug** (see Fig. 17-11*C*). Late in the fetal period, the central cells of this plug degenerate, forming a cavity that becomes the internal part of the external acoustic meatus (see Fig. 17-11*D*). The primordium of the **tympanic membrane** is the first pharyngeal membrane, which separates the first pharyngeal groove from the first pharyngeal pouch (see Fig. 17-11*A*). The external covering of the tympanic membrane is derived from the surface ectoderm, whereas its internal lining is derived from the endoderm of the tubotympanic recess.

The **auricle** develops from the mesenchymal proliferations in the first and second pharyngeal arches. Prominences, called **auricular hillocks**, surround the first pharyngeal groove (Fig. 17-12*A*). As the auricle grows, the contribution of the first arch is reduced (see Fig. 17-12*B* to *D*). The lobule (earlobe) is the last part to develop. The auricle begins to develop at the base of the neck (see Fig. 17-12*A* and *B*). As the mandible develops, the auricle assumes its normal position at the side of the head (see Fig. 17-12*C* and *D*).

Auricular hillocks derived from the first and second pharyngeal arches

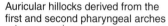

First pharyngeal groove

A

B

C

D

FIGURE 17-12. Development of the auricle of the external ear. **A**, At 6 weeks. Note that three auricular hillocks are located on the first pharyngeal arch and three are situated on the second arch. **B**, At 8 weeks. **C**, At 10 weeks. **D**, At 32 weeks.

FIGURE 17-13. Child with a rudimentary auricle (microtia) and a preauricular tag. The external acoustic meatus is also absent. (Courtesy of A.E. Chudley, MD, Section of Genetics and Metabolism, Department of Pediatrics and Child Health, Children's Hospital, University of Manitoba, Winnipeg, Manitoba, Canada.)

ATRESIA OF THE EXTERNAL ACOUSTIC MEATUS

Atresia, or blockage, of the external acoustic meatus results from failure of the meatal plug to canalize (see Fig. 17-11C). Usually, the deep part of the canal is open, but the superficial part is blocked by bone or fibrous tissue. Most cases are associated with *first arch syndrome* (see Chapter 10). Usually, the auricle is also severely affected, and anomalies of the middle ear, the internal ear, or both may be present. Atresia of the external acoustic meatus can occur bilaterally or unilaterally and usually results from autosomal dominant inheritance.

ABSENCE OF THE EXTERNAL ACOUSTIC MEATUS

Absence of the external acoustic meatus is rare (see Fig. 17-13); usually, the auricle is normal. This anomaly results from failure of inward expansion of the first pharyngeal groove and failure of the meatal plug to disappear.

PREAURICULAR SINUSES

Shallow, pitlike cutaneous sinuses are occasionally located anterior to the auricle. These sinuses usually have pinpoint external openings. Some sinuses contain a vestigial cartilaginous mass. These defects are probably related to abnormal development of the auricular hillocks and defective closure of the dorsal part of the first pharyngeal groove. *Preauricular sinuses* are familial and are frequently bilateral.

CLINICALLY ORIENTED QUESTIONS

1. If a woman has rubella (German measles) during the first trimester of pregnancy, what are the chances that the eyes and ears of the fetus will be affected? What is the most common manifestation of late fetal rubella infection? If a pregnant woman is exposed to rubella, can it be determined if she is immune to the infection?

2. Some believe that a good way of preventing the congenital anomalies caused by rubella is by the purposeful exposure of young girls to rubella. Is this the best way for a woman to avoid having a blind and deaf infant secondary to rubella infection during pregnancy? If not, what can be done to provide immunization against rubella infection?

3. It has been reported that deafness and tooth defects occurring during childhood may result from a condition called *fetal syphilis*. Is this true? If so, how could this happen? Can these congenital defects be prevented?

4. There are reports that blindness and deafness can result from herpesvirus infections. Is this true? If so, which herpesvirus is involved? What are the affected infant's chances of normal development?

5. An article in the newspaper reported that methyl mercury exposure in utero can cause mental deficiency, deafness, and blindness. The article cited the eating of contaminated fish as the cause of the abnormalities. How might these anomalies be caused by methyl mercury?

The answers to these questions are at the back of the book.

18

THE INTEGUMENTARY SYSTEM

The integumentary system consists of the skin and its appendages: sweat glands, nails, hairs, sebaceous glands, and arrector muscles of hairs (Latin [L.] *arrector pili*). The system also includes the mammary glands and teeth.

■ DEVELOPMENT OF THE SKIN

The skin consists of two layers that are derived from two different germ layers (Fig. 18-1): the ectoderm and the mesoderm.

- The **epidermis** is a superficial epithelial tissue that is derived from the surface ectoderm.
- The **dermis** is a deep layer composed of dense connective tissue that is derived from the mesoderm.

Ectodermal (epidermal) and mesenchymal (dermal) interactions involve mutual inductive mechanisms. The embryonic skin at 4 to 5 weeks of development consists of a single layer of surface ectoderm overlying the mesoderm (see Fig. 18-1*A*).

Epidermis

The primordium of the epidermis is the surface ectoderm (see Fig. 18-1*A*). The cells in this layer proliferate and form a layer of squamous epithelium, the **periderm**, and a basal layer (see Fig. 18-1*B*). The cells of the periderm continually undergo keratinization and desquamation and are replaced by cells arising from the **basal layer**. The exfoliated peridermal cells form part of a white, greasy substance—the **vernix caseosa**—that covers the fetal skin. Later, the vernix contains sebum, the secretion from the sebaceous glands in the skin (Fig. 18-2). The vernix protects the developing skin from constant exposure to amniotic fluid during the fetal period.

The basal layer of the epidermis becomes the **stratum germinativum** (see Fig. 18-1*D*), which produces new cells that are displaced into the more superficial layers. By 11 weeks, cells from the stratum germinativum have formed an **intermediate layer** (see Fig. 18-1*C*). Replacement of the peridermal cells continues until approximately the 21st week; thereafter, the periderm disappears and the **stratum corneum** forms (see Fig. 18-1*D*). Proliferation of the cells in the stratum germinativum also produces **epidermal ridges**, which extend into the developing dermis. These ridges begin to appear in embryos of 10 weeks and are permanently established by the 17th week. The pattern of epidermal ridges that develops on the surface of the palms of the hands and the soles of the feet is determined genetically and constitutes the basis for examining fingerprints (**dermatoglyphics**) in criminal investigations and medical genetics. Abnormal chromosome complements affect the development of ridge patterns; for example, infants with Down syndrome have distinctive ridge patterns on their hands and feet that are of diagnostic value.

Late in the embryonic period, **neural crest cells** migrate into the mesenchyme in the developing dermis and differentiate into **melanoblasts** (see Fig. 18-1*B* and *C*). Later, these cells migrate to the **dermoepidermal junction** and differentiate into melanocytes (see Fig. 18-1*D*). The **melanocytes** begin producing **melanin** before birth and

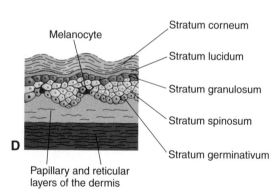

FIGURE 18-1. Successive stages of skin development. **A**, At 4 weeks. **B**, At 7 weeks. **C**, At 11 weeks. The cells of the periderm continually undergo keratinization and desquamation. Exfoliated peridermal cells form part of the vernix caseosa. **D**, Newborn infant. Note the position of the melanocytes in the basal layer of the epidermis. Their processes extend between the epidermal cells to supply them with melanin.

distribute it to the epidermal cells. After birth, increased amounts of melanin are produced in response to ultraviolet light. The relative content of melanin in the melanocytes accounts for the different colors of skin. *Molecular studies indicate that melanocyte-stimulating hormone cell surface receptor and melanosomal P-protein determine the degree of pigmentation by regulating tyrosinase levels and activity.*

Dermis

The dermis develops from the mesenchyme, which is derived from the mesoderm underlying the surface ectoderm (see Fig. 18-1*A* and *B*). The mesenchyme that differentiates into the connective tissue of the dermis originates from the somatic layer of the lateral mesoderm and from the dermatomes of the somites. By 11 weeks, the mesenchymal cells have begun to produce collagenous and elastic connective tissue fibers (see Fig. 18-1C). As the **epidermal ridges** form, the dermis projects into the epidermis, forming dermal ridges. Capillary loops develop in some of the **dermal ridges** and provide nourishment for the epidermis. Sensory nerve endings form in other ridges. The developing afferent nerve fibers apparently play an important role in the spatial and temporal sequence of dermal ridge formation. The blood vessels in the dermis differentiate from the mesenchyme. As the skin grows, new capillaries grow out from the primordial vessels (**angiogenesis**). Some capillaries acquire muscular coats through the differentiation of myoblasts developing in the surrounding mesenchyme, and they become arterioles,

arteries, venules, and veins. By the end of the first trimester, the blood supply of the fetal dermis is well established.

Glands of the Skin

Two kinds of glands, sebaceous glands and sweat glands, are derived from the epidermis and grow into the dermis.

Sebaceous Glands

Most sebaceous glands develop as buds from the sides of the developing **epidermal root sheaths** of the hair follicles (Fig. 18-2). The glandular buds grow into the surrounding connective tissue and branch to form the primordia of the alveoli and their associated ducts. The central cells of the alveoli break down, forming an oily secretion called

FIGURE 18-2. Successive stages in the development of a hair and its associated sebaceous gland and arrector muscle. Note also the successive stages in the development of a sweat gland.

sebum; this is released into the hair follicle and passes to the surface of the skin, where it mixes with desquamated peridermal cells to form the **vernix caseosa**. Sebaceous glands, independent of the hair follicles (e.g., in the glans penis and labia minora), develop in a similar manner as buds from the epidermis.

Sweat Glands

The **eccrine sweat glands** develop as epidermal downgrowths (buds) into the underlying mesenchyme (see Fig. 18-2). As a bud elongates, its end coils to form the primordium of the secretory part of the gland. The epithelial attachment of the developing gland to the epidermis forms the primordium of the sweat duct. The central cells of the primordial ducts degenerate, forming a lumen. The peripheral cells of the secretory part of the gland differentiate into *myoepithelial* and *secretory* cells (see Fig. 18-2). The myoepithelial cells are believed to be specialized smooth muscle cells that assist in expelling sweat from the glands. Eccrine sweat glands begin to function shortly after birth.

The **apocrine sweat glands** develop from downgrowths of the stratum germinativum of the epidermis that give rise to the hair follicles. As a result, the ducts of these glands open, not onto the skin surface as do eccrine sweat glands, but into the upper part of the hair follicles, superficial to the openings of the sebaceous glands. They begin to secrete a protein-rich material during puberty.

■ DEVELOPMENT OF THE HAIRS

Hairs begin to develop during the 9th to 12th weeks, but they do not become easily recognizable until approximately the 23rd week (see Fig. 18-2). Hairs are first recognizable on the eyebrows, upper lip, and chin. A hair follicle begins as a proliferation of the stratum germinativum of the epidermis and extends into the underlying dermis. The **hair bud** soon becomes club-shaped, forming a hair bulb. The epithelial cells of the hair bulb constitute the **germinal matrix**, which later produces the hair. The **hair bulb** is soon invaginated by a small mesenchymal **hair papilla** (see Fig. 18-2). The peripheral cells of the developing hair follicle form the epidermal root sheath, and the surrounding mesenchymal cells differentiate into the **dermal root sheath**. As cells in the germinal matrix proliferate, they are pushed toward the surface, where they keratinize to form the **hair shaft**. The hair grows through the epidermis on the eyebrows and the upper lip by the end of the 12th week of development.

The first hairs that appear—**lanugo** (downy hair)—are fine, soft, and lightly pigmented. Lanugo begins to appear toward the end of the 12th week and is plentiful by 17 to 20 weeks. These hairs help to hold the vernix on the skin. Lanugo is replaced during the perinatal period by coarser hairs that persist over most of the body, except in the axillary and pubic regions, where the lanugo is replaced at puberty by even coarser terminal hairs. In males, similar coarse hairs also appear on the face and often on the chest at puberty.

Melanoblasts migrate into the hair bulbs and differentiate into **melanocytes**. The melanin produced by these cells is transferred to the hair-forming cells in the germinal matrix several weeks before birth. The relative content of melanin accounts for different hair colors. **Arrector muscles of hairs**, small bundles of smooth muscle fibers, differentiate from the mesenchyme surrounding the hair follicle and attach to the dermal root sheath and the papillary layer of the dermis (see Fig. 18-2). The arrector muscles are poorly developed in the hairs of the axilla and in certain parts of the face. The hairs forming the eyebrows and the cilia forming the eyelashes have no arrector muscles.

DISORDERS OF KERATINIZATION

Ichthyosis is a general term for a group of skin disorders resulting from excessive keratinization (Fig. 18-3). The skin is characterized by dryness and fishskin-like scaling, which may involve the entire body surface. A harlequin fetus results from a rare keratinizing disorder that is inherited as an autosomal recessive trait. The skin is markedly thickened, ridged, and cracked. Most of the affected infants die during the first week of life. A collodion infant is covered at birth by a thick, taut membrane that resembles collodion or parchment. This membrane cracks with the first respiratory efforts and begins to fall off in large sheets. Complete shedding of membranes may take several weeks, occasionally leaving normal-appearing skin.

ANGIOMAS OF THE SKIN

Angiomas of the skin is a vascular anomaly in which some transitory primordial blood or lymphatic vessels persist. Similar lesions that are composed of lymphatics are called cystic lymphangiomas, or cystic hygromas (see Chapter 14). True angiomas are benign tumors of the endothelial cells, usually composed of solid or hollow cords; the hollow cords contain blood. Various terms are used to describe angiomatous anomalies ("birthmarks"). Nevus flammeus denotes a flat, pink or red, flamelike blotch that often appears on the posterior surface of the neck. A port wine stain, or hemangioma, is a larger, darker angioma than a nevus flammeus and is nearly always anterior or lateral on the face, neck, or both.

ALBINISM

In *generalized albinism,* an autosomal recessive trait, the skin, hairs, and retina lack pigment; however, the iris usually shows some pigmentation. Albinism occurs when the melanocytes do not produce melanin because of a lack of the enzyme tyrosinase. In *localized albinism—* piebaldism—an autosomal dominant trait, there is a lack of melanin in patches of skin, hair, or both.

and proximally by folds of epidermis called **nail folds.** Cells from the proximal nail fold grow over the nail field and keratinize to form the **nail plate** (see Fig. 18-4B). At first, the developing nail is covered by superficial layers of epidermis called **eponychium** (see Fig. 18-4C). These layers degenerate, exposing the nail, except at its base, where it persists as the **cuticle.** The fingernails reach the fingertips by approximately 32 weeks; the toenails reach the toe tips by approximately 36 weeks.

DEFORMED NAILS

Deformed nails occur occasionally and may be a manifestation of a generalized skin disease or a systemic disease. A number of congenital diseases (e.g., psoriasis) are associated with nail defects.

■ DEVELOPMENT OF THE MAMMARY GLANDS

Mammary glands are modified and highly specialized types of sweat glands. **Mammary buds** begin to develop during the sixth week as solid downgrowths of the epidermis into the underlying mesenchyme (Fig. 18-5C). These changes occur in response to an inductive influence from the mesenchyme. The mammary buds develop from the mammary crests, which are thickened strips of ectoderm extending from the axillary to the inguinal regions (see Fig. 18-5A). The **mammary crests** appear during the fourth week, but normally persist only in the pectoral area, where the breasts develop (see Fig. 18-5B). Each primary mammary bud soon gives rise to several secondary mammary buds that develop into the **lactiferous ducts** and their branches (see Fig. 18-5D and E). Canalization of these buds is induced by maternal sex hormones entering the fetal circulation. This process continues until late gestation, and by term, 15 to 20 lactiferous ducts have formed. The fibrous connective tissue and the fat of the mammary gland develop from the surrounding mesenchyme.

During the late fetal period, the epidermis at the site of origin of the primordial mammary gland becomes depressed, forming a shallow **mammary pit** (see Fig. 18-5E). The nipples are poorly formed and depressed

FIGURE **18-3.** A child with epidermolytic hyperkeratosis. This condition is characterized by severe hyperkeratosis from the time of birth. It has an autosomal dominant inheritance pattern. (Courtesy of Dr. Joao Carlos Fernandes Rodrigues, Servico de Dermatologia, Hospital de Desterro, Lisbon, Portugal.)

■ DEVELOPMENT OF THE NAILS

Toenails and fingernails begin to develop at the tips of the digits at approximately 10 weeks (Fig. 18-4). Development of the **fingernails** precedes that of the **toenails** by approximately 4 weeks. The primordia of the nails appear as thickened areas, or fields, of epidermis at the tip of each digit. Later, these **nail fields** migrate onto the dorsal surface (see Fig. 18-4A), carrying their innervation from the ventral surface. The nail fields are surrounded laterally

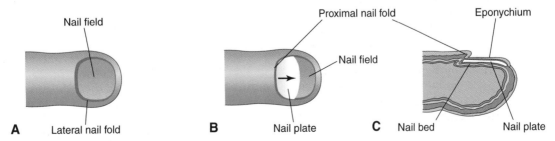

A Nail field   Lateral nail fold   **B** Proximal nail fold   Nail field   Nail plate   **C** Eponychium   Nail bed   Nail plate

FIGURE **18-4.** Successive stages in the development of a fingernail. **A,** The first indication of a nail is a thickening of the epidermis, the nail field, at the tip of the finger. **B,** As the nail plate develops, it slowly grows toward the tip of the finger. **C,** The fingernail normally reaches the end of the digit by 32 weeks.

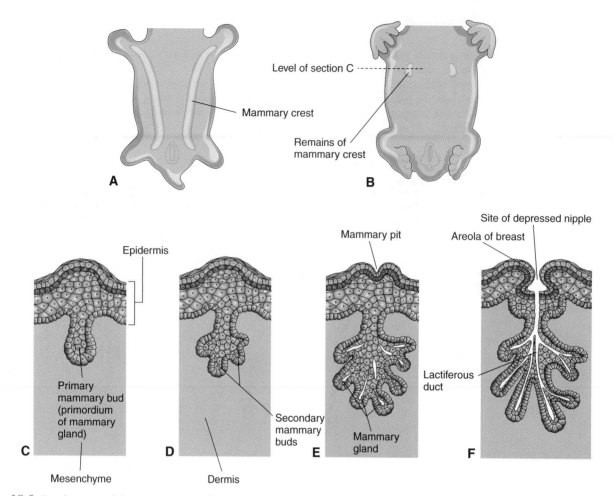

FIGURE 18-5. Development of the mammary glands. **A,** Ventral view of an embryo at approximately 28 days, showing mammary crests (ridges). **B,** Similar view at 6 weeks, showing the remains of these crests. **C,** Transverse section of a mammary crest at the site of a developing mammary gland. **D to F,** Similar sections, showing successive stages of breast development between the 12th week and birth.

GYNECOMASTIA

The rudimentary mammary glands in males normally undergo no postnatal development. **Gynecomastia** refers to excessive development of the male mammary tissue. It occurs in most newborn males because of stimulation of the mammary glands by maternal sex hormones. This effect disappears in a few weeks. During midpuberty, approximately two thirds of boys have varying degrees of hyperplasia of the breasts. Approximately 80% of males with Klinefelter syndrome have gynecomastia (see Chapter 19).

SUPERNUMERARY BREASTS AND NIPPLES

An extra breast (**polymastia**) or nipple (**polythelia**), an inheritable condition, occurs in approximately 1% of the female population. **Supernumerary nipples** are also relatively common in males; often, they are mistaken for moles. Less commonly, **supernumerary breasts** or nipples appear in the axillary or abdominal regions of females. In these positions, the nipples or breasts arise from extra mammary buds that develop along the mammary crests. Approximately one third of affected persons have two extra nipples or breasts.

in newborn infants. After birth, the nipples usually rise from the mammary pits. At birth, the main lactiferous ducts are formed (see Fig. 18-5F); the mammary glands remain underdeveloped until puberty. The mammary glands develop similarly and are of the same structure in both sexes. In females, the glands enlarge rapidly during puberty, mainly because of fat and other connective tissue development in the breasts. Growth of the duct system

also occurs because of the increased levels of circulating estrogens.

■ DEVELOPMENT OF THE TEETH

Two sets of teeth normally develop: the primary dentition, or **deciduous teeth**, and the secondary dentition, or

permanent teeth. Teeth develop from the oral ectoderm, the mesoderm, and the neural crest cells.

The **enamel** is derived from the ectoderm of the oral cavity; all other tissues differentiate from the surrounding mesenchyme and neural crest cells. Experimental evidence indicates that neural crest cells are imprinted with morphogenetic information before or shortly after they migrate from the neural crest. The expression of homeobox *MSX* and *Dlx* genes in the migrating neural crest cells, as well as in the ectoderm and mesenchyme, is essential for the initiation of tooth development.

Odontogenesis (tooth development) is initiated by the inductive influence of the **neural crest** mesenchyme on the overlying ectoderm. The first tooth buds appear in the anterior mandibular region; later tooth development occurs in the anterior maxillary region and progresses posteriorly in both jaws. Tooth development continues for years after birth (Table 18-1). The first indication of tooth development occurs in the sixth week as a thickening of the oral epithelium, a derivative of the surface ectoderm. These U-shaped bands—**dental laminae**—follow the curves of the primordial jaws (Figs. 18-6*A* and 18-7*A*).

Bud Stage of Tooth Development

Each dental lamina develops 10 centers of proliferation from which **tooth buds** grow into the underlying mesenchyme (see Figs. 18-6*B* and 18-7*B*). These tooth buds develop into the first, or **deciduous, teeth**—which are shed during childhood (see Table 18-1). There are 10 tooth buds in each jaw, one for each deciduous tooth. The tooth buds for the **permanent teeth** that have deciduous predecessors—known as *succedaneous teeth*—begin to appear at approximately 10 weeks from deep continuations of the dental laminae (see Fig. 18-7*D*). They develop lingual (toward the tongue) to the **deciduous tooth buds.** The permanent molars that have no deciduous predecessors develop as buds from posterior extensions of the **dental laminae.** The tooth buds for the permanent teeth appear at different times, mostly during the fetal period. The buds for the second and third permanent molars develop after birth.

Cap Stage of Tooth Development

As each tooth bud is invaginated by the mesenchyme—the **primordium of the dental papilla**—the bud becomes cap-shaped (see Fig. 18-7*C*). The ectodermal part of the developing tooth, the **enamel organ**, eventually produces **enamel**. The internal part of each cap-shaped tooth, the **dental papilla**, is the primordium of the dental pulp. Together, the dental papilla and the enamel organ form the **tooth germ** (primordial tooth). The outer cell layer of the enamel organ is the **outer enamel epithelium**, whereas the inner cell layer lining the "cap" is the **inner enamel epithelium** (see Fig. 18-7*D*). The central core of loosely arranged cells between the layers of enamel epithelium is the **enamel (stellate) reticulum** (see Fig. 18-7*E*). As the enamel organ and the dental papilla of the tooth develop, the mesenchyme surrounding the developing tooth condenses to form the **dental sac**, a

TABLE 18-1. The Order and Usual Time of Eruption of Teeth and the Time of Shedding of Deciduous Teeth

TOOTH	USUAL ERUPTION TIME	SHEDDING TIME
Deciduous		
Medial incisor	6–8 mo	6–7 yr
Lateral incisor	8–10 mo	7–8 yr
Canine	16–20 mo	10–12 yr
First molar	12–16 mo	9–11 yr
Second molar	20–24 mo	10–12 yr
Permanent*		
Medial incisor	7–8 yr	
Lateral incisor	8–9 yr	
Canine	10–12 yr	
First premolar	10–11 yr	
Second premolar	11–12 yr	
First molar	6–7 yr	
Second molar	12 yr	
Third molar	13–25 yr	

Modified from Moore KL, Dalley AF: Clinically Oriented Anatomy, 5th ed. Baltimore, Williams & Wilkins, 2006.

*The permanent teeth are not shed. If they are not properly cared for or if disease of the gingiva develops, they may fall out or may have to be extracted.

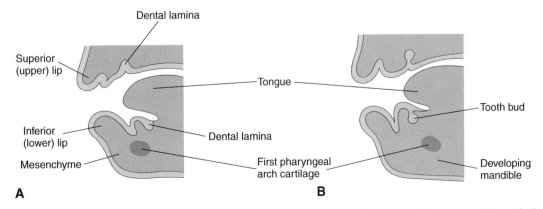

A **B**

Figure **18-6.** Sagittal sections through the developing jaws, showing early development of the teeth. **A,** Early in the sixth week, the dental laminae are evident. **B,** Later in the sixth week, tooth buds arise from the laminae.

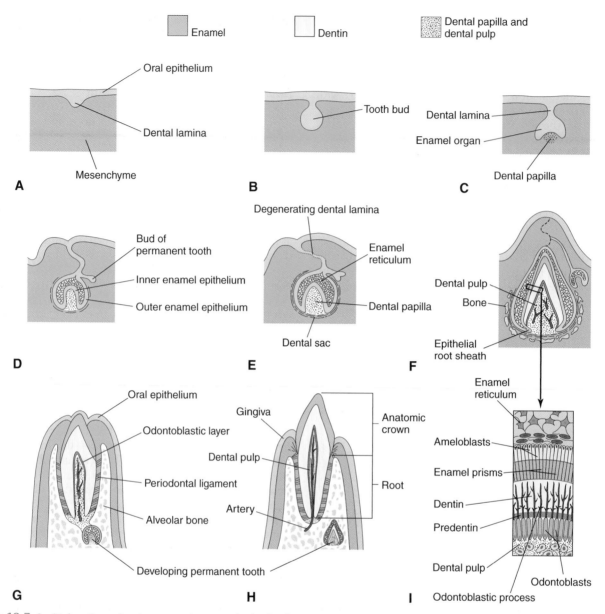

FIGURE 18-7. Sagittal sections, showing successive stages in the development and eruption of an incisor tooth. **A,** At 6 weeks, showing the dental lamina. **B,** At 7 weeks, showing the tooth bud developing from the dental lamina. **C,** At 8 weeks, showing the cap stage of tooth development. **D,** At 10 weeks, showing the early bell stage of a deciduous tooth and the bud stage of a permanent tooth. **E,** At 14 weeks, showing the advanced bell stage of tooth development. Note that the connection (dental lamina) of the tooth to the oral epithelium is degenerating. **F,** At 28 weeks, showing the enamel and dentin layers. **G,** At 6 months postnatally, showing early tooth eruption. **H,** At 18 months postnatally, showing a fully erupted deciduous incisor tooth. The permanent incisor tooth now has a well-developed crown. **I,** Section through a developing tooth, showing ameloblasts (enamel producers) and odontoblasts (dentin producers).

vascularized capsular structure (see Fig. 18-7E). The dental sac is the primordium of the cement and the periodontal ligament. The cement is the bonelike, rigid connective tissue covering the root of the tooth. The **periodontal ligament** is the fibrous connective tissue that surrounds the root of the tooth, separating it from and attaching it to the alveolar bone (see Fig. 18-7G).

Bell Stage of Tooth Development

As the enamel organ differentiates, the developing tooth becomes bell-shaped (see Figs. 18-7D and 18-8). The mesenchymal cells in the dental papilla adjacent to the inner enamel epithelium differentiate into **odontoblasts,** which produce **predentine** and deposit it adjacent to the epithelium. Later, the predentin calcifies and becomes **dentin.** As the dentin thickens, the odontoblasts regress toward the center of the dental papilla; however, their cytoplasmic processes—**odontoblastic processes,** or *Tomes processes*—remain embedded in the dentin (see Fig. 18-7F and I). The brittle enamel is the hardest tissue in the body. It overlies the yellowish dentin, the second hardest tissue in the body, and protects it from being fractured. The cells of the inner enamel epithelium differentiate into **ameloblasts,** which produce enamel in the form of

FIGURE 18-8. Photomicrograph (×17) of a section of the crown and neck of a tooth. Observe the enamel (E), dentin (D), dental pulp (P), and odontoblasts (O). (From Gartner LP, Hiatt JL: Color Textbook of Histology, 2nd ed. Philadelphia, WB Saunders, 2001.)

FIGURE 18-9. Cranium of a 4-year-old child. Bone has been removed from the jaws to show the relation of the developing permanent teeth to the erupted deciduous teeth.

the bony wall of the alveolus. The periodontal ligament is located between the cementum of the root and the bony alveolus.

Tooth Eruption

As the teeth develop, they begin a continuous slow movement in toward the oral cavity (see Fig. 18-7F and G). The mandibular teeth usually erupt before the maxillary teeth, and girls' teeth usually erupt sooner than boys' teeth. A child's dentition contains **20 deciduous teeth**. As the root of the tooth grows, its crown gradually erupts through the oral epithelium. The part of the oral mucosa around the erupted crown becomes the **gingiva** (gum). Usually, eruption of the deciduous teeth occurs between 6 and 24 months after birth (see Table 18-1). The mandibular medial incisors—or **central incisors**—usually erupt 6 to 8 months after birth, but this process may not begin until 12 or 13 months in some children. Despite this, all 20 deciduous teeth are usually present by the end of the second year in healthy children. Delayed eruption of all teeth may indicate a systemic or nutritional disturbance, such as hypopituitarism or hypothyroidism.

The **permanent teeth** develop in a manner similar to that described for deciduous teeth. As a permanent tooth grows, the root of the corresponding deciduous tooth is gradually resorbed by **osteoclasts**. Consequently, when the deciduous tooth is shed, it consists only of the crown and the cervical, or uppermost, part of the root. The permanent teeth usually begin to erupt during the sixth year and continue to appear until early adulthood (Fig. 18-9; see also Table 18-1).

prisms (rods) over the dentin. As the enamel increases, the ameloblasts regress toward the outer enamel epithelium. The **root of the tooth** begins to develop after dentin and enamel formation is well advanced. The inner and outer enamel epithelia come together in the neck region of the tooth, where they form a fold, the **epithelial root sheath** (see Fig. 18-7F). This sheath grows into the mesenchyme and initiates root formation. The odontoblasts adjacent to the epithelial root sheath form dentin that is continuous with that of the crown. As the dentin increases, it reduces the pulp cavity to a narrow **root canal** through which the vessels and nerves pass. The inner cells of the dental sac differentiate into **cementoblasts**, which produce cement that is restricted to the root. Cement is deposited over the dentin of the root and meets the enamel at the neck of the tooth (cementoenamel junction).

As the teeth develop and the jaws ossify, the outer cells of the dental sac also become active in bone formation. Each tooth soon becomes surrounded by bone, except over its crown. The tooth is held in its **alveolus** (bony socket) by the strong **periodontal ligament**, a derivative of the dental sac (see Fig. 18-7G and *H*). Some fibers of this ligament are embedded in the cement; other fibers are embedded in

NATAL TEETH

Natal teeth are those that are erupted at birth. There are usually two in the position of the mandibular incisors. Natal teeth, which are observed in approximately 1 in 2000 newborn infants, may produce maternal discomfort during breast-feeding. In addition, the teeth may lacerate the infant's tongue, or may detach and be aspirated; for these reasons, natal teeth are sometimes extracted.

ENAMEL HYPOPLASIA

Defective enamel formation causes pits, fissures, or both in the enamel. These defects result from temporary disturbances of enamel formation. Various factors may injure ameloblasts (the enamel builders), such as nutritional deficiency, tetracycline therapy, and infectious diseases. **Rickets** arising during the critical period of permanent tooth development (6–12 weeks) is the most common known cause of enamel hypoplasia. Rickets is a disease affecting children who are deficient in vitamin D.

VARIATIONS OF TOOTH SHAPE

Abnormally shaped teeth are relatively common. Occasionally, there are spheric masses of enamel—**enamel pearls**—attached to the tooth (Fig. 18-10*E*). They are formed by **aberrant groups of ameloblasts.** In other children, the maxillary lateral incisor teeth may have a slender, tapered shape (peg-shaped incisors). **Congenital syphilis** affects the differentiation of the permanent teeth, resulting in screwdriver-shaped incisors, with central notches in the incisive edges.

NUMERIC ABNORMALITIES OF TEETH

One or more **supernumerary teeth** may develop, or the normal number of teeth may not form (see Fig. 18-10*D*). Supernumerary teeth usually develop in the area of the maxillary incisors (called a **mesiodens**) and may disrupt the position and the eruption of normal teeth. The extra teeth commonly erupt posterior to the normal teeth. In **partial anodontia**, one or more teeth are absent. Congenital absence of one or more teeth is often a familial trait. In **total anodontia**, no teeth develop; this very rare condition is usually associated with congenital ectodermal dysplasia (disorders involving tissues that are ectodermal in origin).

FIGURE 18-10. Some common tooth anomalies. **A,** Amelogenesis imperfecta. **B,** Dentinogenesis imperfecta. **C,** Tetracycline-stained teeth. **D,** Midline supernumerary tooth (M, mesiodens), located near the root apex of the central incisor. The prevalence of supernumerary teeth is 1% to 3%. **E,** Molar tooth with an enamel pearl (*arrow*). (**A,** Courtesy of Dr. Blaine Cleghorn, Faculty of Dentistry, Dalhousie University, Halifax, Nova Scotia, Canada; **B** to **D,** Courtesy of Dr. Steve Ahing, Faculty of Dentistry, University of Manitoba, Winnipeg, Manitoba, Canada.)

FUSION OF TOOTH GERMS

Fusion is a single large (macrodontia) tooth caused by the union of two adjacent tooth germs. The crowns of the two teeth can be partially or completely fused. The same applies to roots. Occasionally, a tooth bud divides or two buds partially fuse to form fused teeth. This condition is commonly observed in the mandibular incisors of the primary dentition, but can also occur in the permanent dentition.

AMELOGENESIS IMPERFECTA

In amelogenesis imperfecta, the tooth enamel is soft and friable because of hypocalcification, and the teeth are yellow to brown (see Fig. 18-10A). The teeth are covered with only a thin layer of abnormally formed enamel through which the yellow underlying dentin is visible. This gives the teeth a darkened appearance. This autosomal dominant condition affects approximately 1 in 7000 newborn infants.

DENTINOGENESIS IMPERFECTA

Dentinogenesis imperfecta is relatively common in white children (see Fig. 18-10B). In affected children, the teeth are brown to gray-blue, with an opalescent sheen, caused by failure of the odontoblasts to differentiate normally, producing poorly calcified dentin. Both the deciduous and the permanent teeth are usually involved. The enamel tends to wear down rapidly, exposing the dentin. This anomaly is inherited as an autosomal dominant trait.

CLINICALLY ORIENTED QUESTIONS

1. An infant was reportedly born without skin. Is this possible? If so, could such an infant survive?

DISCOLORED TEETH

Foreign substances incorporated into the developing enamel and dentin discolor the teeth. The hemolysis (liberation of hemoglobin) associated with hemolytic disease of the newborn (see Chapter 8) may produce blue to black discoloration of the teeth. *All tetracyclines are extensively incorporated into the teeth.* The critical period of risk is from approximately 14 weeks of fetal life to the 10th postnatal month for deciduous teeth, and from approximately 14 weeks of fetal life to the 16th postnatal year for permanent teeth. Tetracyclines produce brownish-yellow discoloration (mottling) and enamel hypoplasia because they interfere with the metabolic processes of the ameloblasts (see Fig. 18-10C). The enamel is completely formed on all but the third molars by approximately 8 years of age. For this reason, *tetracyclines should not be administered to pregnant women or to children younger than 8 years.*

2. A dark-skinned person presented with patches of white skin on the face, chest, and limbs. He even had a white forelock. What is this condition called, and what is its developmental basis? Is there any treatment for these skin defects?
3. Some boys have enlarged breasts at birth. Is this an indication of abnormal sex development? Some boys develop breasts during puberty. Are they intersexes?
4. A girl developed a breast in the axilla during puberty. She also had extra nipples on her chest. What is the embryologic basis for these anomalies?
5. An infant was born with two teeth. Would these be normal teeth? Is this a common occurrence? Are they usually extracted?

The answers to these questions are at the back of the book.

HUMAN BIRTH DEFECTS

*C*ongenital anomalies, *birth defects*, and *malformations* are terms currently used to describe developmental disorders that are present at birth. **Birth defects** are the leading cause of infant mortality and may be structural, functional, metabolic, behavioral, or hereditary. A **congenital anomaly** is a structural abnormality of any type; however, *not all variations are anomalies.* Anatomic variations are common. Congenital anomalies are of four clinically significant types: malformation, disruption, deformation, and dysplasia.

■ TERATOLOGY: THE STUDY OF ABNORMAL DEVELOPMENT

Teratology is the branch of science that studies the causes, mechanisms, and patterns of abnormal development. A fundamental concept in teratology is that certain stages of embryonic development are more vulnerable to disruption than others.

More than 20% of infant deaths in North America are attributable to birth defects. Major structural anomalies, such as spina bifida cystica—a severe type of defect in which part of the neural tube does not fuse—are observed in approximately 3% of newborn infants. Additional anomalies may only be detected after birth; thus, the incidence of birth defects approaches 6% in 2-year-old children and 8% in 5-year-old children.

Congenital anomalies may be caused by *genetic factors*, such as chromosomal abnormalities, as well as by *environmental factors*, such as drugs and viruses. However, many common congenital anomalies are the result of **multifactorial inheritance**; that is, they are caused by genetic and environmental factors acting together. Yet, for 50% to 60% of congenital anomalies, the causes are unknown (Fig. 19-1). Congenital anomalies may be single or multiple and of major or minor clinical significance. Single **minor anomalies** are present in approximately 14% of neonates. Anomalies of the external ear, for example, are of no serious medical significance, but they indicate the possible presence of associated major anomalies. For example, the presence of a single umbilical artery alerts the clinician to the possible presence of cardiovascular and renal anomalies. Major developmental defects are much more common in early embryos (10%–15%), but most embryos abort spontaneously during the first 6 weeks. Chromosomal abnormalities are present in more than 50% of spontaneously aborted conceptuses.

■ ANOMALIES CAUSED BY GENETIC FACTORS*

In terms of the sheer number of cases, genetic factors are the most important cause of congenital anomalies. It has been estimated that they cause approximately one third of all birth defects (see Fig. 19-1) and nearly 85% of anomalies with known causes. Any mechanism as complex as mitosis or meiosis may occasionally malfunction; thus, *chromosomal aberrations are common and are present in 6% to 7% of zygotes.* Many of these early embryos never undergo normal cleavage to become blastocysts. The changes may affect the sex chromosomes, the autosomes, or both (chromosomes other than sex chromosomes). In some instances, both kinds of chromosome are affected. Persons with chromosomal abnormalities usually have characteristic phenotypes, such as the physical characteristics of infants with Down syndrome. *Numerical and structural changes occur in chromosome complements.*

Numerical Chromosomal Abnormalities

Numeric aberrations of chromosomes usually result from **nondisjunction**, an error in cell division in which a chromosome pair or two chromatids of a chromosome do not disjoin during mitosis or meiosis. As a result, the chromosome pair or the chromatids pass to one daughter cell, and the other daughter cell receives neither (Fig. 19-2). Nondisjunction may occur during maternal or paternal gametogenesis (see Chapter 2). The chromosomes in somatic (body) cells are normally paired;

---

*The authors are grateful to Dr. A.E. Chudley, MD, FRCPC, FCCMG, Professor of Pediatrics and Child Health, and Head, Section of Genetics and Metabolism, Children's Hospital, Health Sciences Centre, University of Manitoba, Winnipeg, Manitoba, Canada, for assistance with the preparation of this section.

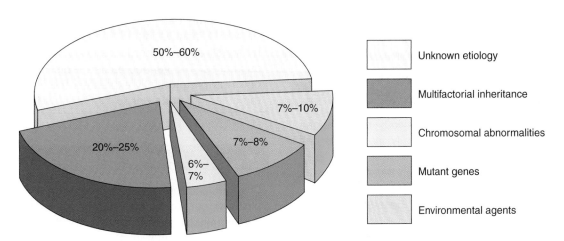

FIGURE 19-1. The causes of human birth defects. Note that the causes of most anomalies are unknown and that 20% to 25% of them are caused by a combination of genetic and environmental factors (multifactorial inheritance).

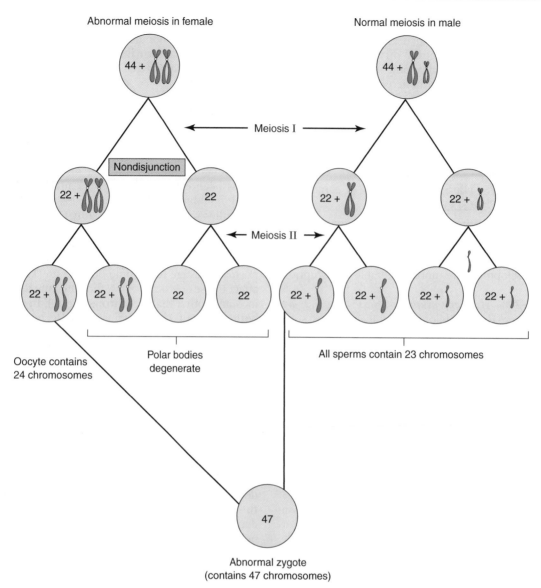

FIGURE 19-2. Nondisjunction of chromosomes during the first meiotic division of a primary oocyte, resulting in an abnormal oocyte with 24 chromosomes. Subsequent fertilization by a normal sperm produces a zygote with 47 chromosomes—**aneuploidy**—a deviation from the human diploid number of 46.

the *homologous chromosomes* making up a pair are homologs. Normal human females have 22 pairs of autosomes plus two X chromosomes, whereas normal males have 22 pairs of autosomes plus one X and one Y chromosome.

INACTIVATION OF GENES

During embryogenesis, one of the two X chromosomes in female somatic cells is randomly inactivated and appears as a mass of **sex chromatin**. Inactivation of the genes on one X chromosome in the somatic cells of female embryos occurs during implantation. *X-inactivation is important clinically* because it means that each cell from a carrier of an X-linked disease has the mutant gene causing the disease, either on the active X chromosome or on the inactivated X

chromosome that is represented by sex chromatin. Uneven X-inactivation in monozygotic twins is one reason given for discordance in a variety of congenital anomalies. The genetic basis for discordance is that one twin preferentially expresses the paternal X and the other, the maternal X.

ANEUPLOIDY AND POLYPLOIDY

Changes in chromosome number result in either aneuploidy or polyploidy. **Aneuploidy** is any deviation from the human diploid number of 46 chromosomes. An *aneuploid* is an individual or a cell that has a chromosome number that is not an exact multiple of the haploid number of 23 (e.g., 45 or 47). The principal cause of aneuploidy is nondisjunction during cell division (see Fig. 19-2), resulting in an unequal distribution of one pair of homologous chromosomes to the daughter cells. One cell has two chromosomes, and the other has neither chromosome of the pair. As a result, the embryo's cells may be *hypodiploid* (45, X, as in *Turner syndrome*) (see Fig. 19-3) or *hyperdiploid* (usually 47, as in trisomy 21, or *Down syndrome*) (see Fig. 19-4). Embryos with **monosomy**—missing a chromosome—usually die. Monosomy of an autosome is extremely uncommon, and approximately 99% of embryos lacking a sex chromosome (45, X) abort spontaneously.

FIGURE 19-3. Turner syndrome in a 14-year-old girl. Note the classic features of the syndrome: short stature; webbed neck; absence of sexual maturation; broad, shieldlike chest with widely spaced nipples; and lymphedema of the hands and feet. (Courtesy of Dr. F. Antoniazzi and Dr. V. Fanos, Department of Pediatrics, University of Verona, Verona, Italy.)

Turner Syndrome

Approximately 1% of female embryos with monosomy X survive. The incidence of 45, X—or Turner syndrome—in newborn females is approximately 1 in 8000 live births. Half of the affected individuals have 45, X; the other half have a variety of abnormalities affecting a sex chromosome. *The phenotype of Turner syndrome is female* and is shown in Figure 19-3. **Phenotype** refers to the morphologic characteristics of an individual, as determined by the genotype and the environment in which it is expressed. Secondary sexual characteristics do not develop in 90% of girls with Turner syndrome, necessitating hormone replacement therapy. *The monosomy X chromosomal abnormality is the most common cytogenetic abnormality observed in live-born humans and in fetuses that abort spontaneously*, and it accounts for approximately 18% of all abortions caused by chromosomal abnormalities. The error in gametogenesis (nondisjunction) that causes monosomy X, when it can be traced, is in the paternal gamete in approximately 75% of cases; that is, it is the paternal X chromosome that is usually missing.

If three chromosomes are present instead of the usual pair, the abnormality is known as *trisomy*. Trisomies are the most common abnormalities of chromosome number. The usual cause of this numeric error is **meiotic nondisjunction of chromosomes** (see Fig. 19-2), resulting in a gamete with 24 instead of 23 chromosomes and, subsequently, a zygote with 47 chromosomes.

Trisomy of the Autosomes

Trisomy of the autosomes is associated mainly with three syndromes (Table 19-1):
● Trisomy 21, or Down syndrome (Fig. 19-4)
● Trisomy 18, or Edwards syndrome (Fig. 19-5)
● Trisomy 13, or Patau syndrome (Fig. 19-6)
    Infants with trisomy 13 and trisomy 18 are severely malformed and mentally retarded. They usually die early in infancy. More than 50% of trisomic conceptions abort early in pregnancy. *Trisomy of the autosomes occurs with increasing frequency as maternal age increases* (Table 19-2).
    Mosaicism—two or more cell types containing different numbers of chromosomes (normal and abnormal)—leads to a less severe phenotype, and the affected individuals may have a nearly normal IQ.

Trisomy of the Sex Chromosomes

Trisomy of the sex chromosomes is a common condition (Table 19-3); however, because no characteristic physical findings are seen in infants or children, this disorder is not usually detected before puberty (Fig. 19-7). The diagnosis is best established by chromosomal and molecular analysis.

Structural Chromosomal Abnormalities

Most abnormalities of chromosome structure result from chromosome breakage followed by reconstitution in an abnormal combination (Fig. 19-8). **Chromosome breaks** may be induced by various environmental factors, such as

TABLE 19-1. Trisomy of the Autosomes

CHROMOSOMAL ABERRATION/ SYNDROME	INCIDENCE	USUAL MORPHOLOGIC CHARACTERISTICS	FIGURE
Trisomy 21, or Down syndrome*	1:800	Mental deficiency; brachycephaly; flat nasal bridge; upward slant to palpebral fissures; protruding tongue; simian crease; clinodactyly of 5th digit; congenital heart defects	19-4
Trisomy 18 syndrome†	1:8000	Mental deficiency; growth retardation; prominent occiput; short sternum; ventricular septal defect; micrognathia; low-set, malformed ears; flexed digits; hypoplastic nails; rocker-bottom feet	19-5
Trisomy 13 syndrome†	1:25,000	Mental deficiency; severe central nervous system malformations; sloping forehead; malformed ears; scalp defects; microphthalmia; bilateral cleft lip or palate; polydactyly; posterior prominence of heels	19-6

*The importance of this disorder in the overall problem of mental deficiency (retardation) is indicated by the fact that persons with Down syndrome represent 10% to 15% of institutionalized, mentally defective individuals. The incidence of trisomy 21 at fertilization is greater than that at birth; however, 75% of affected embryos are spontaneously aborted and at least 20% are stillborn.
†Infants with this syndrome rarely survive beyond 6 months of age.

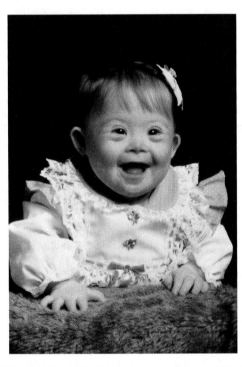

FIGURE 19-4. An infant with Down syndrome (trisomy 21). Note the round face, upslanted palpebral fissures, and short digits with incurving of the fifth digit (clinodactyly). (Courtesy of A.E. Chudley, MD, Section of Genetics and Metabolism, Department of Pediatrics and Child Health, Children's Hospital and University of Manitoba, Winnipeg, Manitoba, Canada.)

FIGURE 19-5. Female neonate with trisomy 18. Note the growth retardation, clenched fists with characteristic positioning of the fingers (second and fifth digits overlapping the third and fourth), short sternum, and narrow pelvis. (Courtesy of A.E. Chudley, MD, Section of Genetics and Metabolism, Department of Pediatrics and Child Health, Children's Hospital and University of Manitoba, Winnipeg, Manitoba, Canada.)

irradiation, drugs, chemicals, and viruses. The resulting abnormality in chromosome structure depends on what happens to the broken pieces. The only two aberrations of chromosome structure that are likely to be transmitted from parent to child are structural rearrangements, such as inversion and translocation.

Translocation

Translocation is the transfer of a piece of one chromosome to a nonhomologous chromosome. If two nonhomologous chromosomes exchange pieces, it is called a *reciprocal translocation* (see Fig. 19-8*A* and *G*). Translocation does not necessarily cause abnormal development. Persons with a translocation between chromosome 21 and chromosome 14, for example (see Fig. 19-8*G*), are phenotypically normal. Such persons are called *balanced translocation carriers*. They have a tendency, independent of age, to produce germ cells

TABLE 19-2. Incidence of Down Syndrome in Newborn Infants

MATERNAL AGE (YEARS)	INCIDENCE
20–24	1:1400
25–29	1:1100
30–34	1:700
35	1:350
37	1:225
39	1:140
41	1:85
43	1:50
45+	1:25

FIGURE 19-7. A boy with Klinefelter syndrome (XXY trisomy). Note the presence of developed breasts; approximately 40% of males with this syndrome have gynecomastia (excessive development of the male mammary glands) and small testes. (Courtesy of Children's Hospital and University of Manitoba, Winnipeg, Manitoba, Canada.)

FIGURE 19-6. Female neonate with trisomy 13. Note, in particular, the bilateral cleft lip; low-set, malformed ears; and polydactyly (extra digits). A small omphalocele (herniation of the viscera into the umbilical cord) is also present. (Courtesy of A.E. Chudley, MD, Section of Genetics and Metabolism, Department of Pediatrics and Child Health, Children's Hospital and University of Manitoba, Winnipeg, Manitoba, Canada.)

MOSAICISM

A person who has at least two cell lines with *two or more different genotypes* (genetic constitutions) is known as a **mosaic**. Either the autosomes or the sex chromosomes may be involved. Usually, the anomalies are less serious than in persons with monosomy or trisomy. Mosaicism usually results from nondisjunction during early cleavage of the zygote (see Chapter 3). Mosaicism resulting from loss of a chromosome by *anaphase lagging* also occurs; the chromosomes separate normally, but one of them is delayed in its migration and is eventually lost.

TABLE 19-3. Trisomy of the Sex Chromosomes

CHROMOSOME COMPLEMENT*	SEX	INCIDENCE[†]	USUAL CHARACTERISTICS
47, XXX	Female	1:1000	Normal appearance; usually fertile; 15% to 25% have mild mental retardation
47, XXY	Male	1:1000	Klinefelter syndrome; small testes; hyalinization of seminiferous tubules; aspermatogenesis; often tall, with disproportionately long lower limbs; intelligence is less than in normal siblings; gynecomastia in approximately 40%
47, XYY	Male	1:1000	Normal appearance; usually tall; often show aggressive behavior

*The numbers designate the total number of chromosomes, including the sex chromosomes (shown after the comma).
[†]See Nussbaum RL, McInnes RR, Willard HF: Thompson & Thompson Genetics in Medicine, 6th ed (revised reprint). Philadelphia, WB Saunders, 2004.

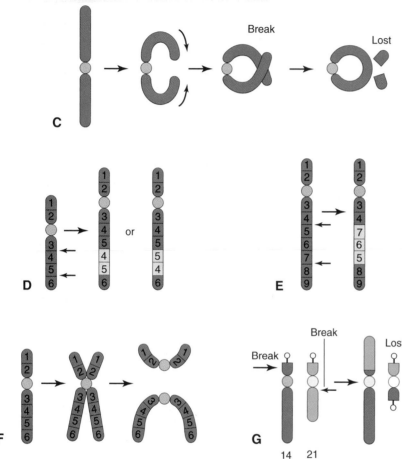

FIGURE 19-8. Various structural abnormalities of chromosomes. **A,** Reciprocal translocation. **B,** Terminal deletion. **C,** Ring chromosome. **D,** Duplication. **E,** Paracentric inversion. **F,** Isochromosome. **G,** Robertsonian translocation. *Arrows* indicate how the structural abnormalities are produced.

TRIPLOIDY

The most common type of polyploidy is **triploidy** (69 chromosomes). Triploid fetuses have severe intrauterine growth restriction (IUGR), with a disproportionately small trunk as well as other anomalies. Triploidy can result if the second polar body does not separate from the oocyte during the second meiotic division (see Chapter 2); more likely, however, triploidy results when an oocyte is fertilized by two sperms (dispermy) almost simultaneously. Triploidy occurs in approximately 2% of embryos, but most of them abort spontaneously. Triploid fetuses account for approximately 20% of chromosomally abnormal miscarriages. In rare cases, triploid fetuses have been born alive, but none have survived more than a few days after birth.

TETRAPLOIDY

Doubling the diploid chromosome number to 92 (tetraploidy) probably occurs during the first cleavage division. Division of this abnormal zygote would subsequently result in an embryo with cells containing 92 chromosomes. Tetraploid embryos abort very early; often, all that is recovered is an empty chorionic sac.

TETRASOMY AND PENTASOMY

Tetrasomy and pentasomy of the sex chromosomes also occur. Persons with these abnormalities have four or five sex chromosomes. The following chromosome complexes have been reported in females: 48, XXXX and 49, XXXXX. The following chromosome complexes have been reported in males: 48, XXXY; 48, XXYY; 49, XXXYY; and 49, XXXXY. The extra sex of chromosomes does not accentuate sexual characteristics; however, usually, the greater the number of sex chromosomes present, the greater the severity of mental retardation and physical impairment.

with an abnormal translocation chromosome. Between 3% and 4% of persons with Down syndrome have translocation trisomies; that is, the extra chromosome 21 is attached to another chromosome.

Deletion

When a chromosome breaks, a portion of it may be lost (see Fig. 19-8*B*). A partial terminal deletion from the short arm of chromosome 5 causes **cri du chat syndrome**. Affected infants have a weak, catlike cry at birth; growth delay with microcephaly (an abnormally small head); hypertelorism (wide-set eyes); low-set ears; micrognathia (a small jaw); severe mental deficiency (retardation); and congenital heart disease. A **ring chromosome** is a type of deletion chromosome from which both ends have been lost and the broken ends have rejoined to form a ring-shaped chromosome (see Fig. 19-8*C*). Ring chromosomes are very rare, but they have been found for all chromosomes. These abnormal chromosomes have been described in persons with Turner syndrome, trisomy 18, and other abnormalities.

MICRODELETIONS AND MICRODUPLICATIONS

High-resolution banding techniques have allowed the detection of very small interstitial and terminal deletions in a number of disorders. Normal-resolution chromosome banding shows 350 bands per haploid set, whereas high-resolution chromosome banding shows up to 1300 bands per haploid set. Because the deletions span several contiguous genes, these disorders, as well as those with microduplications, are referred to as **contiguous gene syndromes**. Two examples are:

- Prader-Willi syndrome (PWS), a sporadically occurring disorder associated with short stature, mild mental retardation, obesity, hyperphagia (overeating), and hypogonadism (inadequate gonadal function)
- Angelman syndrome (AS), characterized by severe mental retardation, microcephaly, brachycephaly (shortness of the head), seizures, and ataxic (jerky) movements of the limbs and trunk

The clinical phenotype is determined by the parental origin of the deleted chromosome 15. If the deletion arises in the mother, AS occurs; if it is passed on by the father, the child exhibits the PWS phenotype. This suggests the phenomenon of **genetic imprinting**, whereby differential expression of genetic material depends on the sex of the transmitting parent.

MOLECULAR CYTOGENETICS

Several new methods for merging classic cytogenetics with DNA technology have facilitated a more precise definition of chromosomal abnormalities, location, or origins, including unbalanced translocations, accessory or marker chromosomes, and *gene mapping*. One new approach to chromosome identification is based on *fluorescent in situ hybridization*, whereby chromosome-specific DNA probes can adhere to complementary regions located on specific chromosomes. This allows improved identification of chromosome location and number in metaphase spreads or even in interphase cells. The fluorescent in situ hybridization techniques using interphase cells may soon obviate the need to culture cells for specific chromosomal analysis, as in the case of prenatal diagnosis of fetal trisomies.

DUPLICATIONS

Duplications may be manifested as a duplicated part of a chromosome located within a chromosome (see Fig. 19-8*D*), attached to a chromosome, or as a separate fragment. *Duplications are more common than deletions, and they are less harmful because no loss of genetic material occurs.* Duplication may involve part of a gene, a whole gene, or a series of genes.

INVERSION

Inversion is a chromosomal aberration in which a segment of a chromosome is reversed. *Paracentric inversion* is confined to a single arm of the chromosome (see Fig. 19-8*E*), whereas pericentric inversion involves both arms and includes the centromere. Carriers of *pericentric inversions* are at risk for having offspring with abnormalities because of unequal crossing over and malsegregation at meiosis.

ISOCHROMOSOMES

The abnormality resulting in isochromosomes occurs when the centromere divides transversely instead of longitudinally (Fig. 19-8*F*). An *isochromosome is* a chromosome in which one arm is missing and the other is duplicated. It appears to be the *most common structural abnormality of the X chromosome*. Persons with this chromosomal abnormality are often short in stature and have other stigmata of Turner syndrome. These characteristics are related to the loss of an arm of an X chromosome.

Anomalies Caused by Mutant Genes

Between 7% and 8% of congenital anomalies are caused by gene defects (see Fig. 19-1). A mutation usually involves a loss or a change in the function of a gene, and is any permanent, heritable change in the sequence of genomic DNA. Because a random change is unlikely to lead to an improvement in development, *most mutations are deleterious and some are lethal.* The mutation rate can be increased by a number of environmental agents, such as large doses of radiation. Anomalies resulting from gene mutations are inherited according to mendelian laws; consequently, predictions can be made about the probability of their occurrence in the affected person's children and other relatives. An example of a *dominantly inherited congenital anomaly* is **achondroplasia** (Fig. 19-9), which results from a *mutation of the complementary DNA in the fibroblast growth factor receptor 3 (FGFR-3) gene on chromosome 4p.* Other congenital anomalies are attributable to *autosomal recessive inheritance.* Autosomal recessive genes manifest themselves only when homozygous; as a consequence, many carriers of these genes (heterozygous persons) are not identified.

Fragile X syndrome is the most common inherited cause of moderate mental retardation (Fig. 19-10), and

FIGURE 19-9. A boy with achondroplasia. Note the short stature, short limbs and fingers, normal length of the trunk, relatively large head, prominent forehead, and depressed nasal bridge. (Courtesy of A.E. Chudley, MD, Section of Genetics and Metabolism, Department of Pediatrics and Child Health, Children's Hospital and University of Manitoba, Winnipeg, Manitoba, Canada.)

FIGURE 19-10. Fragile X syndrome. **A,** An 8-year-old, mentally deficient boy exhibiting a relatively normal appearance, with a long face and prominent ears. **B,** His 6-year-old sister also has this syndrome. She has a mild learning disability and similar features of long face and prominent ears. Note the strabismus (crossed right eye). (Courtesy of A.E. Chudley, MD, Section of Genetics and Metabolism, Department of Pediatrics and Child Health, Children's Hospital and University of Manitoba, Winnipeg, Manitoba, Canada.)

is second only to Down syndrome among all causes of moderate mental retardation in males. Fragile X syndrome has a frequency of 1 in 1500 male births and may account for much of the predominance of males in the mentally deficient population. The diagnosis can be confirmed by chromosomal analysis, which will show the fragile X chromosome, or by DNA studies, which will indicate an expansion of CGG nucleotides in a specific region of the fragile mental retardation I (FMRI) gene.

Several genetic disorders have been linked to the expansion of trinucleotides in specific genes. Examples include myotonic dystrophy, Huntington chorea, spino-bulbar atrophy (Kennedy disease), and Friedreich ataxia. X-linked recessive genes are usually manifested in affected (homozygous) males and occasionally in carrier (heterozygous) females (e.g., fragile X syndrome).

The **human genome** comprises an estimated 30,000 to 40,000 genes per haploid set, or 3 billion base pairs. Because of the *Human Genome Project* and international research collaboration, many disease- and birth defect–causing mutations in genes have been and will continue to be identified. Most genes will be sequenced and their specific function determined. Understanding the cause of birth defects will require an improvement in our understanding of gene expression during early development. Most genes that are expressed in a cell are expressed in a wide variety of cells and are involved in basic cellular metabolic functions, such as nucleic acid and protein synthesis, cytoskeleton and organelle biogenesis, and nutrient transport and mechanisms. These genes are referred to as *housekeeping genes*. The *specialty genes* are expressed at specific times in specific cells and define the hundreds of different cell types that make up the human organism. An essential aspect of developmental biology is the regulation of gene expression. Regulation is often achieved by transcription factors, which bind to regulatory or promoter elements of specific genes.

Genomic imprinting is an epigenetic process whereby the female and male germ lines confer a sex-specific mark on a chromosome subregion, so that only the paternal or the maternal allele of a gene is active in the offspring. In other words, the sex of the transmitting parent influences the expression or nonexpression of certain genes in the offspring. This is the reason for PWS and AS, in which the phenotype is determined by whether the microdeletion is transmitted by the father (PWS) or the mother (AS).

Homeobox genes are a group of genes found in all vertebrates. They have highly conserved sequences and order, and they are involved in early embryonic development and specify the identity and spatial arrangements of body segments. Protein products of these genes bind to DNA and form transcriptional factors that regulate gene expression.

■ ANOMALIES CAUSED BY ENVIRONMENTAL FACTORS

Although the human embryo is well protected in the uterus, certain environmental agents, called **teratogens**, may cause developmental disruptions after maternal exposure to them (Table 19-4). *A* teratogen *is any agent that can produce a congenital anomaly or increase the incidence of an anomaly in a population.* Environmental factors, such as infection and drugs, may simulate genetic conditions, such as when two or more children of normal parents are affected. The important principle to remember is that "not everything that is familial is genetic." The organs and parts of an embryo are most sensitive to teratogenic agents during periods of rapid differentiation (Fig. 19-11). *Environmental factors cause 7% to 10% of congenital anomalies* (see Fig. 19-1). Because molecular signaling and embryonic induction precede morphologic differentiation, the period during which structures are sensitive to interference by teratogens often precedes the stage of their visible development. Teratogens do not appear to be effective in causing anomalies until cellular differentiation has begun; however, their early actions may cause the death of an embryo, for example, during the first 2 weeks of development. The exact mechanisms by which drugs, chemicals, and other environmental factors disrupt embryonic development and induce abnormalities are unclear.

Rapid progress in molecular biology is providing additional information on the genetic control of differentiation, as well as the cascade of molecular signals and factors controlling gene expression and pattern formation. Researchers are now directing increasing attention to the molecular mechanisms of abnormal development in an attempt to understand better the pathogenesis of congenital anomalies.

Principles in Teratogenesis

When considering the possible teratogenicity of an agent, such as a drug or a chemical, three factors are important to consider:

● Critical periods of development
● Dose of the drug or chemical
● Genotype (genetic constitution) of the embryo

Critical Periods of Human Development

An embryo's susceptibility to a teratogen depends on its stage of development when an agent, such as a drug, is present (see Fig. 19-11). The most critical period in development is when cell differentiation and morphogenesis are at their peak. Table 19-5 indicates the relative frequencies of anomalies for certain organs. *The most critical period for brain development is from 3 to 16 weeks,* but its development may be disrupted after this time because the brain is differentiating and growing rapidly at birth, and it continues to do so throughout the first 2 years after birth. Teratogens (e.g., alcohol) may produce mental retardation during the embryonic and fetal periods. *Tooth development continues long after birth* (see Chapter 18); hence, the development of the permanent teeth may be disrupted by *tetracyclines* from 18 weeks (prenatal) to 16 years. *The skeletal system has a prolonged critical period of development,* extending into childhood; hence, the growth of skeletal tissues provides a good gauge of general growth. Environmental disturbances during the first 2 weeks after fertilization may interfere with cleavage of the zygote and implantation of the blastocyst, and may cause early death and spontaneous abortion of the embryo (see Fig. 19-11). In some cases, teratogens acting during the first 2 weeks of development kill the embryo; in other cases,

TABLE 19-4. Teratogens Known to Cause Human Birth Defects

AGENTS	MOST COMMON CONGENITAL ANOMALIES
Drugs	
Alcohol	Fetal alcohol syndrome: intrauterine growth restriction (IUGR); mental retardation; microcephaly; ocular anomalies; joint abnormalities; short palpebral fissures
Androgens and high doses of progestogens	Varying degree of musculinization of female fetuses; ambiguous external genitalia manifested by labial fusion and clitoral hypertrophy
Methotrexate	IUGR; skeletal and renal defects
Cocaine	IUGR; prematurity; microcephaly; cerebral infarction; urogenital anomalies; neurobehavioral disturbances
Diethylstilbestrol	Abnormalities of the uterus and vagina; cervical erosion and ridges
Isotretinoin (13-cis-retinoic acid)	Craniofacial abnormalities; neural tube defects, such as spina bifida cystica; cardiovascular defects; cleft palate; thymic aplasia
Lithium carbonate	Various anomalies, usually involving the heart and great vessels
Methotrexate	Multiple anomalies, especially skeletal, involving the face, cranium, limbs, and vertebral column
Phenytoin (Dilantin)	Fetal hydantoin syndrome: IUGR; microcephaly; mental retardation; ridged metopic suture; inner epicanthal folds; eyelid ptosis; broad, depressed nasal bridge; phalangeal hypoplasia
Tetracycline	Stained teeth; hypoplasia of enamel
Thalidomide	Abnormal development of the limbs; meromelia (partial absence of limb) and amelia (complete absence of limb); facial anomalies; systemic anomalies (e.g., cardiac and kidney defects)
Trimethadione	Developmental delay; V-shaped eyebrows; low-set ears; cleft lip or palate
Valproic acid	Craniofacial anomalies; neural tube defects; often hydrocephalus; heart and skeletal defects
Warfarin	Nasal hypoplasia; stippled epiphyses; hypoplastic phalanges; eye anomalies; mental retardation
Chemicals	
Methylmercury	Cerebral atrophy; spasticity; seizures; mental retardation
Polychlorinated biphenyls	IUGR; skin discoloration
Infections	
Cytomegalovirus	Microcephaly; chorioretinitis; sensorineural loss; delayed psychomotor and mental development; hepatosplenomegaly; hydrocephaly; cerebral palsy; brain (periventricular) calcification
Herpes simplex virus	Skin vesicles and scarring; chorioretinitis; hepatomegaly; thrombocytopenia; petechiae; hemolytic anemia; hydranencephaly
Human immunodeficiency virus	Growth failure; microcephaly; prominent, boxlike forehead; flattened nasal bridge; hypertelorism; triangular philtrum and patulous lips
Human parvovirus B19	Eye defects; degenerative changes in fetal tissues
Rubella virus	IUGR; postnatal growth retardation; cardiac and great vessel abnormalities; microcephaly; sensorineural deafness; cataract; microphthalmos; glaucoma; pigmented retinopathy; mental retardation; neonatal bleeding; hepatosplenomegaly; osteopathy; tooth defects
Toxoplasma gondii	Microcephaly; mental retardation; microphthalmia; hydrocephaly; chorioretinitis; cerebral calcifications; hearing loss; neurologic disturbances
Treponema pallidum	Hydrocephalus; congenital deafness; mental retardation; abnormal teeth and bones
Varicella virus	Cutaneous scars (dermatome distribution); neurologic anomalies (e.g., limb paresis, hydrocephaly, seizures); cataracts; microphthalmia; Horner syndrome; optic atrophy; nystagmus; chorioretinitis; microcephaly; mental retardation; skeletal anomalies (e.g., hypoplasia of limbs, fingers, and toes); urogenital anomalies
High Levels of Ionizing Radiation	Microcephaly; mental retardation; skeletal anomalies; growth retardation; cataracts

TABLE 19-5. Incidence of Major Malformations in Human Organs at Birth

ORGAN	INCIDENCE OF MALFORMATIONS
Brain	10:1000
Heart	8:1000
Kidneys	4:1000
Limbs	2:1000
All other	6:1000
Total	30:1000

Data from Connor JM, Ferguson-Smith MA: Essential Medical Genetics, 2nd ed. Oxford, Blackwell Scientific Publications, 1987.

their disruptive effects are mitigated by powerful regulatory properties of the early embryo.

Development of the embryo is most easily disrupted when the tissues and organs are forming (see Fig. 19-11). During this **organogenetic period**, teratogenic agents may induce major congenital anomalies. Physiologic defects—minor morphologic anomalies of the external ear, for example—and functional disturbances, such as mental retardation, are likely to result from disruption of development during the fetal period. *Each part, tissue, and organ of an embryo has a critical period during which its development may be disrupted* (see Fig. 19-11). The type of congenital anomaly produced depends on which parts, tissues, and organs are most susceptible at the time the teratogen is active.

Embryologic timetables, such as the one in Figure 19-11, are helpful when considering the cause of human birth defects. However, it is incorrect to assume that anomalies always result from a single event occurring during the critical period of development or that it is possible to determine from these tables the day on which an anomaly was produced. What is known is that the teratogen would have to disrupt development of the tissue, part, or organ before the end of the critical period. *The critical period for limb development, for example, is 24 to 36 days after fertilization.*

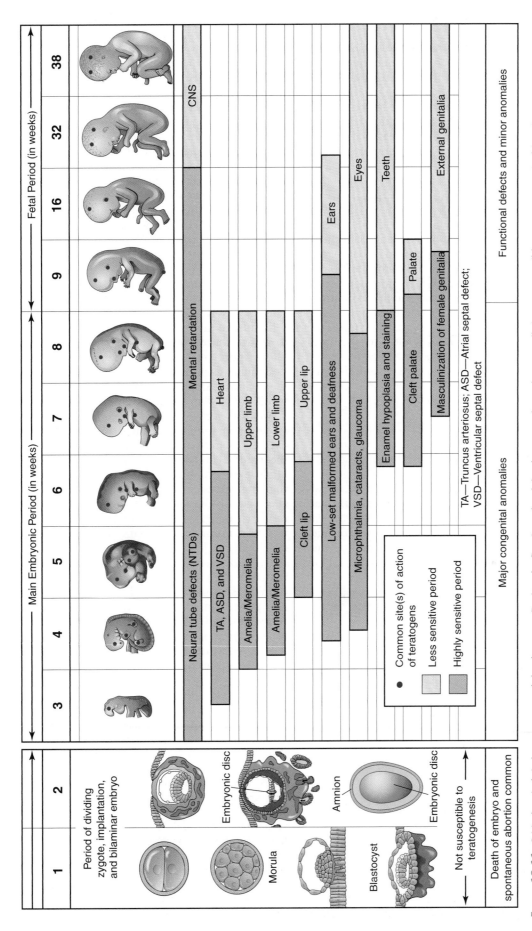

FIGURE 19-11. Critical periods in human prenatal development. During the first 2 weeks of development, the embryo usually is not susceptible to teratogens. At this point, a teratogen damages all or most of the cells, resulting in death of the embryo, or damages only a few cells, allowing the conceptus to recover and the embryo to develop without birth defects. The mauve areas denote highly sensitive periods, when major defects may be produced (e.g., amelia, absence of limbs). The green sections indicate stages that are less sensitive to teratogens, when minor defects may be induced (e.g., hypoplastic thumbs).

Dose of the Drug or Chemical

Animal research has shown a dose-response relationship for teratogens; however, the dose used to produce anomalies in animals is often much higher than the typical human dose exposure. Consequently, *animal studies are not readily applicable to human pregnancies.* For a drug to be considered a human teratogen, a dose-response relationship must be observed; that is, it must be shown that the greater the exposure during pregnancy, the more severe the phenotypic effect.

Genotype (Genetic Constitution) of the Embryo

Numerous studies in experimental animals and several suspected cases in humans have shown genetic differences in the way individual subjects respond to a teratogen. **Phenytoin,** for example, is a well-known human teratogen (see Table 19-4). Between 5% and 10% of embryos exposed to this anticonvulsant medication have **fetal hydantoin syndrome.** However, approximately one third of exposed embryos have only some of the associated congenital anomalies, and more than half of the embryos are unaffected. It appears, therefore, that the genotype of the embryo determines whether a teratogenic agent disrupts its development.

Human Teratogens

Awareness that certain agents can disrupt prenatal development offers the opportunity to prevent some congenital anomalies. For example, if women are made aware of the harmful effects of drugs (e.g., alcohol), environmental chemicals (e.g., polychlorinated biphenyls), and viruses, most pregnant women will avoid exposure to these teratogenic agents. See Table 19-4 for additional information on the topics discussed in the following sections.

PROOF OF TERATOGENICITY

To prove that an agent is a teratogen, it is necessary to show either that the frequency of anomalies is increased above the spontaneous rate in pregnancies in which the mother is exposed to the agent *(prospective approach)* or that malformed infants have a history of maternal exposure to the agent more often than normal children *(retrospective approach).* Both types of data are difficult to obtain in an unbiased form. *Case reports* are not convincing unless both the causative agent and the type of anomaly are so uncommon that their association in several cases can be judged not to be coincidental.

Drugs as Teratogens

Drugs vary considerably in their teratogenicity. Some teratogens, such as thalidomide, cause severe disruption of development if administered during the organogenetic period of certain parts of the embryo. Other teratogens cause mental and growth restriction and other anomalies, if used excessively throughout development.

The use of prescription and nonprescription drugs during pregnancy is surprisingly high. Most pregnant women consume at least one drug during pregnancy. Drug consumption also tends to be higher during the critical period of development among heavy smokers and drinkers. Despite this, *fewer than 2% of congenital anomalies are caused by drugs and chemicals.* Only a few drugs have been positively implicated as human teratogenic agents. Although only 7% to 10% of anomalies are caused by recognizable teratogens (see Fig. 19-1), new agents continue to be identified. It is best for women to avoid using all medication during the first trimester unless a strong medical reason exists for its use, and then it should be used only if the medication is recognized as reasonably safe for the human embryo.

CIGARETTE SMOKING

Maternal smoking during pregnancy is a well-established cause of IUGR. Despite warnings that cigarette smoking is harmful to the fetus, more than 25% of women continue to smoke during pregnancy. In heavy cigarette smokers (20 or more cigarettes daily), premature delivery is twice as frequent as in mothers who do not smoke. In addition, the infants of smokers weigh less than normal. **Low birth weight** (< 2000 g) is the chief predictor of infant death.

Nicotine constricts the uterine blood vessels, thereby causing a decrease in uterine blood flow and reducing the supply of oxygen and nutrients available to the embryo or fetus from the maternal blood in the intervillous space of the placenta. High levels of *carboxyhemoglobin,* resulting from cigarette smoking, appear in the maternal and fetal blood, and may alter the capacity of the blood to transport oxygen. As a result, chronic fetal hypoxia (a decrease in the oxygen level to below normal) may occur, affecting fetal growth and development.

CAFFEINE

Caffeine is the most popular drug in North America because it is present in several widely consumed beverages (e.g., coffee, tea, and cola drinks), chocolate products, and some drugs. *Caffeine is not known to be a human teratogen;* however, there is no assurance that heavy maternal consumption of it is safe for the embryo.

ALCOHOL

Alcoholism is a drug abuse problem that affects 1% to 2% of women of childbearing age. Both moderate and high levels of alcohol intake during early pregnancy may result in alterations in the growth and morphogenesis of the fetus; the greater the intake, the more severe the signs. Infants born to mothers with chronic alcoholism exhibit a specific pattern of defects, including prenatal and postnatal growth and mental deficiency and other anomalies (Fig. 19-12). This pattern of anomalies, called **fetal alcohol syndrome,** is detected in 1 in 1000 to 2 in 1000 live births. *Maternal alcohol abuse is now believed to be the most common cause of mental deficiency.* Even moderate maternal alcohol consumption (e.g., 1–2 ounces daily) may produce **fetal alcohol effects—** children with behavioral and learning difficulties, for

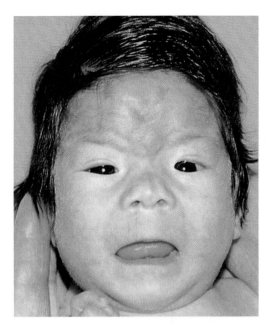

FIGURE 19-12. Infant with fetal alcohol syndrome. Note the thin upper lip, short palpebral fissures, flat nasal bridge, short nose, and elongated and poorly formed philtrum (vertical groove in the median part of the upper lip). Maternal alcohol abuse is believed to be the most common environmental cause of mental deficiency. (Courtesy of A.E. Chudley, MD, Section of Genetics and Metabolism, Department of Pediatrics and Child Health, Children's Hospital and University of Manitoba, Winnipeg, Manitoba, Canada.)

FIGURE 19-13. Masculinized external genitalia of a female infant with a 46, XX chromosome constitution. Observe the enlarged clitoris and the fused labia majora. The *arrow* indicates the single orifice of a urogenital sinus. The virilization was caused by excessive androgens produced by the suprarenal (adrenal) glands during the fetal period (congenital adrenal hyperplasia). (Courtesy of Dr. Heather Dean, Department of Pediatrics and Child Health and University of Manitoba, Winnipeg, Canada.)

example—especially if the drinking is associated with malnutrition. **Binge drinking** (heavy consumption of alcohol for 1–3 days during pregnancy) is very likely to produce fetal alcohol effects. The susceptible period of brain development spans the major part of gestation; therefore, the safest advice is total abstinence from alcohol during pregnancy.

ANDROGENS AND PROGESTOGENS
Androgens and progestogens may affect the female fetus, producing masculinization of the external genitalia (Fig. 19-13). The preparations that should be avoided are the *progestins, ethisterone, and norethisterone*. From a practical standpoint, the teratogenic risk of these hormones is low. However, progestin exposure during the critical period of development is also associated with an increased prevalence of cardiovascular abnormalities, and exposure of male fetuses during this period may double the incidence of *hypospadias* in the offspring (see Chapter 13). Obviously, the administration of testosterone also produces masculinizing effects in female fetuses.

Oral contraceptive (birth control) *pills* containing progestogens and estrogens, when taken during the early stages of an unrecognized pregnancy, are believed to be teratogenic agents. Many infants of mothers who took *progestogen-estrogen birth control pills* during the critical period of development have been found to exhibit VACTERL syndrome—**V**ertebral, **A**nal, **C**ardiac, **T**racheal, **E**sophageal, **R**enal, and **L**imb anomalies. As a precaution, the use of oral contraceptives should be discontinued as soon as pregnancy is detected because of the risk of possible teratogenic effects.

Diethylstilbestrol (DES, or stilbestrol) is recognized as a human teratogen. Vaginal adenosis, cervical erosions, and transverse vaginal ridges have been detected in women exposed to DES in utero. Moreover, a number of young women with a common history of exposure to this synthetic estrogen in utero have been found to have *adenocarcinoma of the vagina*. However, the probability of cancers developing at this early age in females exposed to DES in utero now appears to be low. In males exposed to DES in utero before the 11th week, an increased incidence of genital tract anomalies has been reported.

ANTIBIOTICS
Tetracyclines cross the placental membrane and are deposited in the embryo's bones and teeth at sites of active calcification. As little as 1 g daily of **tetracycline** during the third trimester of pregnancy can produce yellow staining of the primary, or deciduous, teeth. Tetracycline therapy during the fourth to ninth months of pregnancy may also cause tooth defects (e.g., enamel hypoplasia), yellow to brown **discoloration of the teeth,** and diminished growth of the long bones. Moreover, more than 30 cases of hearing deficit and eighth cranial nerve damage have been reported in infants exposed to **streptomycin** derivatives in utero. By contrast, *penicillin* has been used extensively during pregnancy and appears to be harmless to the human embryo and fetus.

ANTICOAGULANTS
All anticoagulants except heparin cross the placental membrane and may cause hemorrhage in the embryo or fetus. Warfarin, an anticoagulant, is definitely a

Figure 19-14. Fetal hydantoin syndrome. **A,** This young girl has a learning disability. Note the unusual ears, the wide spacing of the eyes, the epicanthal folds, the short nose, and the long philtrum. Her mother has epilepsy and took Dilantin throughout her pregnancy. **B,** Right hand of an infant with severe digital hypoplasia (short fingers), born to a mother who took Dilantin throughout her pregnancy. (**A,** Courtesy of A.E. Chudley, MD, Section of Genetics and Metabolism, Department of Pediatrics and Child Health, Children's Hospital and University of Manitoba, Winnipeg, Manitoba, Canada. **B,** From Chodirker, BN, Chudley AE, Persaud TVN: Possible prenatal hydantoin effect in child born to a nonepileptic mother. Am J Med Genet 27:373, copyright (c) 1987. Reprinted by permission of Wiley-Liss, a division of John Wiley and Sons, Inc.)

teratogen. The period of greatest sensitivity is 6 to 12 weeks after fertilization, or 8 to 14 weeks after the last normal menstrual period. Second- and third-trimester exposure may result in mental retardation, optic atrophy, and microcephaly. Heparin does not cross the placental membrane, and so is the drug of choice for pregnant women requiring anticoagulant therapy.

ANTICONVULSANTS

Epilepsy affects approximately 1 in 200 pregnant women, and these women require treatment with an anticonvulsant. Of the anticonvulsant drugs available, phenytoin has been definitively identified as a teratogen. **Fetal hydantoin syndrome** occurs in 5% to 10% of children born to mothers treated with phenytoins or hydantoin anticonvulsants (Fig. 19-14).

Valproic acid has been the drug of choice for the management of different types of epilepsy; however, its use by pregnant women has led to a pattern of anomalies consisting of craniofacial, heart, and limb defects. There is also an increased risk of **neural tube defects.** Phenobarbital is considered a safe antiepileptic drug for use during pregnancy.

ANTINAUSEANTS

Teratologists consider Bendectin (a combination of doxylamine succinate and pyridoxine hydrochloride; known by the trade names Debendox, Lenotan, Diclectin, and others) nonteratogenic in humans because large-scale epidemiologic studies of infants have not shown an increased risk of birth defects after its administration to pregnant women. There has been extensive debate in the lay press and in the courts as to whether this antinauseant is a teratogenic drug in humans.

ANTINEOPLASTIC AGENTS

Tumor-inhibiting chemicals are highly teratogenic. This is not surprising because these agents inhibit mitosis in rapidly dividing cells. It is recommended that they be avoided, especially during the first trimester of pregnancy.

Methotrexate, *a folic acid antagonist* and a derivative of *aminopterin,* is a known potent teratogen that produces major congenital anomalies. It is most often used as a single agent or in combination therapy for neoplastic diseases; however, it may also be indicated in patients with severe rheumatic diseases, including rheumatoid arthritis.

CORTICOSTEROIDS

The teratogenic risk of corticosteroids is minimal to nonexistent.

ANGIOTENSIN-CONVERTING ENZYME INHIBITORS

Exposure of the fetus to angiotensin-converting enzyme inhibitors, used as antihypertensive agents, causes oligohydramnios, fetal death, long-lasting hypoplasia of the bones of the calvaria, IUGR, and renal dysfunction. During early pregnancy, the risk to the embryo is apparently diminished, so there is no indication in such a case to terminate a wanted pregnancy.

INSULIN AND HYPOGLYCEMIC DRUGS

Insulin is not teratogenic in human embryos, except possibly in maternal insulin coma therapy. Hypoglycemic drugs (e.g., tolbutamide) have been implicated in some cases, but evidence of their teratogenicity is very weak. No convincing evidence exists that oral hypoglycemic agents are teratogenic in human embryos. The incidence of congenital anomalies is increased two- to threefold in the offspring of mothers with diabetes. Women with insulin-dependent diabetes mellitus may significantly decrease their risk of having infants with birth defects by achieving good control of their disease before conception.

RETINOIC ACID (VITAMIN A)

Isotretinoin (13-cis-retinoic acid), used for the oral treatment of severe cystic acne, is teratogenic in humans, even at very low doses. The critical period for exposure appears to be from the third week to the fifth week (5–7 weeks after the last normal menstrual period). The risk of spontaneous abortion and birth defects after exposure to **retinoic acid** is high. Postnatal follow-up studies of children exposed to isotretinoin in utero showed significant **neuropsychological impairment.** Vitamin A is a valuable and necessary nutrient during pregnancy, but long-term exposure to large doses of vitamin A is unwise because of insufficient evidence to rule out a teratogenic risk.

SALICYLATES

Some evidence indicates that large doses of *acetylsalicylic acid*, or **aspirin,** the most commonly ingested drug during pregnancy, are potentially harmful to the embryo or fetus. However, epidemiologic studies indicate that aspirin is not a teratogenic agent, but large doses should be avoided.

THYROID DRUGS

Iodides readily cross the placental membrane and interfere with thyroxin production. They may also cause thyroid enlargement and **cretinism** (arrested physical and mental development and dystrophy of the bones and soft tissue). Maternal iodine deficiency may cause *congenital cretinism.* The administration of antithyroid drugs for the treatment of maternal thyroid disorders may cause *congenital goiter* if the dose administered exceeds that required to control the disease.

TRANQUILIZERS

Thalidomide is a potent teratogen. Nearly 12,000 infants have been born with defects caused by this drug. The characteristic feature of thalidomide syndrome is **meromelia**—*phocomelia,* or "seal limbs" (Fig. 19-15). It has been well established clinically that the period when thalidomide causes congenital anomalies is from 24 to 36 days after fertilization (38–50 days after the last normal menstrual period). This sensitive period coincides with the critical periods for the development of the affected parts and organs (see Fig. 19-11). *Thalidomide is absolutely contraindicated in women of childbearing age.* With appropriate precautions, thalidomide is now used for the treatment of leprosy and other disorders because of its immunosuppressive properties.

PSYCHOTROPIC DRUGS

Lithium is the drug of choice for long-term maintenance therapy in patients with the mental illness known as *bipolar disorder;* however, it has been known to cause congenital anomalies, mainly of the heart and great vessels, in infants born to mothers given the drug early in pregnancy. Although lithium carbonate is a human teratogen, the Food and Drug Administration has stated that the agent may be used during pregnancy if "in the opinion of the physician the potential benefits outweigh the possible hazards." **Benzodiazepine** *derivatives* are psychoactive drugs that are frequently used by pregnant women. These include *diazepam* and *oxazepam,* which readily cross the placental membrane. The use of these

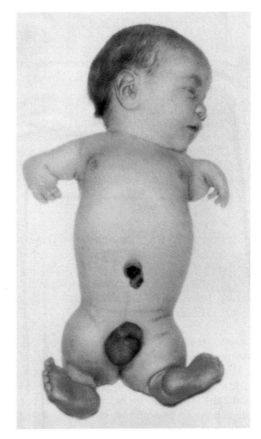

FIGURE 19-15. Newborn male infant with malformed limbs (meromelia—limb reduction) caused by maternal ingestion of thalidomide during the critical period of limb development. (From Moore KL: The vulnerable embryo. Causes of malformation in man. Manitoba Med Rev 43:306, 1963.)

drugs during the first trimester of pregnancy is associated with transient withdrawal symptoms and craniofacial anomalies in the neonate.

ILLICIT DRUGS

Cocaine is one of the most commonly abused illicit drugs in North America, and its increasing use by women of childbearing age is of major concern. Many reports deal with the prenatal effects of cocaine. These include spontaneous abortion, prematurity, and diverse anomalies in the offspring.

There is little evidence that *marijuana* is a human teratogen, although there is some indication that marijuana use during the first 2 months of pregnancy affects fetal length and birth weight. In addition, alterations in sleep and electroencephalogram patterns have been noted in newborn infants exposed prenatally to marijuana.

Methadone, used for the treatment of heroin addiction, is considered a "behavioral teratogen," as is heroin. Infants born to narcotic-dependent women receiving maintenance methadone therapy have been found to have central nervous system dysfunction, lower birth weights, and smaller head circumferences than nonexposed infants. There is also concern about the long-term postnatal developmental effects of methadone.

Environmental Chemicals as Teratogens

In recent years, there has been increasing concern about the possible teratogenicity of environmental, industrial, and agricultural chemicals, pollutants, and food additives.

ORGANIC MERCURY

Infants of mothers whose main diet during pregnancy consists of fish containing abnormally high levels of organic mercury acquire fetal **Minamata disease** and exhibit neurologic and behavioral disturbances resembling those associated with cerebral palsy. *Methylmercury is a teratogen* that causes cerebral atrophy, spasticity, seizures, and mental retardation.

LEAD

Lead crosses the placental membrane and accumulates in fetal tissues. Prenatal exposure to lead is associated with an increased incidence of abortions, fetal anomalies, IUGR, and functional deficits. Children born to mothers exposed to subclinical levels of lead exhibit neurobehavioral and psychomotor disturbances.

POLYCHLORINATED BIPHENYLS

Polychlorinated biphenyls are teratogenic chemicals that produce IUGR and skin discoloration in infants exposed to these agents in utero. The main dietary source of polychlorinated biphenyls in North America is probably sport fish caught in contaminated waters. In Japan and Taiwan, the teratogenic chemical has been detected in contaminated cooking oil.

Infectious Agents as Teratogens

Throughout prenatal life, the embryo and fetus are endangered by a variety of microorganisms. In most cases, the microbial assault is resisted; however, in some cases, abortion or stillbirth occurs, and in other cases, the infants are born with IUGR, congenital anomalies, or neonatal diseases.

RUBELLA (GERMAN, OR THREE-DAY, MEASLES)

The **rubella virus** crosses the placental membrane and infects the embryo or fetus. In cases of primary maternal infection during the first trimester of pregnancy, the overall risk of embryonic or fetal infection is approximately 20%. The clinical features of **congenital rubella syndrome** are *cataracts, cardiac defects,* and *deafness;* however, other abnormalities are occasionally observed (Fig. 19-16). The earlier in pregnancy that maternal rubella infection occurs, the greater the danger that the embryo will be malformed.

CYTOMEGALOVIRUS

Cytomegalovirus is the most common viral infection of the human fetus. Because the disease seems to be fatal when it affects the embryo, most pregnancies likely end in spontaneous abortion when the infection occurs during the first trimester. Newborn infants infected during the early fetal period usually show no clinical signs and are identified through screening programs. Later in pregnancy, *cytomegalovirus infection may result in IUGR and severe fetal anomalies.* Of particular concern are cases of asymptomatic cytomegalovirus infection, which are often associated with audiologic, neurologic, and neurobehavioral disturbances in infancy.

HERPES SIMPLEX VIRUS

Maternal infection with **herpes simplex virus** in early pregnancy increases the abortion rate threefold, and infection after the 20th week is associated with an increased rate of prematurity as well as with congenital anomalies. Infection of the fetus with herpes simplex virus usually occurs very late in pregnancy, probably most often during delivery.

VARICELLA (CHICKENPOX)

Varicella and herpes zoster (shingles) are caused by the same virus, **varicella-zoster virus.** There is convincing evidence that maternal varicella infection during the first 4 months of pregnancy causes congenital anomalies. There is a 20% incidence of these or other anomalies when the infection occurs during the critical period of development (see Fig. 19-11). After 20 weeks of gestation, there is no proven teratogenic risk.

HUMAN IMMUNODEFICIENCY VIRUS

Human immunodeficiency virus (HIV) is the retrovirus that causes acquired immune deficiency syndrome. Infec-

FIGURE 19-16. **A,** Typical bilateral congenital cataracts caused by the rubella virus. Cardiac defects and deafness are other congenital defects common to this syndrome. **B,** Severe congenital glaucoma caused by the rubella virus. Observe the dense corneal haze, enlarged corneal diameter, and deep anterior chamber. (**A,** Courtesy of Dr. Richard Bargy, Department of Ophthalmology, Cornell-New York Hospital, New York, New York. **B,** Courtesy of Dr. Daniel I. Weiss, Department of Ophthalmology, New York University College of Medicine, New York, New York. From Cooper LA, Green RH, Krugman S, et al: Neonatal thrombocytopenic purpura and other manifestations of rubella contracted in utero. Am J Dis Child 110:416, 1965. Copyright 1965, American Medical Association.)

tion of pregnant women with HIV is now a prevalent and serious health problem. Information is conflicting on the fetal effects of in utero infection with HIV. Preventing the transmission of the virus to women and their infants is important because of the potential embryopathic effects.

TOXOPLASMOSIS

Maternal infection with the intracellular parasite *Toxoplasma gondii* is usually through one of the following routes:

● Eating raw or poorly cooked meat (usually pork or lamb containing *Toxoplasma* cysts)
● Close contact with infected domestic animals (usually cats) or infected soil

The T. gondii organism crosses the placental membrane and infects the fetus, causing destructive changes in the brain and the eyes that result in *mental deficiency* and other anomalies. Mothers of infants with congenital defects are often unaware of having had **toxoplasmosis,** the disease caused by the parasitic organism. Because animals (cats, dogs, rabbits, and other domestic and wild animals) may be infected with this parasite, pregnant women should avoid contact with them. In addition, eggs from domestic fowl should be well cooked, and unpasteurized milk should be avoided.

CONGENITAL SYPHILIS

Syphilis infection affects approximately 3 in 10,000 liveborn infants in the United States. *Treponema pallidum,* the small, spiral microorganism that causes syphilis, rapidly crosses the placental membrane as early as 9 to 10 weeks of gestation. The fetus can become infected at any stage of the disease or at any stage of pregnancy. **Primary maternal infections** (acquired during pregnancy and left untreated) nearly always cause serious fetal infection and congenital anomalies. However, adequate treatment of the mother kills the organism. **Secondary maternal infections** (acquired before pregnancy) seldom result in fetal disease and anomalies. If the mother remains untreated, stillbirths occur in approximately 25% of cases.

Radiation as a Teratogen

Exposure to **high levels of ionizing radiation** may injure embryonic cells, resulting in cell death, chromosomal injury, and retardation of mental development and physical growth. The severity of the embryonic damage is related to the absorbed dose, the dose rate, and the stage of embryonic or fetal development when the exposure occurs. Accidental exposure of pregnant women to radiation is a common cause for anxiety.

No conclusive proof exists that human congenital anomalies have been caused by diagnostic levels of radiation. Scattered radiation from a radiographic (x-ray) examination of a part of the body that is not near the uterus (e.g., thorax, sinuses, teeth) produces a dose of only a few millirads, which is not teratogenic to the embryo. If the embryonic radiation exposure is 5 rad or less, the radiation risks to the embryo are minuscule. The recommended limit of maternal exposure of the whole body to radiation from all sources is 500 mrad for the entire gestational period.

ELECTROMAGNETIC FIELDS

No evidence exists that the risk of IUGR or other developmental defects is increased by maternal exposure to low-frequency electromagnetic fields (e.g., electric blankets, video display terminals).

ULTRASONIC WAVES

Ultrasonography is widely used during pregnancy for fetal diagnosis and prenatal care. There are no confirmed biologic effects in patients and their fetuses from the use of diagnostic ultrasound evaluation. Moreover, the benefits to patients exposed to prudent use of this modality outweigh the risks, if any.

Maternal Factors as Teratogens

Poorly controlled *diabetes mellitus* in the mother with persisting hyperglycemia and ketosis, particularly during embryogenesis, is associated with a two- to threefold higher incidence of birth defects. The infant of a diabetic mother is usually large (**macrosomia**). The common anomalies include *holoprosencephaly* (failure of the forebrain to divide into hemispheres), *meroencephaly* (partial absence of the brain), sacral agenesis, vertebral anomalies, congenital heart defects, and limb anomalies. If left untreated, women who are homozygous for phenylalanine hydroxylase deficiency—**phenylketonuria**—and those with **hyperphenylalaninemia** are at increased risk for having off-spring with microcephaly, cardiac defects, mental retardation, and IUGR. The congenital anomalies can be prevented if the mother with phenylketonuria follows a phenylalanine-restricted diet before and during pregnancy.

Mechanical Factors as Teratogens

The amniotic fluid absorbs mechanical pressures, thereby protecting the embryo from most external trauma. It is generally accepted that congenital abnormalities caused by external injury to the mother are extremely rare, but possible. *Clubfoot and congenital dislocation of the hip* may be caused by mechanical forces, particularly in an otherwise malformed uterus. Such deformations may be caused by any factor that restricts the mobility of the fetus, thereby causing prolonged compression in an abnormal posture. A significantly reduced quantity of amniotic fluid (*oligohydramnios*) may result in mechanically induced deformation of the limbs (see Chapter 8), such as hyperextension of the knee. Intrauterine amputations or other anomalies caused by local constriction during fetal growth may result from **amniotic bands,** rings formed as a result of rupture of the amnion during early pregnancy (see Fig. 8-15).

■ ANOMALIES CAUSED BY MULTIFACTORIAL INHERITANCE

Many common congenital anomalies (e.g., cleft lip, with or without cleft palate) have familial distributions consistent with multifactorial inheritance (see Fig. 19-1). Multifactorial inheritance may be represented by a model in which one's "liability" for a disorder is a continuous variable determined by a combination of genetic and environmental factors, with a developmental threshold dividing individuals with the anomaly from those without it. Multifactorial *traits are often single major anomalies*, such as cleft lip, isolated cleft palate, and neural tube defects. Some of these anomalies may also occur as part of the phenotype in syndromes determined by single-gene inheritance, chromosomal abnormality, or an environmental teratogen. The recurrence risks used for genetic counseling of families having congenital anomalies that have been determined by multifactorial inheritance are *empirical risks* based on the frequency of the anomaly in the general population and in different categories of relatives. In individual families, such estimates may be inaccurate because they are usually averages for the population rather than precise probabilities for the individual family.

CLINICALLY ORIENTED QUESTIONS

1. If a pregnant woman takes aspirin in normal doses, will it cause congenital anomalies?
2. If a woman is a drug addict, will her child show signs of drug addiction?
3. Are all drugs tested for teratogenicity before they are marketed? If the answer is "yes," why are these teratogens still sold?
4. Is cigarette smoking during pregnancy harmful to the embryo or fetus? If the answer is "yes," would refraining from inhaling cigarette smoke be safer?
5. Are any drugs safe to take during pregnancy? If so, what are they?

The answers to these questions are at the back of the book.

REFERENCES AND SUGGESTED READING

■ CHAPTER 1

Evans MI: Stem cell therapy: Moving towards reality. Am J Obstet Gynecol 194:662, 2006.

Gasser R: Atlas of Human Embryos. Hagerstown, Md, Harper & Row, 1975.

Gasser R: Virtual Human Embryo DREM Project. Baltimore, NICHD, 2007.

Gibbs N: Stem cells: The hope and the hype. Time 168:26, 2006.

Jirásek JE: An Atlas of Human Prenatal Developmental Mechanics: Anatomy and Staging. London and New York, Taylor & Francis, 2004.

Meyer AW: The Rise of Embryology. Palo Alto, Calif, Stanford University Press, 1939.

Moore CA, Khoury MJ, Bradley LA: From genetics to genomics: Using gene-based medicine to prevent disease and promote health in children. Semin Perinatol 29:135, 2005.

O'Rahilly R, Müller F: Developmental Stages in Human Embryos. Washington, DC, Carnegie Institution of Washington, 1987.

Streeter GL: Developmental horizons in human embryos: Description of age group XI, 13 to 20 somites, and age group XII, 21 to 29 somites. Contrib Embryol Carnegie Inst 30:211, 1942.

■ CHAPTER 2

Guraya SS: Cellular and molecular biology of capacitation and acrosome reaction in spermatozoa. Int Rev Cytol 199:1, 2000.

Hampton T: Researchers discover a range of factors undermine sperm quality, male fertility. JAMA 294:2829, 2005.

Hillier SG: Gonadotropic control of ovarian follicular growth and development. Mol Cell Endocrinol 179:39, 2001.

Horne AW, White JO, Lalani E: The endometrium and embryo implantation. Br Med J 321:1301, 2000.

Moore KL, Agur AMR: Essential Clinical Anatomy, 3rd ed. Baltimore, Williams & Wilkins, 2006.

Nussbaum RL, McInnes RR, Willard HF: Thompson & Thompson Genetics in Medicine, 6th ed (revised reprint). Philadelphia, WB Saunders, 2004.

Oehninger S, Hodgen GD: Hypothalamic-pituitary-ovary-uterine axis. In Copeland LJ, Jarrell J, McGregor J (eds): Textbook of Gynecology, 2nd ed. Philadelphia, WB Saunders, 2000.

■ CHAPTER 3

Carr DH, Gedeon M: Population cytogenetics of human abortuses. In Hook EB, Porter IH (eds): Population Cytogenetics: Studies in Humans. New York, Academic Press, 1977.

Doody, KJ: Advances in assisted reproduction. Semin Reprod Med 23:299, 2005.

Rock J, Hertig AT: The human conceptus during the first two weeks of gestation. Am J Obstet Gynecol 55:6, 1948.

Shevell T, Malone FD, Vidaver J, et al: Assisted reproductive technology and pregnancy outcome. Obstet Gynecol 106:1039, 2005.

Sjoberg NO, Hamberger L (eds): Blastocyst development and early implantation. Hum Reprod 15(Suppl 6): 1–80, 2000.

Trounson A: Developments in infertility therapy: Diagnosis of genetic disease in embryos. Aust Fam Physician 34:123, 2005.

■ CHAPTER 4

Attar E: Endocrinology of ectopic pregnancy. Obstet Gynecol Clin North Am 31:779, 2004.

Bianchi DW, Wilkins-Haug LE, Enders AC, Hay ED: Origin of extra-embryonic mesoderm in experimental animals: Relevance to chorionic mosaicism in humans. Am J Med Genet 46:542, 1993.

Hertig AT, Rock J, Adams EC: A description of 34 human ova within the first seventeen days of development. Am J Anat 98:435, 1956.

Kodaman PH, Taylor HS: Hormonal regulation of implantation. Obstet Gynecol Clin North Am 31:745, 2004.

Lipscomb GH: Ectopic pregnancy. In Copeland LJ, Jarrell JF (eds): Textbook of Gynecology, 4th ed. Philadelphia, WB Saunders, 2000.

Luckett WP: Origin and differentiation of the yolk sac and extraembryonic mesoderm in presomite human and rhesus monkey embryos. Am J Anat 152:59, 1978.

■ CHAPTER 5

Barembaum M, Bronner-Fraser M: Early steps in neural crest specification. Semin Cell Dev Biol 16:642, 2005.

Dale KJ, Pourquié O: A clock-work somite. BioEssays 22:72, 2000.

Flake AW: The fetus with sacrococcygeal teratoma. In Harrison MR, Evans MI, Adzick NS, Holzgrev W (eds): The Unborn Patient: The Art and Science of Fetal Therapy, 3rd ed. Philadelphia, WB Saunders, 2001.

Gasser RF: Evidence that some events of mammalian embryogenesis can result from differential growth, making migration unnecessary. Anat Rec Part B (New Anat) 289B:53, 2006.

Hardin J, Walston T: Models of morphogenesis: The mechanisms and mechanics of cell rearrangement. Curr Opin Genet Dev 14:399, 2004.

Kalcheim C, Ben-Yair R: Cell rearrangements during development of the somite and its derivatives. Curr Opin Genet Dev 15:371, 2005.

Le Douarin NM, Kalcheim C: The Neural Crest, 2 nd ed. Cambridge, Cambridge University Press, 1999.

Pourquié O: Vertebrate segmentation: Is cycling the rule? Curr Opin Cell Biol 12:747, 2000.

Seckl MJ, Fisher RA, Salerno G, et al: Choriocarcinoma and partial hydatidiform moles. Lancet 356:36, 2000.

Tam PPL, Kanai-Azuma M, Kanai Y: Early endoderm development in vertebrates: Lineage differentiation and morphogenetic function. Curr Opin Genet Dev 13:393, 2003.

■ CHAPTER 6

Das UG, Sysyn GD: Abnormal fetal growth: Intrauterine growth retardation, small for gestational age, large for gestational age. Pediatr Clin North Am 51:639, 2004.

Gasser R: Virtual Human Embryo DREM Project. New Orleans, Louisiana State University, 2007.

Gibbs N: Stem cells: The hope and the hype. Time 168:26, 2006.

Jirásek JE: An Atlas of Human Prenatal Developmental Mechanics: Anatomy and Staging. London and New York, Taylor & Francis, 2004.

Kliegman RM: Intrauterine growth restriction. In Martin RJ, Fanaroff AA, Walsh MC (eds): Fanaroff and Martin's Neonatal-Perinatal Medicine: Diseases of the Fetus and Infant, 8th ed. Philadelphia, Mosby, 2006.

Lyons EA, Levi CS: Ultrasound of the normal first trimester of pregnancy. Syllabus: Special Course Ultrasound. Oak Brook, Ill, Radiological Society of North America, 1991.

O'Rahilly R, Müller F: Development Stages in Human Embryos. Publication 637. Washington, DC, Carnegie Institution of Washington, 1987.

Persaud TVN, Hay JC: Normal embryonic and fetal development. In Reece EA, Hobbins JC (eds): Clinical Obstetrics: The Fetus and Mother, 3rd ed. Oxford, Blackwell, 2006.

Sawin SW, Morgan MA: Dating of pregnancy by trimesters: A review and reappraisal. Obstet Gynecol Surv 51:261, 1996.

■ CHAPTER 7

Anderson MS, Hay WW: Intrauterine growth restriction and the small-for-gestational-age infant. In MacDonald MG, Seshia MMK, Mullett MD (eds): Avery's Neonatology: Pathophysiology & Management of the Newborn, 6th ed. Philadelphia, Lippincott Williams & Wilkins, 2005.

Brigatti KW, Malone FD: First trimester screening for aneuploidy. Obstet Gynecol Clin North Am 31:1, 2004.

Crombleholme TM: Surgical treatment of the fetus. In Martin RJ, Fanaroff AA, Walsh MC (eds): Fanaroff and Martin's Neonatal-Perinatal Medicine: Diseases of the Fetus and Infant, 8th ed. Philadelphia, Mosby, 2005.

Das UG, Sysyn GD: Abnormal fetal growth: Intrauterine growth retardation, small for gestational age, large for gestational age. Pediatr Clin North Am 51:639, 2004.

Drugan A, Isada NB, Evans MI: Prenatal diagnosis in the molecular age: Indications, procedures, and laboratory techniques. In MacDonald MG, Seshia MMK, Mullett MD (eds): Avery's Neonatology: Pathophysiology & Management of the Newborn, 6th ed. Philadelphia, Lippincott Williams & Wilkins, 2005.

Jirásek JE: An Atlas of Human Prenatal Developmental Mechanics: Anatomy and Staging. London and New York, Taylor & Francis, 2004.

Lyons EA, Levi CS: Ultrasound of the normal first trimester of pregnancy. Syllabus: Special Course Ultrasound. Oak Brook, Ill, Radiological Society of North America, 1991.

Needlman RD: Fetal growth and development. In Behrman RE, Kliegman RM, Jenson HB (eds): Nelson Textbook of Pediatrics, 17th ed. Philadelphia, Elsevier-Saunders, 2004.

Nicolaides KH: First-trimester screening for chromosomal abnormalities. Semin Perinatol 29:190, 2005.

■ CHAPTER 8

Alexander GR, Wingate MS, Salihu H, et al: Fetal and neonatal mortality risks of multiple births. Obstet Gynecol Clin North Am 32:1, 2005.

Brace RA: Amniotic fluid dynamics. In Creasy RK, Resnik RJD: Maternal-Fetal Medicine, 5th ed. Philadelphia, WB Saunders, 2004.

Collins JH: Umbilical cord accidents: Human studies. Semin Perinatol 26:79, 2002.

Liao JB, Buhimschi CS, Norwitz ER: Normal labor: Mechanism and duration. Obstet Gynecol Clin North Am 32:145, 2005.

Lockwood CJ: The initiation of parturition at term. Obstet Gynecol Clin North Am 31:935, 2004.

Marino T: Ultrasound abnormalities of the amniotic fluid, membranes, umbilical cord, and placenta. Obstet Gynecol Clin North Am 31:177, 2004.

Mundy CA: Intravenous immunoglobulin in the management of hemolytic disease of the newborn. Neonatal Netw 24:17, 2005.

Redline RW: Placental pathology. In Martin RJ, Fanaroff AA, Walsh MC (eds): Fanaroff and Martin's Neonatal-Perinatal Medicine: Diseases of the Fetus and Infant, 8th ed. Philadelphia, Mosby, 2006.

■ CHAPTER 9

Cass DL: Fetal surgery for congenital diaphragmatic hernia: The North American experience. Semin Perinatol 29:104, 2005.

Graham G, Devine PC: Antenatal diagnosis of congenital diaphragmatic hernia. Semin Perinatol 29:69, 2005.

Kays DW: Congenital diaphragmatic hernia and neonatal lung lesions. Surg Clin North Am 86:329, 2006.

Rottier R, Tibboel D: Fetal lung and diaphragm development in congenital diaphragmatic hernia. Semin Perinatol 29:86, 2005.

Slavotinek AM: The genetics of congenital diaphragmatic hernia. Semin Perinatol 29:77, 2005.

Wells LJ: Development of the human diaphragm and pleural sacs. Contr Embryol Carneg Inst 35:107, 1954.

Yang W, Carmichael SL, Harris JA, Shaw GM: Epidemiologic characteristics of congenital diaphragmatic hernia among 2.5 million California births, 1899–1997. Birth Defects Res A Clin Mol Teratol 76:170, 2006.

■ CHAPTER 10

Berkovitz BKB, Holland GR, Moxham B: Oral Anatomy, Histology, and Embryology, 3rd ed. Edinburgh, Mosby, 2005.

Gasser RF: Evidence that some events of mammalian embryogenesis can result from differential growth, making migration unnecessary. Anat Rec Part B (New Anat) 289B:53, 2006.

Goldmuntz E: DiGeorge syndrome: New insights. Clin Perinatol 32:963, 2005.

Gross E, Sichel J-Y: Congenital neck lesions. Surg Clin North Am 86:383, 2006.

Helms JA, Cordero D, Tapadia MD: New insights into craniofacial morphogenesis. Development 132:851, 2005.

Hinrichsen K: The early development of morphology and patterns of the face in the human embryo. Adv Anat Embryol Cell Biol 98:1, 1985.

Jirásek JE: An Atlas of Human Prenatal Developmental Mechanics: Anatomy and Staging. London and New York, Taylor & Francis, 2004.

Jones KL: Smith's Recognizable Patterns of Human Malformation, 6th ed. Philadelphia, Elsevier-Saunders, 2005.

Marazita ML, Mooney MP: Current concepts in the embryology and genetics of cleft lip and cleft palate. Clin Plast Surg 31:125, 2004.

Moxham BJ: The development of the palate: A brief review. Eur J Anat 7 (Suppl 1):53, 2003.

Noden DM, Trainor PA: Relations and interactions between cranial mesoderm and neural crest populations. J Anat 207:575, 2005.

Wyszynski DF, Sarkozi A, Czeizel AE: Oral clefts with associated anomalies: Methodological issues. Cleft Palate Craniofac J 43:1, 2006.

■ CHAPTER 11

Abel R, Bush A, Chitty RS, et al: Congenital lung disease. In Chernick V, Boat T, Wilmott R, Bush A (eds): Kendig's Disorders of the Respiratory Tract in Children, 7th ed. Philadelphia, Saunders-Elsevier, 2006.

Haddad GG, Fontán JJP: Development of the respiratory system. In Behrman RE, Kliegman RM, Jenson HB (eds): Nelson Textbook of Pediatrics, 17th ed. Philadelphia, Elsevier-Saunders, 2004.

Jobe AH: Lung development and maturation. In Martin RJ, Fanaroff AA, Walsh MC (eds): Fanaroff and Martin's Neonatal-Perinatal Medicine: Diseases of the Fetus and Infant, 8th ed. Philadelphia, Mosby, 2006.

O'Rahilly R, Boyden E: The timing and sequence of events in the development of the human respiratory system during the embryonic period proper. Z Anat Entwicklungsgesch 141:237, 1973.

Wells LJ, Boyden EA: The development of the bronchopulmonary segments in human embryos of horizons XVII and XIX. Am J Anat 95:163, 1954.

Whitsett JA, Wert SE: Molecular determinants of lung morphogenesis. In Chernick V (ed): Kendig's Disorders of the Respiratory Tract in Children, 7th ed. Philadelphia, Elsevier-Saunders, 2006.

■ CHAPTER 12

Bates MD, Balistreri WF: Development and function of the liver and biliary system. In Behrman RE, Kliegman RM, Jenson HB (eds): Nelson Textbook of Pediatrics, 17th ed. Philadelphia, Elsevier-Saunders, 2004.

Beck F, Tata F, Chawengsaksophak K: Homeobox genes and gut development. BioEssays 22:431, 2000.

Gosche JR, Vick L, Boulanger SC, Islam S: Midgut abnormalities. Surg Clin North Am 86:285, 2006.

Lau ST, Caty MG: Hindgut abnormalities. Surg Clin North Am 86:285, 2006.

Ledbetter DJ: Gastroschisis and omphalocele. Surg Clin North Am 86:249, 2006.

Martucciello G, Ceccherinil, Lerone M, et al: Pathogenesis of Hirschsprung's disease. J Pediatr Surg 35:1017, 2000.

Naik-Mathuria B, Olutoye OO: Foregut abnormalities. Surg Clin North Am 86:261, 2006.

Wyllie R: Pyloric stenosis and other congenital anomalies of the stomach; intestinal atresia, stenosis, and malformations; intestinal duplications; Meckel diverticulum, and other remnants of the omphalomesenteric duct. In Behrman RE, Kliegman RM, Jenson HB (eds): Nelson Textbook of Pediatrics, 17th ed. Philadelphia, WB Saunders, 2004.

■ CHAPTER 13

Haynes JH: Inguinal and scrotal disorders. Surg Clin North Am 86:371, 2006.

Hyun SJ: Cloacal exstrophy. Neonatal Netw 25:101, 2006.

McElreavey K, Fellous M: Sex determination and the Y chromosome. Am J Med Genet 89:176, 1999.

Palmert MR, Dahms WT: Abnormalities of sexual differentiation. In Martin RJ, Fanaroff AA, Walsh MC (eds): Fanaroff and Martin's Neonatal-Perinatal Medicine: Diseases of the Fetus and Infant, 8th ed. Philadelphia, Mosby, 2006.

Persaud TVN: Embryology of the female genital tract and gonads. In Copeland LJ, Jarrell J (eds): Textbook of Gynecology, 2nd ed. Philadelphia, WB Saunders, 2000.

Sobel V, Zhu Y-S, Imperato-McGinley J: Fetal hormones and sexual differentiation. Obstet Gynecol Clin North Am 31:837, 2004.

Woolf AS: A molecular and genetic view of human renal and urinary tract malformations. Kidney Int 58:500, 2000.

Yamada G, Suzuki K, Haraguchi R, et al: Molecular genetic cascades for external genitalia formation: An emerging organogenesis program. Dev Dyn 235:1738, 2006.

■ CHAPTER 14

Bernstein E: The cardiovascular system. In Behrman RE, Kliegman RM, Jenson HB (eds): Nelson Textbook of Pediatrics, 17th ed. Philadelphia, WB Saunders, 2004.

Gruber PJ: Cardiac development: New concepts. Clin Perinatol 32:845, 2005.

Männer J: Extracardiac tissues and the epigenetic control of myocardial development in vertebrate embryos. Ann Anat 188:199, 2006.

Solloway M, Harvey RP: Molecular pathways in myocardial development: A stem cell perspective. Cardiovasc Res 58:264, 2006.

Srivastava D, Olson EN: A genetic blueprint for cardiac development. Nature 407:221, 2000.

Stoller JZ, Epstein JA: Cardiac neural crest. Semin Cell Dev Biol 16:704, 2005.

Szwast A, Rychik J: Current concepts in fetal cardiovascular disease. Clin Perinatol 32:857, 2005.

Watanabe M, Schaefer KS: Cardiac embryology. In Martin RJ, Fanaroff AA, Walsh MC (eds): Fanaroff and Martin's Neonatal-Perinatal Medicine: Diseases of the Fetus and Infant, 8th ed. Philadelphia, Mosby, 2006.

■ CHAPTER 15

Ambler CA, Nowicki JL, Burke AC, et al: Assembly of trunk and limb blood vessels involves extensive migration and vasculogenesis of somite-derived angioblasts. Dev Biol 234:352, 2001.

Birchmeier C, Brohmann H: Genes that control the development of migrating muscle precursor cells. Curr Opin Cell Biol 12:725, 2000.

Cohen MM Jr, MacLean RE (eds): Craniosynostosis: Diagnosis, Evaluation, and Management, 2nd ed. New York, Oxford University Press, 2000.

Cooperman DR, Thompson GH: Musculoskeletal disorders. In Martin RJ, Fanaroff AA, Walsh MC (eds): Fanaroff and Martin's Neonatal-Perinatal Medicine: Diseases of the Fetus and Infant, 8th ed. Philadelphia, Mosby, 2006.

Franz-Odendaal TA, Hall, BK, Witten PE: Buried alive: How osteoblasts become osteocytes. Dev Dyn 235:176, 2006.

Hall BK: Bones and Cartilage: Developmental Skeletal Biology. Philadelphia, Elsevier, 2005.

Hinrichsen KV, Jacob HJ, Jacob M, et al: Principles of ontogenesis of leg and foot in man. Ann Anat 176:121, 1994.

Kablar B, Krastel K, Ying C, et al: Myogenic determination occurs independently in somites and limb buds. Dev Biol 206:219, 1999.

Kablar B, Tajbakhsh S, Rudnick MA: Transdifferentiation of esophageal smooth muscle is myogenic bHLH factor-dependent. Development 127:1627, 2000.

Kalcheim C, Ben-Yair R: Cell rearrangements during development of the somite and its derivatives. Curr Opin Genet Dev 15:371, 2005.

Maldjian C, Hofkin S, Bonakdarpour A, et al: Abnormalities of the pediatric foot. Acad Radiol 6:191, 1999.

O'Rahilly R, Gardner E: The timing and sequence of events in the development of the limbs of the human embryo. Anat Embryol 148:1, 1975.

Van Heest AE: Congenital disorders of the hand and upper extremity. Pediatr Clin North Am 43:1113, 1996.

■ CHAPTER 16

Barkovich AJ, Kuzniecky RI, Jackson GD, et al: A developmental and genetic classification for malformations of cortical development. Neurology 65:1873, 2005.

Botto LD, Lisi A, Robert-Gnansia E, et al: International retrospective cohort study of neural tube defects in relation to folic acid recommendations: Are the recommendations working? BMJ 330:571, 2005.

Gasser RF: Evidence that some events of mammalian embryogenesis can result from differential growth, making migration unnecessary. Anat Rec Part B (New Anat) 289B:53, 2006.

Gressens P, Hüppi PS: Normal and abnormal brain development. In Martin RJ, Fanarof AA, Walsh MC (eds): Fanaroff and Martin's Neonatal-Perinatal Medicine: Diseases of the Fetus and Infant, 8th ed. Philadelphia, Mosby, 2006.

Johnston MV, Kinsman, S: Congenital anomalies of the central nervous system. In Behrman RE, Kliegman RM, Jenson HB (eds): Nelson Textbook of Pediatrics, 17th ed. Philadelphia, Elsevier-Saunders, 2004.

LeDouarin N, Kalcheim C: The Neural Crest, 2nd ed. Cambridge, UK, Cambridge University Press, 1999.

O'Rahilly R, Müller F: Embryonic Human Brain: An Atlas of Developmental Stages, 2nd ed. New York, Wiley-Liss, 1999.

Zhu X, Lin CR, Prefontaine GG, et al: Genetic control of pituitary development and hypopituitarism. Curr Opin Genet Dev 15: 332, 2005.

■ CHAPTER 17

Barald KF, Kelley MW: From placodes to polarization: New tunes in inner ear development. Development 131:4119, 2004.

Barishak YR: Embryology of the Eye and Its Adnexa, 2nd ed. Basel, Karger, 2001.

Bauer PW, MacDonald CB, Melhem ER: Congenital inner ear malformation. Am J Otol 19:669, 1998.

FitzPatrick DR, van Heyningen V: Developmental eye disorders. Curr Opin Genet Dev 15:348, 2005.

Haddad J Jr: The ear. In Behrman RE, Kliegman RM, Jenson HB (eds): Nelson Textbook of Pediatrics, 17th ed. Philadelphia, Elsevier-Saunders, 2004.

Jones KL: Smith's Recognizable Patterns of Human Malformation, 6th ed. Philadelphia, WB Saunders, 2005.

Mallo M: Formation of the middle ear: Recent progress on the developmental and molecular mechanisms. Dev Biol 231:410, 2001.

O'Rahilly R: The prenatal development of the human eye. Exp Eye Res 21:93, 1975.

Porter CJW, Tan SW: Congenital auricular anomalies: Topographic anatomy, embryology, classification, and treatment strategies. Plast Reconstr Surg 115:1701, 2005.

■ CHAPTER 18

Buhimschi CS: Endocrinology of lactation. Obstet Gynecol Clin North Am 31:963, 2004.

Cobourne MT: The genetic control of early odontogenesis. Br J Orthod 26:21, 1999.

Darmstadt GL, Sidbury R: The skin. In Behrman RE, Kliegman RM, Jenson HB (eds): Nelson Textbook of Pediatrics, 17th ed. Philadelphia, Elsevier-Saunders, 2004.

Osborne MP: Breast anatomy and development. In Harris JR (ed): Diseases of the Breast, 2nd ed. Philadelphia, Lippincott Williams & Wilkins, 2000.

Paller AS, Mancini AJ: Hurwitz Clinical Pediatric Dermatology: A Textbook of Skin Disorders of Childhood and Adolescence, 3rd ed. Philadelphia, WB Saunders, 2006.

Smolinski KN: Hemangiomas of infancy: Clinical and biological characteristics. Clin Pediatr 44:747, 2005.

Ten Cate AR: Development of the tooth. In Ten Cate AR (ed): Oral Histology: Development, Structure, and Function, 5th ed. St. Louis, CV Mosby, 1998.

Winter GB: Anomalies of tooth formation and eruption. In Welbury RR (ed): Paediatric Dentistry, 2nd ed. Oxford, Oxford University Press, 2001.

■ CHAPTER 19

Baley JE, Toltzis P: Viral infections. In Martin RJ, Fanaroff AA, Walsh MC (eds): Fanaroff and Martin's Neonatal-Perinatal Medicine: Diseases of the Fetus and Infant, 8th ed. Philadelphia, Mosby, 2006.

Boyer KM, Holfels E, Roizen N, et al: Risk factors for *Toxoplasma gondii* infection in mothers of infants with congenital toxoplasmosis: Implications for prenatal management and screening. Am J Obstet Gynecol 192:564, 2005.

Briggs GG, Freeman RK, Yaffe SJ: Drugs in Pregnancy and Lactation, 7th ed. Baltimore, Williams & Wilkins, 2005.

Centers for Disease Control and Prevention (CDC): Improved national prevalence estimates for selected major birth defects—United States, 1999–2001 (MMWR 54:1301, 2006). JAMA 295:618, 2006.

Galerneau F, Inzucchi SE: Diabetes mellitus in pregnancy. Obstet Gynecol Clin North Am 31:907, 2004.

Hall JG: Chromosomal clinical abnormalities. In Behrman RE, Kliegman RM, Jenson HB (eds): Nelson Textbook of Pediatrics, 17th ed. Philadelphia, WB Saunders, 2004.

Hudgins L, Cassidy SB: Congenital anomalies. In Martin RJ, Fanaroff AA, Walsh MC (eds): Fanaroff and Martin's Neonatal-Perinatal Medicine: Diseases of the Fetus and Infant, 8th ed. Philadelphia, Mosby, 2006.

Jones KL: Smith's Recognizable Patterns of Human Malformation, 6th ed. Philadelphia, Elsevier-Saunders, 2005.

Kriebs JM: Changing the paradigm: HIV in pregnancy. J Perinat Neonat Nurs 20:71, 2006.

Medicodes' Hospital and Payer: International Classification of Diseases, 9th Revision. Clinical Modification, 4th ed, Volumes 1–3. Salt Lake City, Medicode, Inc., 1995.

Mills JL: Depressing observations on the use of selective serotonin-reuptake inhibitors during pregnancy. N Engl J Med 354:636, 2006.

Nussbaum RL, McInnes RR, Willard HF: Thompson & Thompson Genetics in Medicine, 6th ed (revised reprint). Philadelphia, WB Saunders, 2004.

Persaud TVN: Environmental Causes of Human Birth Defects. Springfield, Ill, Charles C Thomas, 1990.

Robertson J, Polifka JE, Avner M, et al: A survey of pregnant women using isotretinoin. Birth Defects Res A Clin Mol Teratol 73:881, 2005.

Schiller C, Allen PJ: Follow-up of infants prenatally exposed to cocaine. Pediatr Nurs 31:427, 2005.

Schwarz EB, Maselli J, Norton M, Gonzales R: Prescription and teratogenic medications in United States ambulatory practices. Am J Med 118:1240, 2005.

Stewart TL: Screening for aneuploidy: The genetic sonogram. Obstet Gynecol Clin North Am 31:21, 2004.

ANSWERS TO CLINICALLY ORIENTED QUESTIONS

■ CHAPTER 1

1. The term *conceptus* refers to the embryo and its membranes (amnion, chorion, umbilical vesicle, and allantois). A *conceptus* refers to the products of conception, that is, everything that develops from the zygote. The *embryo* is the embryonic part of the conceptus.

2. Everyone, especially those in the health sciences, should know about conception, contraception, and how people develop, both normally and abnormally. Health professionals are expected to give intelligent answers to the questions people ask, such as, "When does the baby's heart start to beat?" "When does it move its limbs?" "When is the fetus most at risk for effects from alcohol?"

3. Physicians date pregnancies from the last normal menstrual period because this date is usually remembered by women. It is not usually possible to detect the precise time of ovulation or of fertilization (when development begins). Laboratory tests and ultrasound imaging can be performed to detect when ovulation is likely to occur and when pregnancy has occurred, but they are not routinely performed because of the costs involved.

■ CHAPTER 2

1. Pregnant women do not menstruate, even though there may be some bleeding at the usual time of menstruation. This blood may be leaking from the intervillous space because of partial separation of the placenta. Because there is no shedding of the endometrium, this blood is not menstrual fluid.

2. It depends on when she forgot to take the oral contraceptive. If it was at midcycle, ovulation might occur and pregnancy could result. Taking two doses the next day would not prevent ovulation.

3. *Coitus interruptus* refers to withdrawal of the penis from the vagina before ejaculation occurs. This method is not reliable. Often, a few sperms are expelled from the penis with the secretions of the auxiliary sex glands (e.g., seminal glands) before ejaculation occurs. One of these sperms may fertilize the oocyte.

4. *Spermatogenesis* refers to the complete process of sperm formation. *Spermiogenesis* is the transformation of a spermatid into a sperm. Therefore, spermiogenesis is the final stage of spermatogenesis.

5. A copper-releasing intrauterine device may inhibit the capacitation of sperms and their transport through the uterus to the fertilization site in the uterine tube; in this case, it would be a *contraceptive device*. A hormone-releasing intrauterine device (e.g., levonorgestrel) may cause changes that alter the morphologic features of the endometrium; as a result, the blastocyst does not implant. In this case, the intrauterine device would be a *contra-implantation device*.

■ CHAPTER 3

1. The ovarian and endometrial (menstrual) cycles cease between 47 and 55 years of age, with the average age being 48 years. Menopause results from the gradual cessation of gonadotropin production by the pituitary gland; however, it does not mean that the ovaries have exhausted their supply of oocytes. The risk of Down syndrome and other trisomies is increased in the children of women who are 35 years or older (see Chapter 19). Spermatogenesis also decreases after the age of 45 years, and the number of nonviable and abnormal sperms increases. Nevertheless, sperm production continues until old age. The risk of producing abnormal gametes is much less common in men than in women; however, older men may accumulate mutations that the child might inherit. Mutations may produce congenital anomalies (see Chapter 19).

2. Considerable research on new contraceptive methods is being conducted, including the development of oral contraceptives for men. This research includes experimental work on hormonal and nonhormonal prevention of spermatogenesis and the stimulation of immune responses to sperms. Arresting the development of millions of sperms on a continuous basis has proven much more difficult than arresting the monthly development of a single oocyte monthly.

3. It is not known whether polar bodies are ever fertilized; however, it has been suggested that *dispermic chimeras* result from the fusion of a fertilized oocyte with a fertilized polar body. Chimeras are rare individuals who are composed of a mixture of cells from two zygotes. More likely, dispermic chimeras result from the fusion of dizygotic twin zygotes early in development. Dizygotic twins are derived from two zygotes. If a polar body were fertilized and remained separate from the normal zygote, it could form an embryo.

4. The most common cause of spontaneous abortion during the first week of development is chromosomal abnormality, such as the abnormalities resulting from nondisjunction (see Chapter 2). Failure of the chorion to produce an adequate amount of human chorionic gonadotrophin to maintain the corpus luteum in the ovary could also result in early spontaneous abortion.

5. Yes, it is possible; however, this phenomenon is extremely rare. The term *superfecundation* indicates fertilization (during separate acts of coitus) of two or more oocytes that are ovulated at approximately the same time. The possibility of this process occurring in humans cannot be discounted because evidence exists from dizygotic (nonidentical) twins belonging to different blood groups, which cannot be accounted for in any other way.

6. Essentially, they do mean the same thing. *Mitosis* is the usual process of cell reproduction that results in the formation of daughter cells of the zygote. *Cleavage* is the series of mitotic cell divisions of the zygote. This process results in the formation of daughter cells, or *blastomeres*. The expressions *cleavage division* and *mitotic division* have the same meaning when referring to the dividing zygote.

7. The nutritional requirements of the dividing zygote are not great. The blastomeres may be nourished partly by the sparse yolk granules in these cells; however, the nutrients are derived mainly from the secretions of the uterine tubes and, later, from the uterine glands.

8. Yes. One of the blastomeres could be removed, and a Y chromosome could be identified by fluorescence staining

with quinacrine mustard or by molecular techniques (see Chapter 7). This technique could be made available to couples with a family history of sex-linked genetic diseases (e.g., hemophilia, muscular dystrophy) and to women who have already given birth to a child with such a disease and are reluctant to have more children. In these cases, only female embryos developing in vitro would be transferred to the uterus.

■ CHAPTER 4

1. *Implantation bleeding* refers to the loss of small amounts of blood from the implantation site of a blastocyst that occurs a few days after the expected time of menstruation. Women unfamiliar with this possible occurrence may interpret the bleeding as a light menstrual flow; in such cases, they would give the physician the wrong date for their last normal menstrual period. This blood is not menstrual fluid; it is blood from the intervillous space of the developing placenta. Blood loss could also result from the rupture of chorionic arteries, veins, or both (see Chapter 8).

2. Drugs or other agents may cause abortion of the embryo, but they do not cause congenital anomalies if taken during the first 2 weeks of development. A drug or other agent either damages all of the embryonic cells, killing the embryo, or injures only a few cells, in which case the embryo recovers to develop normally.

3. Intrauterine devices are typically very effective at preventing pregnancy by altering sperm capacitation or motility or by altering, for instance, the morphologic features of the endometrium. However, an intrauterine device does not physically block a sperm from entering the uterine tube and fertilizing an oocyte, if one is present. Although the endometrium could be hostile to implantation, a blastocyst could develop and implant in the uterine tube (i.e., ectopic tubal pregnancy). If fertilization occurs in a woman who is using an intrauterine device, the risk of ectopic pregnancy is approximately 15% to 20%.

4. Abdominal pregnancies are very uncommon. Although such a pregnancy can result from primary implantation of a blastocyst in the abdomen, in most cases, it is believed to result from ectopic implantation of a blastocyst that spontaneously aborts from the uterine tube and enters the peritoneal cavity. The risk of severe maternal bleeding and fetal mortality is high in cases of abdominal pregnancy. However, if the diagnosis is made late in pregnancy and the patient (mother) is free of symptoms, the pregnancy may be allowed to continue until the viability of the fetus is ensured (e.g., 32 weeks), at which time it would be delivered by cesarean section.

5. Yes, it can occur, but it is very rare. An intrauterine and ectopic tubal pregnancy is most common.

■ CHAPTER 5

1. Yes, certain drugs can produce congenital anomalies if administered during the third week after the last normal menstrual period (see Chapter 19). For instance, antineoplastic agents (chemotherapy, or antitumor drugs) can produce severe skeletal and neural tube defects in the embryo, such as acrania and meroencephaly (partial absence of the brain), if administered during the third week.

2. Yes, risks to the mother 40 years or older and the embryo are increased. Increased maternal age is a predisposing factor to certain medical conditions. Preeclampsia, a hypertensive disorder of pregnancy characterized by increased blood pressure and edema, for example, occurs more frequently in older pregnant women than in younger ones. Advanced maternal age is also associated with a significantly increased risk to the embryo or fetus. The most common risks are birth defects associated with chromosomal abnormalities, such as Down syndrome and trisomy 13 (see Chapter 19); however, women older than 40 years may have normal children.

■ CHAPTER 6

1. Early in the eighth week, embryos have webbed toes and stubby, tail-like caudal eminences and look different from 9-week fetuses; however, by the end of the eighth week, embryos and early fetuses appear similar. The name change is made to indicate that a new phase of development (rapid growth and differentiation) has begun and that the most critical period of development has been completed.

2. The question of when an embryo becomes a human being is difficult to answer because opinions are affected by religious and personal views. The scientific answer is that, from the time of fertilization, the embryo has human potential, and no other, because of its human chromosomal constitution.

3. No, it cannot. During the embryonic period, more similarities than differences exist in the external genitalia (see Chapter 13). It is impossible to tell by ultrasound examination whether the primordial sexual organ (genital tubercle at 5 weeks and phallus at 7 weeks) will become a penis or a clitoris. Sexual differences are not clear until the early fetal period (10th to 12th week). Sex chromatin patterns and chromosomal analysis (fluorescence in situ hybridization) of embryonic cells obtained during amniocentesis can show the chromosomal sex of the embryo (see Chapter 7).

■ CHAPTER 7

1. Ultrasound examinations have shown that mature embryos (8 weeks) and young fetuses (9 weeks) show spontaneous movements, such as twitching of the trunk and limbs. Although the fetus begins to move its back and limbs during the 12th week, the mother cannot feel the fetus move until the 16th to 20th week. Women who have had several children usually detect this movement, called *quickening*, sooner than women who are pregnant for the first time because they know what fetal movements feel like. Quickening is often perceived as a faint flutter or a quivering motion.

2. Folic acid supplementation before conception and during early pregnancy is effective in reducing the incidence of neural tube defects (e.g., spina bifida). It has been shown that the risk of having a child with neural tube defect is significantly lower when a vitamin supplement containing 400 μg of folic acid is consumed daily. However, no consensus exists that vitamins are helpful in preventing these defects in most at-risk pregnancies.

3. Direct injury to the fetus from the needle during amniocentesis is very uncommon when ultrasound guidance is used to locate the position of the fetus and monitor needle insertion. The risk of inducing an abortion is slight (approximately 0.5%) in second-trimester pregnancies. Maternal or fetal infection is also an uncommon complication.

■ CHAPTER 8

1. A *stillbirth* is the birth of an infant that was dead before delivery, weighs at least 500 g, and is at least 20 weeks old. The incidence of having a stillborn infant is approximately three times greater among mothers older than 40 years than among women 20 to 30 years. It is true that more male fetuses than female fetuses are stillborn. The reason for this is unknown.

2. Sometimes the umbilical cord is abnormally long and wraps around part of the fetus, such as the neck or a limb. This *cord accident* may obstruct blood flow in the umbilical vein to the fetus and in the umbilical arteries from the fetus to the placenta. If this obstruction causes the fetus to receive insufficient oxygen and nutrients, then the fetus dies. A true knot in the umbilical cord, formed when the fetus passes through a loop in the cord, also obstructs blood flow through the cord. Prolapse of the umbilical cord into the cervix at the level of a presenting part (often the head) may also be considered a cord accident. This creates pressure on the cord and prevents the fetus from receiving adequate oxygen. Entanglement of the cord around the fetus can also cause congenital defects (e.g., absence of a forearm).

3. Most over-the-counter pregnancy tests are based on the detection of relatively large amounts of human chorionic gonadotrophin in the woman's urine. The results of such tests are positive a short time (approximately 1 week) after the first missed menstrual period. Human chorionic gonadotrophin is produced by the syncytiotrophoblast of the chorion. These tests usually give an accurate diagnosis of pregnancy; however, a physician should be consulted as soon as possible to confirm pregnancy because some tumors (choriocarcinomas) also produce this hormone.

4. The *bag of waters* is a colloquial term for the amniotic sac, which contains amniotic fluid (largely composed of water). Sometimes the amniochorionic sac ruptures before labor begins, allowing fluid to escape. Premature rupture of the membranes is the most common event leading to premature labor (birth). Premature rupture of the membranes may complicate the birth process or may allow a vaginal infection to spread to the fetus.

Sometimes sterile saline is infused into the uterus by way of a catheter—amnioinfusion—to alleviate fetal distress. The term *dry birth* is used to describe a low volume of amniotic fluid.

5. *Fetal distress* is synonymous with *fetal hypoxia*, indicating decreased oxygenation to the fetus as a result of a general decrease of the maternal oxygen content of the blood, decreased oxygen-carrying capacity, or diminished blood flow. Fetal distress exists when the fetal heart rate is less than 100 beats per minute. Pressure on the umbilical cord may also cause fetal distress secondary to impairment of the blood supply to the fetus in approximately 1 in 200 deliveries. In these cases, the fetal body compresses the umbilical cord as it passes through the cervix and the vagina.

6. The incidence of dizygotic twins increases with maternal age. Dizygotic twinning is an autosomal recessive trait that is carried by the daughters of mothers of twins; hence, dizygotic twinning is hereditary. Monozygotic twinning, on the other hand, is a random occurrence that is not genetically controlled.

■ CHAPTER 9

1. Yes, it is. When an infant is born with a congenital diaphragmatic hernia, part of its stomach and liver may be in its thorax (chest); however, this is uncommon. Usually, the abnormally placed viscera are the intestines. The viscera enter the thorax through a posterolateral defect in the diaphragm, usually on the left side.

2. An infant born with a congenital diaphragmatic hernia may survive; however, the mortality rate is high (approximately 76%). Treatment must be given immediately. A feeding tube is inserted into the stomach, and the air and the gastric contents are aspirated with continuous suction. The displaced viscera are replaced into the abdominal cavity, and the defect in the diaphragm is surgically repaired. Infants with large diaphragmatic hernias who are operated on within 24 hours after birth have survival rates of 40% to 70%. Intrauterine surgical repair of a congenital diaphragmatic hernia has been attempted; however, this intervention carries considerable risk to the fetus and the mother. The developing use of minimally invasive surgical techniques may reduce this risk.

3. It depends on the degree of herniation of the abdominal viscera. With a moderate hernia, the lungs may be mature, but small. With a severe degree of herniation, lung development is impaired. Most infants with a congenital diaphragmatic hernia die, but not because of the defect in the diaphragm or viscera in the thorax (chest); they die because the lung on the affected side is hypoplastic (underdeveloped).

4. Yes, it is possible to have a small congenital diaphragmatic hernia and not be aware of it. Some small diaphragmatic hernias may remain asymptomatic into adulthood and may be discovered only during routine radiographic or ultrasound examination of the thorax. The lung on the affected side would probably develop normally because there would be little or no pressure on it during prenatal development.

■ CHAPTER 10

1. *Harelip* is the obsolete term for the clinical entity known as *cleft lip*. The term was adopted because the hare (a mammal resembling a large rabbit) has a divided upper lip. It is not an accurate comparison, however, because the cleft in the hare's lip is in the median part of the upper lip, whereas most human clefts are lateral to the median plane.

2. No, both statements are inaccurate. All embryos have grooves in their upper lips where the maxillary prominences meet the merged medial nasal prominences; however, normal embryos do not have cleft lips. When lip development is abnormal, the tissue in the floor of the labial groove breaks down, forming a cleft lip.

3. The risk in this case is the same as in the general population, approximately 1 in 1000.

4. Although environmental factors may be involved, it is reasonable to assume that the son's cleft lip and cleft palate were hereditary and recessive in their expression. This would mean that the father also carried a concealed gene for cleft lip and that his family genetics were equally responsible for the son's anomalies.

5. Minor anomalies of the auricle of the external ear are common, and usually they are of no serious medical or cosmetic consequence. Approximately 14% of newborn infants have minor morphologic abnormalities; fewer than 1% of them have other defects. The child's abnormal ears could be considered branchial anomalies because the six small auricular hillocks (swellings) of the first two pairs of pharyngeal arches contribute to the auricles; however, such minor abnormalities of ear shape would not normally be classified in this way.

■ CHAPTER 11

1. Multiple stimuli initiate breathing at birth. Slapping the buttocks used to be a common physical stimulus; however, this action is usually unnecessary. Under normal circumstances, the infant's breathing begins promptly, which suggests that it is a reflex response to the sensory stimuli of exposure to air and touching. The changes in blood gases after interruption of the placental circulation, such as the decrease in oxygen tension and pH and the increase in partial pressure of carbon dioxide, are also important in stimulating breathing.

2. Hyaline membrane disease, a common cause of respiratory distress syndrome, occurs after the onset of breathing in infants with immature lungs and a deficiency of pulmonary surfactant. The incidence of respiratory distress syndrome is approximately 1% of all live births, and it is the leading cause of death in newborn infants. It occurs mainly in infants who are born prematurely. Hyaline membrane disease is caused by environmental factors (mainly surfactant deficiency).

3. A 22-week fetus is viable and, if born prematurely and given special care in a neonatal intensive care unit, may survive. The chances of survival, however, are poor for infants who weigh less than 600 g because the lungs are immature and incapable of adequate alveolar-capillary gas exchange. Furthermore, the fetus's brain is not usually differentiated sufficiently to permit regular respiration.

■ CHAPTER 12

1. Undoubtedly, the infant had congenital hypertrophic pyloric stenosis, a diffuse hypertrophy (enlargement) and hyperplasia of smooth muscle in the pyloric part of the stomach. This condition produces a hard palpable mass; however, it is not a tumor. It is a benign enlargement and is definitely not a malignant tumor. The muscular enlargement causes narrowing of the exit canal (pyloric canal). In response to the outflow obstruction and vigorous peristalsis, the vomiting is projectile, as in the case of the infant described. Surgical relief of the pyloric obstruction is the usual treatment. The cause of pyloric stenosis is not known; however, it is believed to have a multifactorial pattern of inheritance (i.e., genetic and environmental factors are probably involved).

2. It is true that infants with Down syndrome have an increased incidence of duodenal atresia. They are also more likely to have imperforate anus and other congenital defects (e.g., atrial septal defects). These anomalies are likely caused by their abnormal chromosomal constitution (i.e., three instead of two copies of chromosome 21). Duodenal atresia can be corrected surgically by bypassing the pyloric obstruction (duodenoduodenostomy).

3. In very uncommon cases, when the intestines return to the abdomen after physiologic umbilical herniation, they may rotate in a clockwise direction rather than in the usual counterclockwise manner. As a result, the cecum and the appendix are located on the left side, a condition called *situs inversus abdominis*. A left-sided cecum and appendix can also result from a mobile cecum. If the cecum is not fixed to the posterior abdominal wall during the fetal period, the cecum and appendix are freely movable and could migrate to the left side.

4. Undoubtedly, the individual described had an ileal (Meckel) diverticulum, a fingerlike outpouching of the ileum. This common anomaly is sometimes referred to as a *second appendix*, which is a misnomer. An ileal diverticulum produces symptoms that are similar to those of appendicitis. It is also possible, although rare, that the person had a duplication of the cecum, which would result in two appendices.

5. Hirschsprung disease, or congenital megacolon (Greek *megas*, big), is the most common cause of obstruction of the descending colon in newborn infants. The cause of the condition is failure of migration of neural crest cells into the wall of the intestine. The neural crest cells normally form neurons, so there is a deficiency of the nerve cells that innervate the muscular wall of the bowel—congenital aganglionosis. When the bowel wall collapses, obstruction occurs and constipation results. Bowel overdistention and perforation may also occur.

6. If the infant had an umbilicoileal fistula, the abnormal canal connecting the ileum and the umbilicus could permit the passage of the contents of the ileum to the umbilicus. This occurrence would be an important diagnostic clue to the presence of this canal. The fistula

results from the persistence of the intra-abdominal part of the omphaloenteric duct.

CHAPTER 13

1. Most people with a horseshoe kidney have no urinary problems. These abnormal kidneys are usually discovered at autopsy, during diagnostic imaging, or in the dissecting room. Nothing needs to be done with the abnormal kidney unless the person has an uncontrolled infection of the urinary tract. In some cases, the urologist may divide the kidney into two parts and fix them in positions that do not result in urinary stagnation.

2. His developing kidneys probably fused during the sixth to eighth weeks as they "migrated" from the pelvis. The fused kidneys then ascended toward the normal position on one side or the other. Usually, no problems are associated with fused kidneys; however, surgeons must be conscious of the possibility of this condition and recognize it for what it is. This abnormality is called *crossed renal ectopia*.

3. Affected individuals have both ovarian and testicular tissue. Although spermatogenesis is uncommon, ovulation is not. Pregnancy and childbirth have been observed in a few patients; however, this is very unusual.

4. By 48 hours after birth, a definite sex assignment can be made in most cases. The parents are told that their infant's genital development is incomplete and that tests are needed to determine whether the infant is a boy or a girl. They are usually advised against announcing their infant's birth to their friends until the appropriate sex has been assigned. The buccal smear test for the identification of sex chromatin is done as soon as possible. Chromatin-positive cells—those with sex chromatin in their nuclei—almost always indicate a female. Chromatin-negative cells usually indicate a male; however, study of the baby's chromosomes may be required before sex can be assigned. Hormone studies may also be required.

5. Virilization (masculinization) of the female fetus as a result of congenital adrenal hyperplasia is the most common cause of ambiguous external genitalia. In other cases, androgens enter the fetal circulation after maternal ingestion of androgenic hormones. In unusual cases, these hormones are produced by a tumor on one of the mother's suprarenal glands. Partial or complete fusion of the urogenital folds or labioscrotal swellings is the result of exposure to androgens before the 12th week of development. Clitoral enlargement occurs after this point; however, androgens do not cause sexual ambiguity because the other external genitalia are fully formed by this time.

CHAPTER 14

1. Heart murmurs are sounds transmitted to the thoracic wall from turbulence of blood in the heart or great arteries. Loud murmurs often represent stenosis of one of the semilunar valves (aortic or pulmonary valve). A ventricular septal defect or a patent oval foramen (foramen ovale) may also produce a murmur.

2. Congenital heart defects are common. They occur in 6 to 8 in 1000 newborn infants and represent approximately 10% of all congenital anomalies. Ventricular septal defects are the most common type of heart anomaly. They occur more frequently in males than in females, but the reason for this is unknown.

3. The cause of most congenital anomalies of the cardiovascular system is unknown. In approximately 8% of children with heart disease, a genetic basis is clear. Most of these anomalies are associated with obvious chromosomal abnormalities (e.g., trisomy 21) and deletion of parts of chromosomes. Down syndrome is associated with congenital heart disease in 50% of cases. Maternal ingestion of drugs, such as antimetabolites and warfarin sodium (an anticoagulant), has been shown to be associated with a high incidence of cardiac defects. Evidence suggests that heavy consumption of alcohol during pregnancy may cause heart defects; however, it is impossible to say whether excessive use of alcohol by the mother caused the infant's heart condition.

4. Several viral infections are associated with congenital cardiac defects; however, only rubella virus (German measles) is known to cause cardiovascular disease (e.g., patent ductus arteriosus). Rubeola (common measles) does not cause cardiovascular defects. Rubella virus vaccine is available and is effective in preventing the development of rubella infection in a woman who has not had the disease and is planning to have a baby. It will subsequently prevent rubella syndrome from developing in her infant as well. Because of the potential hazard of the vaccine to the embryo, the vaccine is given only if there is assurance that there is no likelihood of pregnancy for the next 2 months.

5. This anomaly is called *transposition of the great arteries* because the positions of the great vessels (aorta and pulmonary trunk) are reversed. Survival after birth depends on mixing between the pulmonary and the systemic circulations (e.g., through an atrial septal defect—patent oval foramen). Transposition of the great arteries occurs in slightly more than 1 in 5000 live births and is more common in male infants than in female infants (by almost 2 to 1). Most infants with this severe cardiac anomaly die during the first months of life; however, corrective surgery can be performed in those who survive for several months. Initially, an atrial septal defect may be created to increase mixing between the systemic and the pulmonary circulations. Later, an arterial switch operation (reversing the aorta and the pulmonary trunk) can be performed. However, more commonly, a baffle is inserted into the atrium to divert systemic venous blood through the mitral valve, left ventricle, and pulmonary artery to the lungs, and to divert pulmonary venous blood through the tricuspid valve, right ventricle, and aorta. This physiologically corrects the circulation.

6. Very likely, one twin has dextrocardia, which usually is of no clinical significance. The heart is simply displaced to the right. In the individual described, the heart presents a mirror image of the normal cardiac structure. This occurs during the fourth week of development, when the heart tube rotates to the left rather than to the right. Dextrocardia is a relatively common anomaly in monozygotic twins.

■ CHAPTER 15

1. A rib associated with the seventh cervical vertebra is of clinical importance because it may compress the subclavian artery, the brachial plexus, or both, producing symptoms of artery and nerve compression. These ribs develop from the costal processes of vertebrae. Lumbar ribs are common and have a similar embryologic basis.

2. A hemivertebra can produce lateral curvature of the vertebral column (scoliosis). A hemivertebra is composed of one half of a body, a pedicle, and a lamina. This anomaly occurs when mesenchymal cells from the sclerotomes on one side do not form the primordium of half of a vertebra. As a result, more growth centers are found on one side of the vertebral column; this imbalance causes the vertebral column to bend laterally.

3. Craniosynostosis indicates premature closure of one or more of the cranial sutures. This developmental abnormality results in cranial malformations. Scaphocephaly, or dolichocephaly—a long, narrow cranium—results from premature closure of the sagittal suture. This type of craniosynostosis accounts for approximately 50% of cases of premature closure of cranial sutures and is more commonly seen in males.

4. The features of Klippel-Feil syndrome are a short neck, a low hairline, and restricted neck movements. In most cases, fewer than normal cervical vertebrae are present.

5. Prune-belly syndrome results from partial or complete absence of the abdominal musculature. Usually, the abdominal wall is thin. This syndrome is usually associated with malformations of the urinary tract, especially the urinary bladder (e.g., exstrophy). In males, almost all patients have cryptorchidism.

6. Absence of the sternocostal part of the left pectoralis major muscle is usually the cause of an abnormally low nipple and areola. Despite its numerous and important actions, absence of all or part of the pectoralis major muscle usually causes no disability. The actions of other muscles associated with the shoulder joint compensate for the partial absence of this muscle.

7. The girl has a prominent sternocleidomastoid muscle. This muscle attaches the mastoid process to the clavicle and sternum; hence, continued growth of the side of the neck results in tilting and rotation of the head. This relatively common condition—congenital torticollis (wry neck)—may occur because of injury to the muscle during birth. Stretching and tearing of some muscle fibers may have occurred during delivery, resulting in bleeding into the muscle. Over several weeks, necrosis of some fibers occurs, and the blood is replaced by fibrous tissue. This results in shortening of the muscle and pulling of the child's head to one side. If the condition is not corrected, the shortened muscle also could distort the shape of the face on the affected side.

8. The young athlete probably had an accessory soleus muscle. It is present in approximately 6% of people. This anomaly probably results from splitting of the primordium of the soleus muscle into two parts.

9. The ingestion of drugs did not cause the child's short limbs. The infant has a skeletal disorder known as *achondroplasia*. This type of short-limbed dwarfism has an incidence of 1 in 10,000 and shows an autosomal dominant inheritance. Approximately 80% of affected infants are born to normal parents and, presumably, the condition results from fresh mutations (changes in the genetic material) in the parents' germ cells. Most people with achondroplasia have normal intelligence and lead normal lives within their physical capabilities. If the parents of an achondroplastic child have more children, the risk of having another child with this condition is slightly higher than the risk in the general population; however, the risk for the achondroplastic person's own children is 50%.

10. Brachydactyly is an autosomal dominant trait. If the woman (likely bb) marries the brachydactylous man (likely Bb), the risk is 50% for a brachydactylous child and 50% for a normal child. It would be best for her to discuss her obvious concern with a medical geneticist.

11. Bendectin, an antinauseant mixture of doxylamine, dicyclomine, and pyridoxine, does not produce limb defects in human embryos. Several epidemiologic studies have not shown an increased risk of birth defects after exposure to Bendectin or its separate ingredients during early pregnancy. In the case described, the mother took the drug more than 3 weeks after the end of the critical period of limb development (24–36 days after fertilization). Most limb reduction defects have a genetic basis.

12. Cutaneous syndactyly is the most common type of limb anomaly. It varies from cutaneous webbing between the digits to synostosis (union of the phalanges, the bones of the digits). This anomaly occurs when separate digital rays do not form in the fifth week or when the tissue between the developing digits does not undergo apoptosis. Simple cutaneous syndactyly is easy to correct surgically. The absence of the sternal head of the pectoralis major muscle caused the nipple to be lower than the other one.

13. The most common type of clubfoot is talipes equinovarus, occurring in approximately 1 in 1000 newborn infants. In this deformity, the soles of the feet are turned medially and the feet are sharply plantar flexed. The feet are fixed in the tiptoe position, resembling the foot of a horse (Latin *equinus*, horse).

■ CHAPTER 16

1. Neural tube defects (NTDs) have a multifactorial inheritance pattern. Although only a few environmental factors have been shown to be directly related (such as folic acid), studies indicate that there are also genetic components. After the birth of one child with an NTD, the risk of a subsequent child having an NTD is much higher. The recurrence risk in the United Kingdom, where NTDs are common (7.6 per 1000 in South Wales and 8.6 per 1000 in Northern Ireland), is approximately 1 in 25. NTDs can be detected prenatally by a combination of ultrasound scanning and measurement of levels of alpha fetoprotein in the amniotic fluid and maternal serum.

2. The condition described is hydranencephaly, an extremely rare anomaly. Most of both cerebral hemispheres are reduced to membranous sacs that contain cerebrospinal fluid. Absence of the cerebral hemispheres can result from different developmental disturbances.

The condition most likely results from vascular occlusion of both internal carotid arteries secondary to a severe intrauterine infection. In some cases, hydranencephaly appears to be a severe type of intrauterine hydrocephalus. These infants usually do not survive longer than 3 months.

3. Mental deficiency and growth restriction are the most serious aspects of fetal alcohol syndrome. Average IQ scores in affected children are 60 to 70. It has been estimated that the incidence of mental deficiency resulting from heavy drinking during pregnancy may be as high as 1 in 400 live births. Heavy drinkers are those who consume five or more drinks on one occasion, with a consistent daily average of 45 mL of absolute alcohol. Currently, no safe threshold for alcohol consumption during pregnancy is known. Physicians recommend complete abstinence from alcohol during pregnancy.

4. No conclusive evidence indicates that maternal smoking affects the mental development of a fetus; however, cigarette smoking compromises the oxygen supply to the fetus because blood flow to the placenta is decreased during smoking. Because it is well established that heavy maternal smoking seriously affects the physical growth of the fetus and is a major cause of intrauterine growth restriction, it is not wise for mothers to smoke during pregnancy. The reduced oxygen supply to the brain could affect fetal intellectual development, even though the effect may be undetectable. Abstinence gives the fetus the best chance for normal development.

5. Most laypeople use the term *spina bifida* in a general way. They are unaware that the common type, spina bifida occulta, is usually clinically insignificant. It is an isolated finding in up to 20% of radiographically examined vertebral columns. Most people are unaware that they have this vertebral defect because it produces no symptoms unless it is associated with a neural tube defect or abnormality of the spinal nerve roots. The various types of spina bifida cystica are of clinical significance. Meningomyelocele is a more severe defect than meningocele because neural tissue is included in the lesion. Because of this, the function of the abdominal and limb muscles may be affected. Meningoceles are usually covered with skin, and motor function in the limbs is usually normal unless associated developmental defects of the spinal cord or brain are present. Management of infants with spina bifida cystica is complex and involves several medical and surgical specialties. Spinal meningocele is easier to correct surgically than spinal meningomyelocele, and the prognosis is also better.

■ CHAPTER 17

1. The chance of significant damage to the embryo or fetus after rubella infection depends primarily on the timing of the viral infection. In cases of primary maternal infection during the first trimester of pregnancy, the overall risk of embryonic or fetal infection is approximately 20%. It is estimated that approximately 50% of such pregnancies end in spontaneous abortion, stillbirth, or congenital anomalies (deafness, cataract, glaucoma, and mental retardation). When infection occurs at the end of the first trimester, the probability of congenital anomalies is only slightly higher than that for an uncomplicated pregnancy. Certain infections occurring late in the first trimester, however, may result in severe eye infections (e.g., chorioretinitis), which may affect visual development. Deafness is the most common manifestation of late fetal rubella infection (i.e., during the second and third trimesters). If a pregnant woman is exposed to rubella, an antibody test can be performed. If she is determined to be immune, she can be reassured that her embryo or fetus will not be affected by the virus. Preventive measures are essential for the protection of the embryo. It is especially important for girls to obtain immunity to rubella (e.g., by active immunization) before they reach childbearing age.

2. The purposeful exposure of young girls to rubella (German measles) is not recommended. Although complications resulting from such infections are uncommon, neuritis and arthritis (inflammation of the nerves and the joints, respectively) occasionally occur. Encephalitis (inflammation of the brain) occurs in approximately 1 in 6000 cases. Rubella infection is often subclinical (difficult to detect), yet children with such infections represent an exposure risk to pregnant women. There is a chance of injury to embryos because the danger period is greatest when the eyes and ears are developing. This occurs early enough in pregnancy that some women might be unaware that they are pregnant. A much better way of providing immunization against rubella is the administration of live vaccine to children older than 15 months and to nonpregnant postpubertal females who can be reasonably relied on not to become pregnant within 3 months of immunization.

3. Congenital syphilis (fetal syphilis) results from transplacental transmission of the microorganism *Treponema pallidum*. Transfer of this microorganism from untreated pregnant women may occur throughout pregnancy; however, it usually takes place during the last trimester. Deafness and tooth deformities commonly develop in these children. These anomalies can be prevented by treating the mother early in pregnancy. The microorganism that causes syphilis is very sensitive to penicillin, an antibiotic that does not harm the fetus.

4. Several viruses in the herpesvirus family can cause fetal blindness and deafness during infancy. Cytomegalovirus can cross the placenta, be transmitted to the infant during birth, and be passed to the infant in breast milk. Herpes simplex viruses (usually type 2, or genital herpes) are usually transmitted just before or during birth. The chances of normal development in infected infants are not good. Some infants have microcephaly, seizures, deafness, and blindness.

5. Methyl mercury is teratogenic in human embryos, especially to the developing brain. Because the eyes and the internal ears develop as outgrowths from the brain, it is understandable that their development is also affected. Besides the methyl mercury that passes from the mother to the embryo or fetus through the placenta, the newborn infant may receive additional methyl mercury from breast milk. Sources of methyl mercury include fish from contaminated water, flour made from methyl mercury–treated seed grain, and meat from animals raised on contaminated food.

■ CHAPTER 18

1. Congenital absence of the skin is very uncommon. Patches of skin may be absent, most often from the scalp, or sometimes from the trunk and the limbs. Affected infants usually survive because healing of the lesions is uneventful and takes 1 to 2 months. A hairless scar persists. The cause of congenital absence of hair, termed *aplasia cutis congenita*, is usually unknown. Most cases are sporadic; however, several well-documented pedigrees show autosomal dominant transmission of this skin defect.

2. The white patches of skin on a dark-skinned person result from partial albinism (piebaldism). This defect, which also affects light-skinned persons, is a heritable disorder transmitted by an autosomal dominant gene. Ultrastructural studies show an absence of melanocytes in the depigmented areas of skin. Presumably, the cause is a genetic defect in the differentiation of melanoblasts. These skin and hair defects are not amenable to treatment; however, they can be covered with cosmetics and hair dyes.

3. The breasts, including the mammary glands within them, of males and females are similar at birth. Breast enlargement in a newborn infant is common and results from stimulation by maternal hormones that enter the infant's blood through the placenta. Therefore, enlarged breasts are a normal occurrence in male infants and do not indicate abnormal sex development. Similarly, physiologic pubertal gynecomastia occurs in some males during their early teens as a result of decreased levels of testosterone. The breast enlargement is usually transitory. Familial gynecomastia is an X-linked, or autosomal dominant sex-linked, trait. Gynecomastia also occurs in approximately 50% of males with Klinefelter syndrome (described in Chapter 19). These boys and men are not intersexes because their external and internal genitalia are normal, except for their testes, which are small because of degeneration of the seminiferous tubules.

4. An extra breast (polymastia) or nipple (polythelia) is common. The axillary breast may enlarge during puberty, or it may not be noticed until pregnancy occurs. The embryologic basis of extra breasts and nipples is the presence of mammary crests (ridges) that extend from the axillary to the inguinal regions. Usually, only one pair of breasts develops; however, breasts can develop anywhere along the mammary crests. The extra breast or nipple is usually just superior or inferior to the normal breast. An axillary breast or nipple is very uncommon.

5. Teeth that are present at birth are termed *natal teeth* and are observed in approximately 1 in 2000 newborn infants. Usually, two mandibular medial (central) incisors are present. The presence of natal teeth usually suggests that early eruption of other teeth may occur. Often, they fall out on their own; however, there is a danger that they may be aspirated. For this reason, natal teeth are sometimes extracted.

■ CHAPTER 19

1. No evidence indicates that the occasional use of aspirin in recommended therapeutic dosages is harmful during pregnancy; however, large doses at subtoxic levels (e.g., for rheumatoid arthritis) have not been proven to be harmless to the embryo and fetus. All pregnant women should discuss the use of over-the-counter medications with their physicians.

2. A woman who is addicted to a habit-forming drug (e.g., heroin) and takes it during pregnancy is almost certain to give birth to a child who shows signs of drug addiction. The fetus's chances of survival until birth, however, are not good; mortality and premature birth rates are high among fetuses of drug-addicted mothers.

3. All drugs prescribed in North America are tested for teratogenicity before they are marketed. The thalidomide tragedy, however, clearly shows the need for improved methods for detecting potential human teratogens. Thalidomide has not been found to be teratogenic in pregnant mice and rats—yet it is a potent teratogen in humans during the fourth to sixth weeks of pregnancy. Because it is unethical to test the effects of drugs on human embryos, no way exists to guarantee that some drugs that may be human teratogens will not be marketed. Human teratologic evaluation depends on retrospective epidemiologic studies and the reports of astute physicians. This is the way that the teratogenicity of thalidomide was detected. Most new drugs contain a disclaimer in the accompanying package insert, such as, "This drug has not been proven safe for pregnant women." Some drugs may be used if, in the opinion of the physician, the potential benefits outweigh the possible hazards. All known teratogenic drugs that may be taken by a pregnant woman are available only through prescription by a physician.

4. Cigarette smoking during pregnancy is harmful to the embryo and fetus. Its most adverse effect is intrauterine growth restriction. Women who stop smoking during the first half of pregnancy have infants with birth weights closer to the birth weights of infants of nonsmokers. Decreased placental blood flow, believed to be a nicotine-mediated effect, is believed to cause decreased intrauterine blood flow. No conclusive evidence exists that maternal smoking causes congenital anomalies. The growth of the fetus of a woman who smokes, but does not inhale is still endangered because nicotine, carbon monoxide, and other harmful substances are also absorbed into the maternal bloodstream through the mucous membranes of the mouth and throat. These substances are then transferred to the embryo or fetus through the placenta. Smoking in any manner during pregnancy is not advisable.

5. Ample evidence indicates that most drugs do not cause congenital anomalies in human embryos; however, a pregnant woman should take only drugs that are essential and are recommended by her physician. A pregnant woman with a severe lower respiratory infection, for example, would be unwise to refuse drugs recommended by her physician to cure her illness; her health and that of her embryo or fetus could be endangered by the infection. Most drugs, including sulfonamides, meclizine, penicillin, antihistamines, and Bendectin, are considered safe drugs. Similarly, local anesthetic agents, dead vaccines, and salicylates (e.g., aspirin) in low doses are not known to cause congenital anomalies.

Index

Note: Page numbers followed by the letter f refer to figures and those followed by the letter t to tables.